D1243260

Common Foot Problems in Primary Care

Second Edition

RICHARD B. BIRRER, MD, FAAFP, FACP

Chairman and Senior Vice President,
Attending, Departments of Family Practice,
Community Medicine, and Emergency Medicine,
Catholic Medical Center of Brooklyn and Queens, Inc.;
Associate Professor of Emergency Medicine,
Albert Einstein College of Medicine;
Associate Professor of Family Medicine,
State University of New York Health
Science Center of Brooklyn

MICHAEL P. DELLACORTE, DPM, FACFAS, FACFAOM

Director of Podiatry, Mary Immaculate Division/
Assistant Director of Podiatric Medical Education,
Catholic Medical Center of Brooklyn and Queens, Inc.;
Associate Clinical Professor of Surgery,
New York College of Podiatric Medicine;
Diplomate, American Board of Podiatric Surgery;
Diplomate, American Board of Podiatric Orthopedics
and Primary Podiatric Medicine

PATRICK J. GRISAFI, DPM, FACFAS

Chief, Division of Podiatric Surgery/
Director of Podiatric Medical Education,
Catholic Medical Center of Brooklyn and Queens, Inc.;
Associate Clinical Professor of Surgery,
New York College of Podiatric Medicine;
Diplomate, American Board of Podiatric Surgery

Common Foot Problems in Primary Care

Second Edition

HANLEY & BELFUS, INC. / Philadelphia

7.98

Publisher: **Hanley & Belfus, Inc.**
               Medical Publishers
               210 S. 13th Street
               Philadelphia, PA 19107
               (215) 546-7293, 800-962-1892
               FAX (215) 790-9330
               Website: http://www.hanleyandbelfus.com

Library of Congress Cataloging-in-Publication Data

Birrer, Richard B.
    Common foot problems in primary care / Richard B. Birrer, Michael
P. DellaCorte, Patrick J. Grisafi.—2nd ed.
        p.   cm.
    Includes bibliographical references and index.
    ISBN 1–56053–222–X
    1. Foot—Diseases. 2. Family medicine.   I. Dellacorte, Michael P.
II. Grisafi, Patrick J.   III. Title.
    [DNLM: 1. Foot—physiopathology.   2. Foot Diseases.   3. Foot
Injuries.   WE 880 B619c 1998]
RD563.C653 1998
617.5′85—dc21   97–41961
                                                                  CIP

Common Foot Problems in Primary Care, 2nd edition

ISBN 1–56053–222–X

Last digit is the print number: 9 8 7 6 5 4 3 2 1

Table of Contents

Contributors

RICHARD B. BIRRER, MD, FAAFP, FACP
Chairman and Senior Vice President,
Attending, Department of Family Practice,
Community Medicine, and Emergency
Medicine, Catholic Medical Center of
Brooklyn and Queens, Inc., Jamaica;
Associate Professor of Emergency Medicine,
Albert Einstein College of Medicine,
Bronx; Associate Professor of Family
Medicine, State University of
New York Health Science Center,
Brooklyn, New York

ROBERT A. CARUSO, MD, FACP
Medical Director, Long Term Care/Chief of
Geriatric Medicine, Catholic Medical
Center of Brooklyn and Queens, Inc.,
Jamaica, New York

**MICHAEL P. DELLACORTE, DPM, FACFAS,
FACFAOM**
Director of Podiatry, Mary Immaculate
Division/Assistant Director of
Podiatric Medical Education, Catholic
Medical Center of Brooklyn and
Queens, Inc., Jamaica, New York;
Associate Clinical Professor of
Surgery, New York College of Podiatric
Medicine, New York; Diplomate,
American Board of Podiatric Surgery;
Diplomate, American Board of Podiatric
Orthopedics and Primary
Podiatric Medicine

HARRISON DONNELLY, MD
Director of Infectious Diseases,
St. Joseph's Hospital, Division of
Catholic Medical Center of
Brooklyn and Queens, Inc.,
Flushing, New York

STEVEN CHARLES GARNER, MD
Director of Radiology, Catholic Medical Center
of Brooklyn and Queens, Inc., Jamaica;
Clinical Instructor of Radiology,
Albert Einstein School of Medicine, Bronx,
New York; Diplomate, American Board of
Radiology; Diplomate, American Board of
Emergency Medicine

PATRICK J. GRISAFI, DPM, FACFAS
Chief, Division of Podiatric
Surgery/Director of Podiatric Medical
Education, Catholic Medical Center of
Brooklyn and Queens, Inc., Jamaica, New York;
Associate Clinical Professor of
Surgery, New York College of Podiatric
Medicine, New York; Diplomate, American
Board of Podiatric Surgery

NEIL MANDAVA, MD, FACS
Director, Department of Surgery, St. John's
Queens Hospital, Division of Catholic Medical
Center of Brooklyn and Queens, Inc., Elmhurst;
Assistant Professor of Medicine,
Albert Einstein College of Medicine,
New York, New York

ELIZABETH MCDONALD, MD
Director, Department of Medicine, St. John's
Queens Hospital, Division of Catholic Medical
Center of Brooklyn and Queens, Inc., Elmhurst;
Assistant Professor of Medicine, Albert Einstein
College of Medicine, Bronx, New York

STUART PLOTKIN, DPM
Diplomate, American Board of Podiatric
Orthopedics and Primary Podiatric Medicine;
Staff Attending, St Joseph's Hospital, Division
of Catholic Medical Center of Brooklyn and
Queens, Inc., Flushing; Staff Attending,
St. Charles Hospital,
Port Jefferson Station, New York

Dedication

To all primary care physicians and health care practitioners
who provide for the foot care needs of their patients.

Acknowledgments

Hernan Alamilla, DPM

Sandy Amador, DPM

Jean Archer, DPM

Elizabeth B. Azueta

Adam Cirlincione, DPM

Carl Conui, DPM

Malin Fonseka

Patricia Farragher, DPM

Howard Kashefsky, DPM

Douglas Livingston, DPM

Jacqueline M. Mahon

David Sands, DPM

Joseph N. Savino, MD

Eileen Schnaue, DPM

Gideon Yoeli, MD

Preface to the First Edition

To him whose feet hurt, everything hurts.

Socrates

"My feet are killing me" and "Oh, my aching feet" are two common American complaints. According to a recent Gallup poll, nearly 75% of individuals over 18 years of age complained that their feet hurt. An incredible 62% of them believed that their feet were supposed to hurt! Women were afflicted more than men. At least one third of women attributed their foot pain to uncomfortable shoes; 45% wore those shoes because they looked good. Twenty percent of these same women would not relinquish style for comfort. In 1986, at least $300 million was spent on insoles, corn remedies, bunion removers, foot powders, and other over-the-counter foot care products. Such problems do not exist in the "non-civilized" populations of the world where shoes are not worn! Ironically, the majority of people consider the foot the ugliest part of their body.

From a medical perspective, the foot is similarly neglected through both omission and commission. How many of us examine the foot as carefully as we examine other parts of the body? Although virtually all health care providers are knowledgeable in examination of the foot, less than 50% perform such examination on a regular basis. Worse still, the foot is overlooked in whole or in part some 66% of the time in the management of patients with diabetes or peripheral vascular disease. Lack of formal clinical rotations in podiatry and the traditional separation of the medical and podiatric specialties are major reasons why medical practitioners overlook the foot care of their patients. The foot can no longer be regarded as an unsophisticated, static appendage joining the leg to the ground. Rather the foot is a dynamically functional, marvelously designed structure that in many ways is even more intricately constructed and specially modified than the hand. Indeed, the human foot is engineered not only to last a lifetime but also to withstand an incredible amount (115,000 miles) of wear along the way.

This text is specifically designed for primary care practitioners, who see the majority of patients with healthy and diseased feet. The comprehensive nature of the primary care specialties (internists, family practitioners, nurse practitioners, physician's assistants, and pediatricians) mandates more than a cursory concern for patients' feet. It is the goal of this text to guide practitioners in the care of healthy and diseased feet, assist them in maintaining preventive vigilance, and, above all, improve the partnership they share with these patients. Lastly, the value of this book transcends basic and clinical sciences and treatment guidelines. The specialties of medicine and podiatry are uniquely blended so that each can share in the wisdom and experience of the other.

Richard B. Birrer, MD
Michael P. DellaCorte, DPM
Patrick J. Grisafi, DPM

Preface to the Second Edition

Like the first edition of *Common Foot Problems in Primary Care,* this second edition is intended to be a resource for all primary care practitioners who see patients with both healthy and ailing feet. It is directed to and designed for students and residents in all related areas of health care, providing them with a foundation in basic and advanced care of common foot problems.

The need for foot care services has grown exponentially. Today, most pharmacies have an aisle dedicated to foot care products. Patients, by virtue of advertisements and public information articles, are more aware of foot problems, especially those associated with infection and biomechanics. Thus, an increasingly mobile public demands of us rapid and successful care of their acute problems, along with precise guidance into a state of perpetual pedal wellness.

Significant changes have been made in this second edition. The primary care practitioner needs a handy reference book for quick information retrieval; thus, we have included more lists and tables to enhance access. New discussions center on medical imaging and nuclear medicine techniques. There is more on pedal sonography, computer tomography, bone scans, and magnetic resonance imaging. There also is an expanded section on basic radiographic techniques, including 26 new figures, for those practitioners with x-ray equipment in their offices.

Text examining infectious disease, verucca, vascular surgery, heel spur syndrome, and prescription writing for shoes and orthoses has been expanded. The trauma chapter has been divided, and a new chapter on sports medicine emerged. While most sports medicine involves management and prevention of trauma, we believe that a separate focus allows more attention to athletic-related foot ailments. Topics such as diabetes and the arthropathies have been streamlined, with more easy reference charts on classification and management.

When we first took on this project, we thought it would be a quick and simple task; we were very wrong. Completion of this edition required the time and dedication of a number of individuals. We extend a special thanks to the Podiatry Resident Staff of the Catholic Medical Center, Malin Fonseka for her endless typing and retyping, and Jacqueline Mahon, our Editor at Hanley & Belfus, for her perseverance and patience in making this text possible.

Richard B. Birrer, MD
Michael P. DellaCorte, DPM
Patrick J. Grisafi, DPM

Foreword

Foot disease in primary care is a "high impact" problem: it is common, often painful and disabling, and sometimes a cause of economic loss to the patient and family as well as society. Many foot problems are seen initially by primary care providers. While some diagnoses will require referral to a podiatrist or orthopedic surgeon, we should be able to care for many of these conditions. With the increasing emphasis on managed care in the United States, primary care providers must be competent in the diagnosis and management of foot problems.

Disorders of the foot often are not as simple as one might think; pedal diseases and injuries are varied. Problems can involve not only the musculoskeletal structures, but also the metabolic (gout), endocrine (diabetes mellitus), vascular (arteriosclerosis), and neurologic (peripheral neuropathy) systems. Foot anatomy is complex, and weight-bearing, ambulatory functions make the feet especially susceptible to trauma.

When I was in medical school, foot problems ranked high on the list of inadequately covered topics. I learned a great deal about lupus erythematosus, amyotrophic lateral sclerosis, and peptic ulcer disease, but not enough about bunions, calluses, and plantar fasciitis.

Common Foot Problems in Primary Care, 2nd edition, examines foot problems typically encountered by primary care providers and serves as an excellent reference for the care of healthy and diseased or injured feet.

Robert B. Taylor, MD
Portland, Oregon

Anatomy of the Foot

Richard B. Birrer, MD

Osteology

The foot consists of 26 bones and 55 articulations and is responsible for transmitting the ground reactive force to the body during standing, ambulation, and other activities (Fig. 1). The bones of the foot can be conveniently divided into three regions: forefoot, midfoot, and rearfoot. The forefoot is represented by the 14 bones of the toes and five metatarsals. The midfoot consists of the three cuneiform bones, the cuboid, and the navicular. Finally, the rearfoot, or the greater tarsus, is composed of the talus and the calcaneus. The foot contains two arches: longitudinal (midpart) and transverse (forepart). The transverse arch forms the convexity of the dorsum of the foot. The tarsal and tarsometatarsal articulations constitute the longitudinal arch, which is maintained primarily by the plantar ligaments and aponeurosis. Just as no two persons are the same, feet differ widely among individuals; additionally, each foot of an individual is distinctive. Often, it is these minor variations in each foot that alter the mechanics of the feet and cause subsequent sequelae.

The phalanges of the foot are similar to the hand in number and distribution, though they are somewhat shorter and broader than their counterparts in the hand. Proximally the five metatarsals articulate with both the lesser tarsus and themselves through broad concavities, whereas distally they taper to join the phalanges through convex heads. The first metatarsal is the shortest and strongest; it contains plantar articulation for the two sesamoid bones (tibial and fibular) located in the tendons of the flexor hallucis brevis. The second metatarsal is the longest and the least mobile and serves as the anatomic touchstone for abduction and adduction of the foot. The fifth metatarsal is noted for its lateral prominence (styloid process) which serves as the insertion site of the tendon of the peroneus brevis. The styloid area often is avulsed during acute inversion injuries of the foot (Jones fracture).

Distally, the three cuneiform bones (medial, intermediate, and lateral) assist in the formation of the transverse arch. The cuneiforms with the cuboid and their articulations to the metatarsals form Lisfranc's joint. The midtarsal joint is formed by the articulations of the navicular to the calcaneus and the calcaneus to the cuboid.

The largest tarsal bone, the calcaneus (os calcis), serves three basic functions. Most of the body's weight, transmitted through the talus, is borne by the calcaneus which is the site for compression fractures because of its high percentage of cancellous bone. Posteriorly, the calcaneus completes the longitudinal arch and, through its articulation with the talus, joins the foot to the leg. The articulation forms a canal or groove termed the sinus tarsi. Finally, the posterior third of the calcaneus serves as the insertion point for the tendoachilles, thus providing an effective lever for the calf muscle insertion. The anterior third of the calcaneus articulates with the cuboid bone (the calcaneal-cuboid joint or the midtarsal joint of Chopart) and a middle facet, termed the sustentaculum tali, for attachment with the talus.

The attachment of the foot to the leg occurs through the talus (astragalus). Medially and laterally, the talus articulates with the tibial and fibular malleoli, and with the talar trachlea

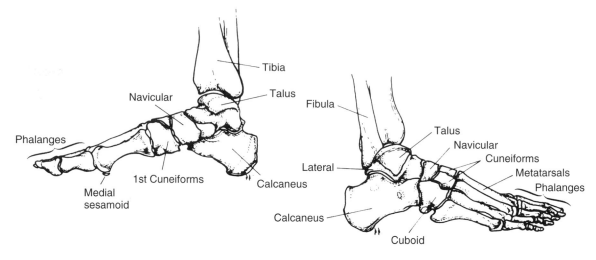

Figure 1. The bones of the foot.

forms the uniaxial ankle joint. The anterior portion of the talar trochlea is wider than the posterior portion and curves slightly, thus providing inherent stability during dorsiflexion but instability in plantar flexion. Both are the principal motions of the ankle joint. The fibrous joint capsule provides additional support, especially medially and laterally. The talus has no muscular attachments and, combined with the high-pressure forces per square inch, is susceptible to vascular damage during trauma. Fractures of the talus, therefore, frequently are associated with avascular necrosis.

There are a number of sesamoids and accessory bones variably present in the foot. The sesamoids usually are present within tendons juxtaposed to articulations and often are incompletely ossified (i.e., contain cartilage, fibrous tissue, and bone). The tibial (medial) and fibular (lateral) sesamoids of the flexor hallucis brevis are always present plantar to the first metatarsal head. The lateral sesamoid usually is single, but the medial one may be bi-, tri-, or quadripartite. It is important to assure that any multipartite sesamoid be present bilaterally before fracture is considered. Other locations where sesamoids may be found are under the heads of the four lateral metatarsals or in the tendons of the tibialis anterior, tibialis posterior, or peroneus longus. Between the ages of 10 and 20, accessory bones appear in the foot. Common examples include an os trigonum at the posterior plantar surface of the talus, an accessory navicular bone (os tibiale externum) located at the medial border, and ossicles at the base of the fifth metatarsal (os vesalianum), intermetatarsal, interphalangeal, and intercuneiform areas.

Syndesmology

The medial collateral ligament, or deltoid ligament, of the ankle joint has both superficial and deep components (Fig. 2). Superficially, the ligament consists of tibionavicular, tibiocalcaneal, and posterior tibiotalar components. The anterior middle component also stabilizes the subtalar joint. The deep portion of the deltoid ligament is the anterior tibiotalar ligament, which is responsible for stabilizing the medial malleolus and talus. Laterally, the ligamentous structure is not as sturdy, consisting of three ligaments: the anterior talofibular, calcaneofibular, and the posterior talofibular ligament. The lateral collateral ligament is torn commonly, by inversion sprains, whereas the deltoid is torn rarely.

The subtalar joint (talocalcaneal) is surrounded by a thin, nonsupportive joint capsule. Stability in the joint is maintained essentially by five sturdy ligaments: the interosseous, medial collateral, lateral collateral, talocalcaneal, and cervical ligaments. The interosseous, medial collateral, and talocalcaneal ligaments prevent excessive eversion, while the cervical and lateral collateral ligaments inhibit inversion.

The spring ligament (inferior calcaneonavicular ligament) serves to articulate the navicular bone with the sustentaculum tali of the calcaneus. The ligaments of the calcaneocuboid joint include the plantar ligaments and a portion of the bifurcate ligament. The plantar ligaments help maintain the longitudinal arch. The bifurcate ligament can be injured during forced inversion.

The plantar aponeurosis consists of a very strong fibrous central portion and a small, thinner medial and lateral section. Each is oriented longitudinally on the plantar aspect of the foot. The central portion runs from the medial calcaneal tuberosity and inserts distally, with the superficial portion attaching the skin to the pads of the toes and a deeper portion blending with flexor tendon sheaths. The medial and lateral components of the plantar aponeurosis provide vertical intermusculature septa for the plantar musculature. This aponeurosis is analogous to the one in the hand.

There are three important ankle retinacula that bind the leg tendons as they enter the foot. The extensor retinaculum consists of two portions: superior and inferior. Continuous with the deep leg fascia and joint (the anterior, lateral, and medial malleolus), the superior extensor retinaculum serves to contain the tendons of the extensor digitorum longus, extensor hallucis longus, tibialis anterior, and the peroneus tertius. The Y-shaped inferior retinaculum consists of upper and lower bands and runs from the lateral calcaneus to the medial tibial malleolus and plantar aponeurosis, thus preventing "bow stringing" of the dorsal tendon at the conjunction with the superior retinaculum. Coursing between the distal fibula and the lateral calcaneus are the peroneal retinacula, which firmly secure the peroneous longus and brevis tendons behind the

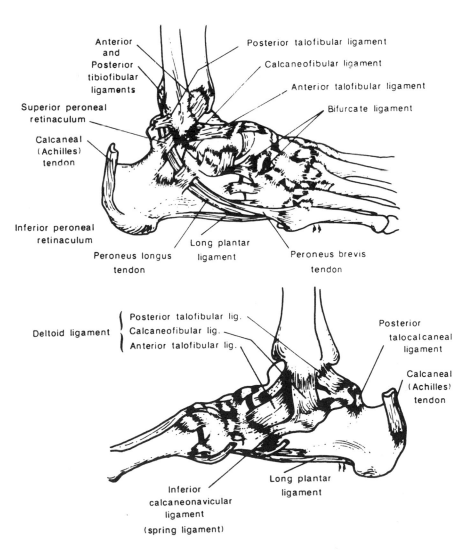

Figure 2. The medial and lateral ligaments of the ankle.

fibular malleolus. Medially, the flexor retinaculum extends from the calcaneus to the tibial malleolus and provides a firm support structure for the neurovascular bundle, flexor digitorum longus, flexor hallucis longus, and the tibialis posterior.

Myology

The muscles of the foot can be divided into extrinsic and intrinsic components (Figs. 3 and 4).

Extrinsic Muscles

The extrinsic muscles consist of muscles from the anterior, posterior, and lateral compartments of the leg. The posterior compartment consists of the posteriorly located flexors of the foot (i.e., gastrocnemius, plantaris, and soleus). The gastrocnemius and plantaris arise from the femur, whereas the soleus originates from the posterior surface of the proximal fibula branches of the tibial nerve. They form the tendocalcaneus (Achilles) as they merge to insert into the posterior calcaneus. The Achilles is the largest and the strongest tendon in the human body because it consists of fibers derived not only from the two heads of the gastrocnemius but also from the soleus and plantaris.

The remaining extrinsic flexors course behind the medial malleolus. They are the tibialis posterior, flexor digitorium longus, and the flexor hallucis longus. The tibialis posterior inserts into the navicular bone, the medial and intermediate cuneiforms, and the bases of the second, third, and fourth metatarsals. The tibialis posterior maintains the longitudinal arch and provides foot inversion.

The anterior compartment of the leg contains the dorsiflexors or extensors of the foot. They are the tibialis anterior, extensor digito-

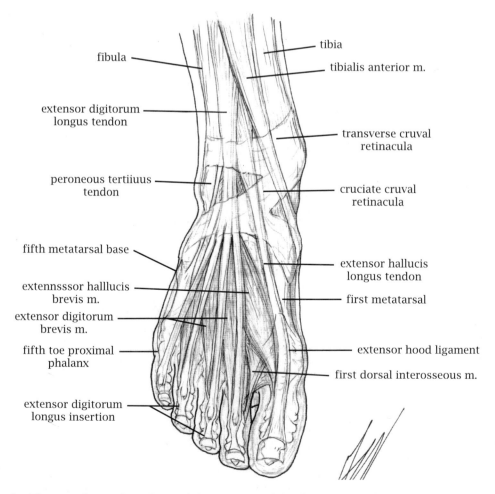

Figure 3. The muscles and tendons of the dorsum of the foot. (Original art by Alan K. Whitney, DPM, Cherry Hill, New Jersey.)

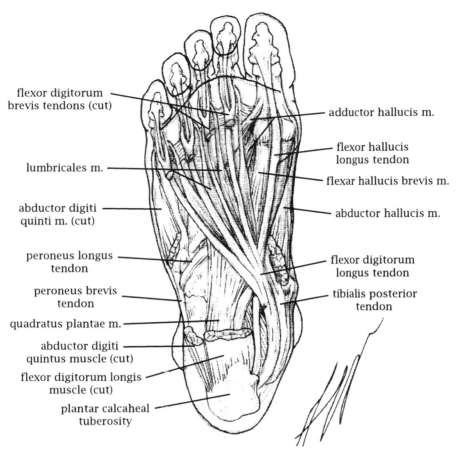

Figure 4. The muscles and tendons of the plantar surface of the foot. (Original art by Alan K. Whitney, DPM, Cherry Hill, New Jersey.)

rum longus, extensor hallucis longus, and the peroneus tertius. The lateral compartment contains the peroneals, both longus and brevis. Both groups are innervated by the common peroneal nerve. With its insertion on the medial cuneiform and adjacent base of the first metatarsal, the tibialis anterior surface is a foot inverter, ankle dorsiflexor, and arch supporter. The extensor tendons aid in extension. The peroneus longus lies posterior to the tendon of the peroneus brevis and inserts into the base of the first metatarsal and the medial cuneiform. The peroneus brevis continues more laterally to attach to the base of the fifth metatarsal. The peroneal group is responsible for foot eversion.

Thus, the integrity of the longitudinal and transverse arches of the foot depends primarily on the bony structures and support derived from the ligaments and aponeurosis. Secondary support is provided by the extrinsic musculature originating in the leg during dynamic activity.

Intrinsic Muscles

The only dorsal intrinsic muscle of the foot is the extensor digitorum brevis, which runs from the anterior region of the superior lateral calcaneus to the dorsum of the first four toes. The lateral terminal branch of the deep peroneal nerve innervates the muscle. There are four layers to the plantar intrinsic muscles, all of which are innervated by the medial or lateral plantar nerves. From medial to lateral, the abductor hallucis, flexor digitorum brevis, and abductor digiti minimi constitute the first layer. The muscles arise from the calcaneal tuberosity and insert into the toes. They are important to the dynamic stability of the longitudinal arch.

The quadratus plantar and the lumbricales make up the second layer, and the tendons of the flexor digitorum longus and flexor hallucis longus pass through this region to their respective insertions. The quadratus plantar arises from two heads on the medial and lateral calcaneal tuberosity and terminates in tendinous slips, joining the long flexor tendons to the second, third, fourth, and occasionally fifth toes. The lumbricales arise from the tendon to the flexor digitorum longus and insert into the dorsal aspect of the proximal phalanges. Their function is to flex the metatarsal phalangeal joint and extend the proximal interphalangeal joint. Paralysis or absence of the lumbricales results in hammer toes.

The third layer consists of the adductor hallucis, flexor hallucis brevis, and adductor digiti quinti. Arising from the cuboid and lateral cuneiform, the flexor hallucis brevis divides into medial and lateral components before its insertion into the corresponding aspects of the base of the proximal phalanx of the first toe. The oblique and transverse heads of the adductor hallucis insert into the lateral border of the flexor hallucis brevis. The bases of the second, third, and fourth metatarsal heads give rise to the oblique head of the adductor hallucis, while the deep transverse metatarsal ligament between the third, fourth, and fifth metatarsals provides site origin for the smaller transverse head. The origin of the flexor digiti minimi is the base of the fifth metatarsal. Together with the tendon of the abductor digiti minimi, it inserts on the lateral side of the base of the proximal phalanx of the fifth toe.

The fourth layer of intrinsic muscles is made up of the plantar and dorsal interossei. The tendons of the peroneus longus and tibialis posterior also are found here. The four dorsal interossei are bipennate and are located in the intermetatarsal areas. Their function is to abduct the second, third, and fourth toes from the axis through the second metatarsal ray. The three plantar interossei are unipennate and function to adduct the three lateral toes by inserting into the medial sides of the bases of the proximal phalanges of the third, fourth, and fifth toes.

Neurology

The sciatic nerve provides the motor and sensory innervation of the foot. It divides into the common peroneal and tibial nerves, both of which are derived from the ventral rami, L4–S3, and lie within a common sheath. The smaller component, the common peroneal nerve, divides into superficial and deep components. The superficial peroneal nerve (musculocutaneous) provides the cutaneous sensory distribution to the dorsum of the foot; the medial portion of the hallux; the lateral side of the sec-

ond toe; the medial surface of the third toe; adjacent sides of the third, fourth, and fifth toes; and the lateral portion of the ankle. The motor portion of the deep peroneal nerve (see Fig. 3) (anterior tibial nerve) supplies the extensor hallucis longus, tibialis anterior, extensor digitorum longus and brevis, peroneus tertius, and sensory innervation of the medial aspect of the second toe and the lateral side of the hallux. The third component of the common peroneal nerve is the sural nerve, which provides sensory distribution to the skin of the lateral malleolus and the fifth toe.

The tibial nerve (posterior tibial or medial popliteal) supplies the heel of the medial sole of the foot, as well as the posterior compartments of the leg. It divides into the medial and lateral plantar nerves (see Fig. 4) and serves the intrinsic muscles of the foot, with the exception of the extensor digitorum brevis. The nerve and its branches provide cutaneous innervation to most of the plantar aspect of the foot. The saphenous, the largest cutaneous branch of the femoral nerve (L2–L4), provides cutaneous innervation to the medial aspect of the foot, often extending as far as the metatarsal phalangeal joint of the hallux. It is the only nerve to the foot that is of nonsciatic origin.

Vascular

Arteries

The anterior and posterior arteries, which are the two terminal branches of the popliteal arteries, supply the foot (see Fig. 3). The anterior tibial arteries, in concert with the venae comitantes, pass beneath the superior and inferior extensor retinacula to the dorsum of the foot as the dorsalis pedis artery. The anterior tibial artery also gives rise to the anterior medial and lateral malleolar arteries. The origin of the anastomotic network is formed by the anterior malleolar arteries. The medial and lateral tarsal branches are derived from the dorsalis pedis, which gives rise to the arcuate artery and the first dorsal and plantar metatarsal arteries.

The larger posterior tibial artery, in accompaniment with the venae comitantes, courses around the medial malleolus, just medial to the medial border of the tendoachilles, and divides into the medial and lateral plantar arteries after passing underneath the flexor retinaculum with its accompanying neurovascular bundle. The smaller medial plantar artery supplies the first and third metatarsal spaces (see Fig. 4). The larger lateral artery anastomoses with the dorsalis pedis to create the plantar vascular arch, which directs the arterial supply to the lateral four toes with a smaller contribution to the hallux. The largest branch of the posterior tibial artery is the peroneal artery, which supplies the lateral and posterior aspects of the calcaneus. It anastomoses with the anterior lateral malleolar branches. Note that there is a wide variation in arterial architecture in the foot and leg. Up to 15% of individuals may be missing a dorsalis pedis artery, though the posterior tibial always is present.

Veins

The venous drainage system of the foot consists of both superficial and deep branches. The greater and lesser saphenous veins are the principal superficial veins of the lower leg, with a deep plantar venous arch serving as a primary deep-drainage system. This arch system empties into the venae comitantes, which ascend to unite in the region of the interosseous membrane to form the popliteal vein, which eventually empties into the femoral vein.

Both the superficial and deep networks of the veins communicate extensively, particularly near the edge of the ankle and the distal and medial portions of the leg. The valvular arrangement in the perforating veins allows for blood to flow from the superficial veins to the deep network, but not in the opposite direction under normal conditions. Incompetence of the valves occurs with varicose veins. The long saphenous vein lies just anterior to the medial malleolus and is subject to less anatomic variation than the veins of the upper extremity.

There are no lymphatic nodes within the foot. The dorsal aspect of the foot receives the lymphatic plexus of the digits, with the lymphatic vessels following the course of the saphenous vein to the nodes of the popliteal fossa and then to the inguinal nodes.

▬▬

References

1. Hunter SC, Powell LD, Seto CK, Zawatsky PD: Foot problems. *In* Mellion MB, Walsh WM, Shelton GL (eds): The Team Physician's Handbook, 2nd ed. Philadelphia, Hanley & Belfus, 1997, pp 605–616.
2. Riegger CL: Anatomy of the foot and ankle. Phys Ther 68:1802–1814, 1988.
3. Williams PL, Warwick R, Dyson M, Bannister LH (eds): Gray's Anatomy, 37th ed. Edinburgh, Churchill Livingstone, 1989.

History and Physical Examination

Richard B. Birrer, MD, Michael P. DellaCorte, DPM,
and Patrick Grisafi, DPM

The foot and ankle are uniquely adapted to transmit the total body weight to the physical environment. The versatility of these structures, coupled with thick heel and toe pads and the resiliency of the longitudinal transverse arches of the foot, allows concentrated stresses to be dissipated over a large variety of terrain and provides the fine adjustments and balance necessary for walking and other ambulatory activities. The foot and ankle are not immune to the long-term effects of microtrauma from the physical environment, nor to general systemic conditions such as arthritis, diabetes, or peripheral vascular disease. Even the shoes that are worn to protect the feet against the ravages of the environment can cause or worsen many foot problems. Thus, during the history-taking and physical examination, it is imperative that not only feet and ankles be examined but also other areas of the body that may give clues to the pathology affecting the feet. The wear of the patient's shoes should be checked, as well.

A thorough and successful evaluation of the foot is contingent upon a solid knowledge of anatomy, physiology, and biomechanics. The history should be taken in four parts: chief complaint/history of the present illness, past medical history, review of systems, and personal history.

Taking the History

The Present Illness

The chief complaint should be described by the patient. The history of the present illness should include the time and type of onset, in-tensity, duration, quality, conditions that relieve or aggravate the symptom(s), and whether the problem is referred to other regions of the foot or lower extremity. As examples, consider the acute, severe, localized pain of gout; the intermittent claudication of peripheral vascular disease associated with walking; the relief of osteoid osteoma pain with aspirin; the burning pain of metatarsalgia with hyperkeratosis; and the pain of initial weight-bearing in the early morning related to plantar heel-spur syndrome.

It often is helpful to categorize complaints as primary or secondary and go through detailed questioning about each. If there is a question of trauma, then the mechanism and injury must be fully elucidated. Was there a direct blow to the dorsum of the foot? Did the foot begin to hurt after a long run on rough surface (e.g., stone bruise)? It is particularly important to determine whether there was forced inversion or eversion of the foot with or without associated plantarflexion or dorsiflexion.

The time at which the injury occurred, whether there was any immediate therapy, and what the outcome was also are very important. If the injury is a chronic one, has there been any rehabilitation, prolonged immobilization, or recurrent instability or symptomatology since the time of the injury? Previous treatment modalities should be investigated, including medications, orthotics, laboratory, and radiographic evaluations, and surgery.

The acronym NLDOCAT may be helpful in determining the history of the present illness. It represents: Nature of symptoms (e.g., burning, aching), Location, Duration, Onset of symptoms (acute onset versus insidious), **C**ourse of symptoms (e.g., progressive, intermittent), **A**ggravating factors, and **T**reatment rendered. When the acronym is used, there is less likelihood that an important component of the history will be overlooked.

Because pain is the final common pathway for a myriad of conditions affecting the foot, the physician should be familiar with its podiatric evaluation (Table 1). While headache, stomachache, and even chest pain have somatic or nonorganic as well as organic causes, foot pain in children and adults almost always is due to underlying organic pathology. The mechanism of the foot and the ankle during normal gait pattern is exquisitely tuned. Consider that about 60 tons of force has been dissipated by each foot of a 150-pound person who has walked a mile. Any alteration affecting the plantigrade position during ground contact produces abnormal stress and results in pain.

Incidence of pain in the toes is 55–65%, in the ball of the foot 25–35%, in the arch 10%, and in the heel 5%. Podiatric pain is more common in females than males, with 80% of women reporting significant foot pain while wearing shoes. Of those individuals with deformities, 71% have bunions, 50% have hammer toes, 18% have tailor's bunions, 13% have prominent metatarsal heads, and 4% have miscellaneous deformities. Pain with associated deformities increases with age in both sexes, but is eight times more common in females compared to males. The frequency of forefoot surgery in both genders peaks in the fourth, fifth, and sixth decades and parallels the frequency, duration, and intensity of pain.

Past Medical History

It is important to get a thorough past medical history, including family background. This history should detail allergies, with care being taken to include specific items used in the treatment of the lower extremity, such as iodine (Betadine preparations), topical anesthetics, and tape. Information on medications including use of tobacco and alcohol, previous hospitalizations, and recent fevers is an essential ingredient for the complete history. The family background should be checked for vascular disease, arthritis, gout, hypertension, cancer, cardiovascular disease, and bleeding problems.

Review of Systems

Since the feet can present the first clinical evidence of systemic pathology, the patient should be asked about thyroid disease, peripheral vascular disease, vasculitis, gout, psoriasis, diabetes, malignancy, collagen vascular disease, and arthritis of any etiology. A number of neurologic problems affecting the back can present only with foot findings. Herniated nucleus pulposus, spina bifida, spinal cord tumors, neurofibromatosis, and Friedreich's ataxia commonly involve the foot before other symptoms become evident. The review of systems also should highlight history of congenital or childhood infectious problems (e.g., Charcot-Marie-Tooth disease, poliomyelitis, club foot) and the presence of edema (e.g., hepatic, renal, or cardiac disease). Finally, during the general systemic review, an attempt should be made to determine the patient's psychological perception of the foot problem. For instance, what is the individual's pain threshold? Is there an element of secondary gain, malingering, or hypochondriasis present?

Personal History

An occupational and hobby history should include the amount of weight bearing that the patient undergoes during the workday, dura-

Table 1. Common Causes of Foot Pain

Forefoot	Hindfoot
Insufficient first ray	Tarsal coalition
	Sever's disease
Arthritis	Contusion
Bunion	Fracture
Hallux valgus	Midfoot
Excessive second ray	Entrapment syndromes
	Fracture
Metatarsalgia	Contusion
Callus formation	Tendinitis
Atrophic planter fat pad	Dislocation
	Heel
Corns	Planter fasciitis
Arthritis	Hypermobility
Neuroma	Excessive pronation
Neuropathy	Impingement
Sesamoiditis	Arthritis
Fracture	Achilles tendinitis
Cavus foot	Trauma
Warts	Cavus foot
Bursitis	Bursitis
Freiberg's disease	Fracture
Dislocation	Contusion

tion of any sitting or desk work involved, and the type of shoe gear worn at work versus the type worn outside of work. Lastly, if the patient is an athlete, a full athletic history should be elicited about the type and amount of sports activity in which the patient participates on a regular basis. Any regimen changes (e.g., increased or decreased distances, change in surface or footwear) are critical. Past injuries and their treatments should be fully reviewed, as should the gear that the patient wears, the athletic surfaces that the patient plays on, and the amount of time per week that the patient spends doing the athletic endeavor.

The Physical Exam
Observation/Vital Signs

The physical exam begins when the patient walks through the physician's door. The patient should be asked to ambulate to and fro, turn 180°, and repeat the movement. The same activities then should be performed on the heels and balls of the feet. During weight-bearing activity, deformities such as differences in the width or length of both feet, heel varus or valgus, calf atrophy, splay foot, varicose veins, and in-toeing or out-toeing (which may suggest internal tibial torsion or anteversion of the femoral necks in children) should be noted. Observe posture and gait, and look for antalgia, shuffling, steppage, or other deformity. The patient's clothing from the waist down should be removed and the exam repeated. Carefully note the position and function of the feet and ankles as the patient undresses. Weight bearing is a useful stress test for underlying pathology. Record the patient's vital signs, and seat the patient on the exam table with shoes and socks off.

General Inspection

In the normally relaxed position there is mild plantarflexion and inversion of the feet. Dorsiflexion and eversion are characteristic of a spastic flat foot. The medial longitudinal arch produces a perceptible dome on the dorsum of the foot which extends from the calcaneous to the first metatarsal head. At rest, while non-weight-bearing, this arch is more prominent. However, when it is excessively high, it is termed per cavus; when absent, pes planus. A collapsed arch is suggestive of neuropathic injury or a Charcot joint. In children there may be some medical inclination of the forefoot on the hindfoot, termed forefoot adductus, or the hindfoot may be in excessive valgus or varus position. Note the number of toes. They should appear straight, flat, and proportional to one another as compared to those of the other foot. Overlapping toes are suggestive of an underlying hammer toe and/or bunion.

Vascular Examination

The evaluation of the vascular network includes the dorsalis pedis, posterior tibialis, and popliteal and femoral pulses. They are graded 0 to 4, with 3 to 4 being normal. The femoral pulse lies just inferior to the inguinal ligament at a point midway between the anterior superior iliac spine and the pubic tubercle. The superficial dorsalis pedis pulse is easily palpated on the dorsum of the foot between the extensor digitorum longus and hallucis longus tendons. The posterior tibial artery is palpated just posterior to the medial malleoli between the tibialis posterior and the flexor digitorum longus tendons. The popliteal pulse can be found by pressing the fingers of both hands up into the popliteal fossa medial to the lateral biceps femoris tendon while the knee is actively extended.

Determine capillary refill time (normally 3–5 seconds) by compressing the toe tufts until they blanch. Prolongation of the time it takes for normal pink coloration to return following release is synonymous with vascular disease. The elevation and dependency test also can be used to assess pedal circulation. Normally there is no pallor (grade 0) after elevating the foot to 60° for 1 minute. Definite pallor in 60 seconds is grade I, pallor in 30–60 seconds is grade II, pallor in less than 30 seconds is grade III, and pallor without elevation is grade IV.

Immediately after the elevation test the patient should sit up and hang the feet over the examining table edge. Severe ischemia is denoted by color return requiring more than 40 seconds of dependency, moderated occlusive disease if 15–25 seconds are necessary, and normal circulation if color returns in 10–15 seconds. If either test is abnormal, further vascular evaluation should include Doppler plus thermography studies.

The retrograde filling (Trendelenburg) test is used to assess valvular competency in the communicating veins as well as in the saphenous systems. The great saphenous vein is occluded by a tourniquet on the upper thigh for 20–25 seconds after the leg has been drained of venous blood through elevation. During standing there should be slow filling of the saphenous vein from below as the femoral artery pushes blood through the capillary bed into the venous system. Rapid filling of the superficial veins indicates incompetent communicating venous valves. The tourniquet is then released. Sudden additional filling of the superficial system suggests incompetent valves of the saphenous vein.

Neurologic Examination

The neurologic exam can be cursory unless there is underlying pathology, such as low back pain or diabetes. The exam should include reflexes of both the Achilles (ankle jerk S1–S2) and prepatellar (knee jerk L2–L4) tendons. It is important to assess vibratory sensations since they usually are the first to be diminished in diabetic neuropathy. With the patient's eyes closed, a tuning fork is successively placed on each digit. The sensation should be the same bilaterally.

Soft touch and pain also should be evaluated. Check the patient's reliability with a nonvibrating tuning fork or the hub of the needle. The L4 dermatome extends from the medial aspect of the leg to the medial malleolus and the medial side of the foot. The L5 dermatome covers the lateral side of the leg and the dorsum of the foot. The S1 dermatome covers the lateral portion of the foot.

Sensory testing includes each peripheral nerve that innervates the dorsum of the foot (saphenous on the medial side, peroneal on the dorsum, sural on the lateral side) and the L4–L5–S1 dermatomes. If gait abnormality is noted upon the patient's arrival in the office, then further function tests should be performed, such as heel-toe gait, balance function, and heel-to-shin testing. Motor testing also can be accomplished, but it is easier to do during the musculoskeletal part of the physical examination.

Dermatologic Examination

Inspect the web spaces for any sign of inflammation or vesicles indicative of a tinea infection. Next, examine the skin of the dorsum of the foot. It should be smooth and nonthickened and contain hair follicles, particularly over the toes. A loss of hair on the toes is indicative of poor arterial supply to the digits (e.g., peripheral vascular disease, diabetes). The plantar surface, especially the ball and the bed, contain thickened areas to accommodate weight bearing. Abnormal lichenification and thickening of the skin over the metatarsal heads or the medial border of the hallux (e.g., tyloma or heloma) occurs in response to bearing of abnormal amounts of weight. The location of such lesions should be carefully noted in the chart.

Skin color typically is dark pink during weight bearing, becoming lighter during nonweight-bearing activity. If, during dependence, the foot becomes deep red, indicating dependent rubor, small vessel disease is suggested. Cyanosis, skin atrophy, and ulceration are suggestive of vascular disease. Medial ulcerations are more common in venous disease, whereas lateral ulcerations are more typical of arterial disease. Both occur principally at the level of the malleoli.

Conclude the inspection by noting whether there is localized or generalized edema of the foot or ankle. Unilateral localized edema is highly suggestive of trauma or infection (e.g., tinea) if there is associated erythema and warmth. Bilateral swelling is more suggestive of hepatic, cardiac, or renal pathology, or pelvic obstruction to venous return. Occasionally, unilateral edema follows congenital absence of lymph glands (Milroy's disease) or obstruction due to primary or secondary carcinoma. Carefully inspect the toenails for dystrophia, erythema, discoloration, pitting, and deformity. Excessive growth of a nail along with its medial or lateral margins (unguis incarnatus) can produce erythema, edema, and secondary infection. Clubbing of the nails suggests cardiopulmonary compromise.

Biomechanical Examination

Biomechanics is the application of mechanical laws to living structures, specifically to the locomotor system of the human body. The biomechanical exam is probably the most difficult part of the lower extremity assessment and must include not only the foot and ankle but also the knee and hip. The anatomic position for lower-extremity biomechanical examination places the patient standing erect, with the feet perpendicular to the body and at the normal angle and base of gait. It is best to start with the patient lying supine on the examination table. Palpate the anterior superior iliac spines, and measure the distance between them and the ipsilateral medial malleolus to determine limb length. A true limb-length discrepancy of 5 mm or more can cause significant functional and structural problems.

Measuring from a nonfixed point (e.g., umbilicus) detects any apparent limb length discrepancy due to pelvic tilt.

It is not necessary to measure joint motion per se, but it is necessary to know if a particular motion is in the abnormal range. Therefore, both sides should be tested for comparison. Note the internal and external rotation of the hip during extension and flexion. This transverse plane motion should be equal in both the extended and flexed position, and both hips should have the same range of motion. The position of the knee also should be noted (i.e., varus, valgus, recurvatum); mild valgus is normal.

There are three body planes in which the foot and ankle function: transverse, sagittal, and frontal. Motion can occur in one plane, two planes, or all three planes. Dorsiflexion is a pure sagittal plane motion. It is described as the top of the foot moving closer to the anterior leg. Plantarflexion, the opposing sagittal plane motion, is when the foot moves away from the anterior leg. The two frontal plane motions are inversion and eversion. Inversion occurs when the bottom of the foot turns toward the midline of the body. Eversion is the opposite action, with the bottom of the foot turning away from the midline of the body. Abduction and adduction are the two pure transverse plane motions. Abduction occurs when the foot rotates away from the midline of the body. Adduction is described as the foot moving toward the midline of the body.

Ankle joint range of motion should be evaluated (Table 2). To assess this motion it is essential to stabilize the subtalar joint by fixating the calcaneus and inverting the forefoot so that it locks into the hindfoot, thus prohibiting forefoot motion. Have the patient sit at the edge of the examination table with the knees bent, relaxing the gastrocnemius and the soleus muscles. Grip the forefoot and manipulate the foot into plantarflexion and dorsiflexion. The relationship of the lateral aspect of the foot and the posterior aspect of the leg are the reference points to determine ankle joint range of motion (Fig. 1).

A small amount of lateral talar tilt between the malleoli can occur in full plantarflexion under normal conditions. This is because the narrow posterior portion of the talus does not fit tightly into the mortise formed by the tibia and fibula. However, in dorsiflexion the talus is held snugly between the two malleoli. Edema of an extra- or intra-articular location reduces or constricts normal ankle motions, and end points feel boggy. Less than 10° of dorsiflexion suggests an equinus condition, and it is important to note if the equinus is soft tissue or osseous in nature. This is done by reducing the stretch of gastrocnemius through knee flexion. No change in dorsiflex-

Table 2. Normal Range of Motion for the Foot and Ankle

Foot	
1st Metacarpophalangeal Joint	
Flexion	45°
Extension	70–90°
1st Interphalangeal Joint	
Flexion	70–90°
Subtalar Joint	
Supination	20°
Pronation	10°
Ankle	
Dorsiflexion	10°
Plantarflexion	70°

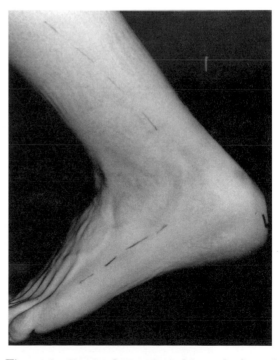

Figure 1. Testing for equinus: bisect the lateral leg and the lateral foot. Place the subtalar joint in neutral position and dorsiflex the foot. Dorsiflexion of 10° or more rules out equinus.

ion suggests an osseous lesion. (See Chapter 12).

Triplanar motion is motion that deviates from all three body planes. Two major joints of the foot—the subtalar and midtarsal—are triplanar joints. Triplanar motion is described as pronation and supination. The pronatory supinatory axis begins posterior, plantar, and lateral, and it ends medial, anterior, and dorsal. Around this axis occur the motions of pronation (Fig. 2A)—consisting of abduction, dorsiflexion, and eversion—and supination (Fig. 2B)—consisting of adduction, plantarflexion, and inversion. The subtalar joint (STJ) has one axis around which triplanar motion exists. Three times more motion occurs in the transverse and frontal planes than in the sagittal plane due to the greater axis deviation from the transverse and frontal planes. The midtarsal joint (MTJ) consists of the talonavicular and calcaneocuboid joints and contains two axes: longitudinal (LMTJ) and oblique (OMTJ). Both axes are triplanar. The LMTJ has more motion in all three planes. Deviation from the triplanar motion, at the STJ, OMTJ, or LMTJ, can occur due to rearfoot or forefoot deformities intrinsically created at birth or by com-

pensation of foot abnormalities in the proximal lower extremity.

For the STJ part of the examination the patient should be rolled into a prone position with the feet hanging over the edge of the examination table. The table should be elevated to a comfortable height for the examiner to manipulate the person's foot. The patient's STJ should be moved into neutral position. An understanding of the STJ neutral position is essential to understanding normal lower extremity function. Neutral position is defined as the position where the joint functions best (Fig. 3). To determine the STJ neutral position, put the joint through its total excursion of motion while palpating the head of the talus anteriorly within the ankle mortise and moving the calcaneus in a pronatory and supinatory direction. When you feel the change of direction of that motion, the joint is in its neutral position.

Generally the STJ has twice as much supination as pronation—20° to 10°, respectively. Subtalar motion derived from the concerted activities of the foot allows functioning on uneven surfaces. Pain as well as restriction of motion are suggestive of possible fracture acutely, or degenerative joint disease or arthri-

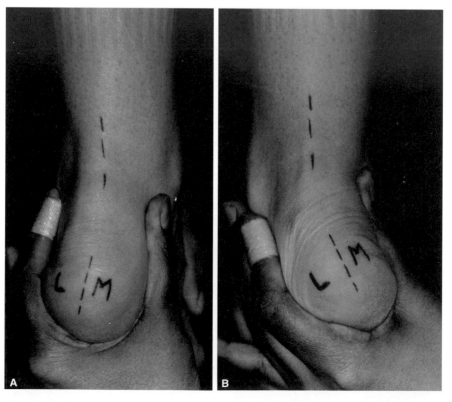

Figure 2. Subtalar joint (L = lateral, M = medial). *A,* Pronation. *B,* Supination.

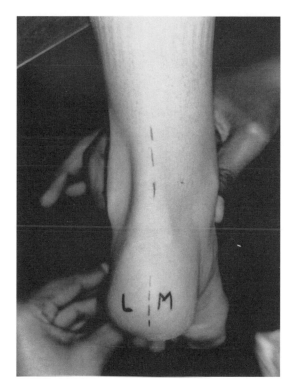

Figure 3. Neutral position of subtalar joint (L = lateral, M = medial). The lines bisecting the posterior leg and the posterior calcaneus should be in line.

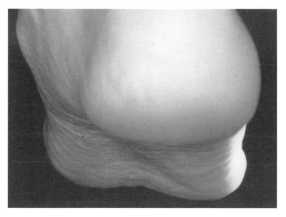

Figure 4. Forefoot varus. Note the inversion of the forefoot in relation to the rearfoot.

tis more chronically. Subtalar mobility is enhanced in the younger patient.

When the foot is in neutral position, the amount of calcaneal varus/valgus should be evaluated off weight bearing. It is highly unusual for the calcaneus to be in a valgus position, but it does occur. Next, the forefoot to rearfoot configuration should be noted for the amount of varus or valgus at the midtarsal joint. This is done by sighting from the rear of the calcaneus down the forefoot along the plane formed by the metatarsals (Fig. 4). The midtarsal joint does not have a neutral position; it is most stable when maximally pronated. Maximal pronation can be achieved by "loading" the lateral column of the foot, which is performed by placing the thumb below the fifth metatarsal head and applying force to simulate weight bearing. Ideally, the patient's foot will exhibit a small amount of rearfoot varus in the calcaneus, maybe 3°, and a parallel midtarsal joint or forefoot to rearfoot position, so that there appears to be no deviation in the inverted or averted position when one sights down the calcaneus.

Once a deformity is identified, determine whether it is fixed or flexible. Fixed deformities of the foot can be uniplanar, triplanar, or a combination of both. Sagittal plane fixed deformities are pes calcaneus (calcaneus in dorsiflexed position) or equinus (rearfoot is plantarflexed). Frontal plane deformities are varus (fixed inversion) or valgus (fixed eversion) and can occur at the forefoot, rearfoot, tibia, or the knee. Transverse fixed deformities include abductus (foot pointing away from the body) or adductus (pointing toward the body). Triplane deformities include supinatus and pronatus.

Reduced motion in the first toe (e.g., hallux limitus or rigidus) usually is reflected in an abnormal gait consisting of a shortened "toe-off/push off" phase that tends to be protective and antalgic. In the four lateral toes only the metatarsophalangeal joints (MTPJs) can actively extend, while the distal and proximal interphalangeal joints (IPJs) are capable of active flexion. Thus, in assessing the range of motion of the lesser toes, passive extension and flexion of the proximal and distal IPJs as well as the MTPJs is essential. Often subtle deformities such as claw or hammer toes are revealed.

The patient should now stand, barefoot and in a comfortable position, for determination of the angle and base of gait. The angle of gait is defined as the angle of the foot to the line of progression (Fig. 5). The line of progression is a straight line in the direction that the patient is walking. The normal angle of gait is 5–10° abducted. Note if the patient is in-toed or out-toed. The base of gait is the distance between the right and left malleoli as one foot swings past the other during gait. Normal base of gait is 1–2 cm during swing phase. Have the patient stand with his or her back to you and evaluate

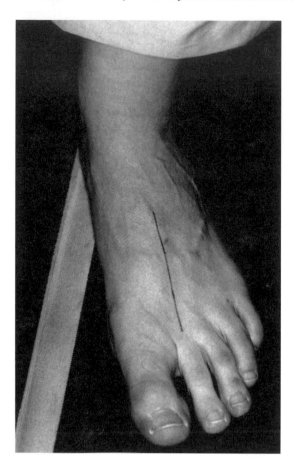

Figure 5. Angle of gait. White tape represents the line of progression; the line on the foot is the center reference point of the foot. Normal angle of gait is 10–15° abducted.

the position of the calcaneus. Neutral calcaneal stance position and resting calcaneal stance position should be determined. Is there significant valgus in stance? Custom-made foot orthotics can be prescribed to reduce or correct abnormalities discovered in the biomechanical exam. The biomechanical goal in treatment of the patient is to decrease the amount of foot and leg compensation secondary to poorly aligned joints or structural deformities.

Another method of assessing foot biomechanics uses the Harris foot mat. The mat is an inked rubber sheet with elevated squares of rubber at various heights so that areas of increasing pressure bring more and more inked rubber edges to the paper. Thus, a printout of the loading pattern can be made. Frequently, excessive loading under the metatarsal heads becomes more noticeable with this test. If this mat is unavailable, Betadine solution can be applied to the plantar aspect of the foot, and the patient can then stand on a white piece of paper to provide a two-dimensional impression of the foot. A plaster of Paris cast of the foot gives a true three-dimensional impression, which is necessary for the fabrication of functional foot orthotics.

The Gait Cycle

The ideal conditions for normal gait are:
- A level pelvis
- Legs of equal length
- Knee joint axis in the frontal plane (i.e., knees facing straight ahead)
- Knees and ankles directly over each other
- Legs straight and perpendicular to the foot
- First and fifth rays in the same plane (i.e., level) with the second, third, and fourth rays
- Ankle joint at a minimum of 10° dorsiflexion when the STJ is in neutral position and the MTJ is maximally pronated.

Abnormalities in these conditions lead to changes in foot function and gait.

The gait cycle describes normal walking and consists of two parts: a swing phase and a stance phase. The swing phase is the time when the foot does not touch the ground and is swinging forward, constituting approximately one-third of the cycle. The stance phase is the time when the foot makes contact with the ground, constituting approximately two-thirds of the cycle.

The stance phase has three divisions, beginning with heel contact and ending with toe-off of the same foot. The first division begins with heel contact and is completed with full forefoot loading. It constitutes the first 27% of the stance phase. At heel strike, the foot is inverted to the ground, the leg internally rotates, and the STJ pronates, allowing the foot to become a "mobile adapter" to the uneven ground. The STJ pronation also allows the knee to flex, enhancing shock absorption (Fig. 6[A]).

The second division of the stance phase is midstance, which occurs when the forefoot and rearfoot are in contact with the ground. Midstance begins with full forefoot loading and ends with heel-off, and it constitutes 40% of the stance phase. During midstance the STJ begins resupination so that the forefoot becomes a rigid lever for propulsion. At the midpoint of midstance, the STJ is in neutral position and the opposite leg is swinging by (Fig. 6[B]).

The third division of the stance phase is propulsion, which begins with heel-off and ends with the toe-off (Fig. 6[C]). Propulsion constitutes 33% of the stance phase. Weight is transferred during contact and midstance from the lateral heel to medial forefoot, so that during propulsion stress is passed out through the first and second toes as a rigid lever for propulsion. Stress then passes to the opposite foot at heel contact, and the cycle starts over again with the swing phase (Fig. 6[D]).

To enhance smooth walking, six elements are needed: (1) Pelvic rotation—the hip of the swinging limb rotates around the stance phase limb, allowing for less drop of the center of gravity and thus decreasing shock at heel contact. (2) Pelvic drop occurs during midstance, so that the swing phase limb is lowered approximately 5° when swinging by the stance phase limb. Hence, the center of gravity need not be raised as high for a smoother walk. (3) Knee flexion occurs at contact to reduce the shock of heel contact and also decrease the amount necessary to raise the center of gravity. (4) The ankle joint plantarflexes, reducing the amount of shock the foot encounters at heel strike. (5) The STJ and MTJ go through their range of motion for smooth walking throughout the gait cycle. (6) The body displaces its weight laterally so that the torso is over the weight-bearing foot. The distal end of the femur is angled inward for less lateral displacement of the body, which leads to a smoother walk. In addition, the upper body rotates 180° opposite that of the lower extremity to reduce the transverse and sagittal motion of the lower extremity.

Deviation from these normal gait cycle components results in abnormalities in foot function, which progress to foot deformities such as bunions, hammer toes, and flatfoot (see Chapter 12).

Running creates a variation in the cycle. During running, the foot is slightly supinated just before the heel strikes. The outside of the heel touches the surface first, followed by loading of the arch, which then flattens. The foot then pronates; together with contraction of the calf muscles, this dissipates the generated forces throughout the entire foot and leg. The longitudinal arch continues to flatten until the arch ligament (plantar aponeurosis) is tightened. During takeoff, the forefoot supinates to stabilize the foot until the great toe leaves the ground. Depending on the runner's speed, the foot is in pronation during 40–70% of the supporting phase.

Musculoskeletal Examination

Palpate the foot beginning with the first toe. The metatarsal and MTP joints are readily palpated. Carefully palpate the soft tissue overlying the joint, noting its angulation and the presence or absence of underlying bursal inflammation, which may be due to pressure, friction, or urate deposition. More proximally along the medial border of the foot is the prominent navicular tubercle. A localized trigger point or tenderness is often associated with antalgia in children and is suggestive

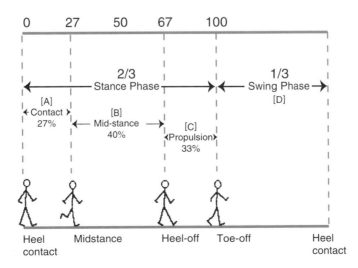

Figure 6. The walking gait cycle.

of osteochondritis dessicans of the navicular (Kohler's). Flexion and inversion of the foot causes the tibialis posterior to stand out (L5 ramus). The flexor digitorum longus tendon directly posterior to the tibialis posterior tendon is best palpated by resisting plantarflexion of the patient's toes while the calcaneus is stabilized. The tendon of the flexor hallucis longus cannot be palpated, but can be tested by opposition of plantarflexion of the great toe. Medially, the large, strong, and wide deltoid ligament usually is not palpable in the space inferior to the medial malleolus. Most proximally, the prominent medial malleolus articulates with one-third of the medial side of the talus.

On the lateral aspect of the foot, the MTP joint and the head of the fifth metatarsal bone are easily palpated. Overlying the head of the fifth metatarsal bone is a bursa which, due to its superficial nature, can easily become inflamed, a condition commonly referred to as "tailor's bunion." As one travels proximally along the shaft of the fifth metatarsal, its flared base, the styloid process, becomes evident. The tendon of the peroneus brevis inserts into the styloid process. Between the styloid process and the cuboid bone is a depression that contains the peroneus longus tendon as it travels to the medial plantar surface of the foot. Moving proximally, the calcaneus' peroneal tubercle, which separates the peroneus longus and brevis tendons, is easily notable. The tubercle is just distal to the lateral malleolus and is usually about 5 cm in length, though there is some variation between patients. The peronei can be assessed by opposing plantarflexion and eversion with pressure against the head and shaft of the fifth metatarsal.

The distal portion of the fibula constitutes the lateral malleolus. It extends more distally than the medial malleolus and is more effective in preventing eversion injury. The dome of the talus can be appreciated by plantarflexing the foot with the examiner's thumb placed on the anterior lateral portion of the malleolus. With the application of a small amount of inversion force, more of the talar dome can be appreciated. The sinus tarsi area can be felt by placing the thumb just anterior to the lateral malleolus and the soft tissue depression, which is filled by a superficial fat pad and the deeper extensor digitorum brevis muscle. With rare exception, as in the case of ankle trauma with diastasis, the inferior portion of the tibiofibular joint can be appreciated. It lies immediately proximal to the talus and is fortified by very strong anterior inferior tibiofibular ligaments. The anterior talofibular ligament transverses the sinus tarsi and is the first ligament torn in inversion ankle sprains. Pathology of the subtalar complex, such as fracture or rheumatoid arthritis, produces deep tenderness on palpation of the sinus tarsi. The extensor digitorium brevis can be appreciated by having the patient voluntarily extend the toes while the sinus tarsi is palpated.

The lateral collateral ligaments (anterior talofibular, calcaneal, fibular, and posterior talofibular) are not distinctly palpable under normal conditions. Their functional integrity can best be assessed through a number of ankle joint stress tests. To test the integrity of the anterior talofibular ligament, plantarflexion and inversion should be performed. The production of pain in the region of the sinus tarsi is highly suggestive of a sprain of the ligament. Greater degrees of pain that are more diffuse suggest that the calcaneofibular ligament also may be involved.

Tibiotalar stability can be assessed by performing the anterior draw test (Fig. 7). With one hand on the anterior aspect of the tibia and the calcaneus in the palm of the other hand, the calcaneus and talus are drawn anteriorly while the distal tibia is pushed posteriorly. There is no pain and only imperceptible movement under normal conditions. Anterior displacement of the talus and calcaneus by more than 3–5 mm or a difference of greater than 0.5 mm between ankles is highly suggestive of a rupture of the anterior talofibular ligament. A soft end-point or the perception of a "clunk" may be appreciated and also is considered to be a positive sign. Reversing the procedure assesses the stability in the posterior plane. It is important that the exam be performed with the anteroposterior muscles surrounding the ankle completely relaxed and that the ankle be positioned 90° to the leg because it often is impossible to demonstrate even a significantly positive anterior draw sign in the plantarflexed position. The results should always be compared to the normal side. For an acute injury, infiltration of 5–10 cc of 1% lidocaine in the joint opposite to the side of injury, with additional infiltration of the involved ligament(s), can be helpful.

The talar tilt or inversion/eversion stress test can be used to assess the integrity of the lateral as well as the medial ligaments of the ankle (Fig. 8). The normal angle of talar tilt is 3–23°, and a 5–10° difference between ankles is

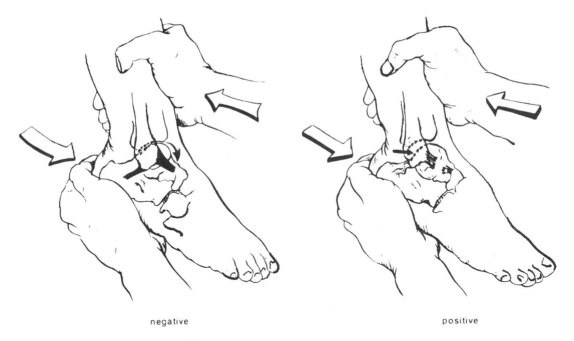

negative   positive

Figure 7. The anterior drawer test.

considered to be within normal limits. In the case of a questionable lateral tear, an inversion force is applied to the talus with the foot in equinus. Opening up of the ankle mortise in this manner is suggestive of tears in two or more of the lateral compartments. If a repeat stress test with the foot in the neutral position produces a tilt, then concomitant rupture of the calcaneofibular ligament is likely. It usually is not necessary to perform a drawer test if the integrity of the deltoid ligament is questionable. In this case an eversion force is applied, and an abnormal gap of the ankle mortise denotes ligament rupture. Each of these clinical tests can be confirmed by simultaneous stress radiographs.

The hindfoot is best examined by placing the heel in the palm of the hand and the thumb and the index finger in the contralateral soft tissue depressions on either side of the Achilles tendon. The posterior third of the calcaneus is easily appreciated. As one moves plantar, the bone normally flares at its outer base. On the medial plantar aspect of the calcaneus, there is a medial tubercle, which tends to be broad and large, that provides attachment for the flexor digitorum brevis and plantar aponeurosis and the abductor hallucis muscle. A tender medial tubercle suggests a heel spur. More posterior tenderness along the calcaneus, especially in children, is suggestive of an apophysitis (Sever's disease).

The large Achilles tendon, which represents the combined tendon of the gastrocnemius and soleus muscles, inserts into the posterior calcaneus. Its integrity can be assessed by direct palpation, having the patient jump up and down on the balls of the feet or walk on the toes, and the squeeze test of Thompson-Doherty-Simpson (Fig. 9). Squeezing the calf, which normally produces plantarflexion, produces markedly decreased motion or none at all. When the tendon has been acutely ruptured, there is often a palpable gap that is painful and tender where the rupture has occurred.

Between the overlying skin and the insertion of the Achilles tendon lies the calcaneal bursa, which can become inflamed following excessive direct pressure or secondary damage to the Achilles tendon. High heels and tight shoes frequently are responsible. Between the Achilles tendon and the posterior superior aspect of the calcaneus lies the retrocalcaneal bursa. As with the calcaneal bursa, it can become inflamed following tendinitis or severe contusion of the calcaneus.

Examination of the plantar surface of the foot is somewhat difficult due to the thickness of the overlying skin, as well as the supportive connective tissue layers of the arches and fat pad. With the lower extremity in extension and the calf of the leg supported by one of the examiner's hands, the sole of the foot is gently

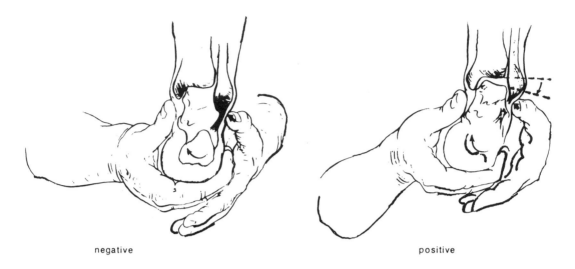

negative   positive

Figure 8.   The talar tilt stress test.

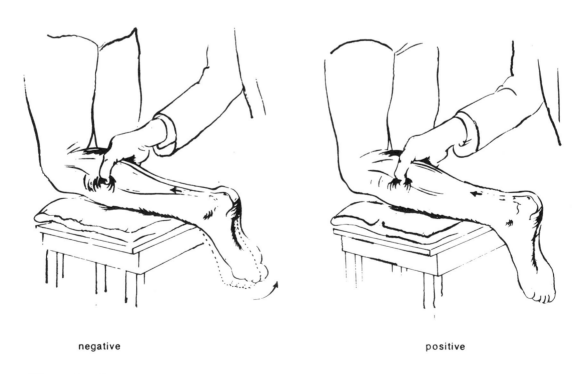

negative   positive

Figure 9.   The Thompson-Doherty-Simpson squeeze test for integrity of the Achilles tendon.

palpated. Firm pressure at the first metatarsal head reveals two small sesamoid bones lying within the tendon of the flexor hallucis brevis. Tenderness suggests sesamoiditis, which can be aggravated during the toe-off portion of normal gait. During palpation, one should assess the presence or absence of tenderness and the size and location of each head.

Proximal to the metatarsal heads lies the plantar fascia, or aponeurosis. It should feel smooth and nontender. Tender trigger points may indicate plantar fasciitis, whereas the palpation of discrete nodules suggests a Dupuytren's type contracture (plantar fibromatosis) in the foot. Such nodules should be distinguished from more superficial ones, typical of corns and warts. Each of the metatarsal interspaces should be carefully palpated for tenderness and swelling. The identification of a tender trigger between metatarsals is suggestive of neuroma, termed Morton's neuroma if in the third interspace.

The most visible portion of the foot is the dorsum or extensor surface. During weight bearing the toes should be straight and flat. MTPJ hyperextension with flexion of the proximal and distal IPJs is termed claw toes, which typically involves all toes and usually is associated with per cavus deformity. Constant frictional irritation of the shoes on the flexed IPJs produces dorsal callosities over the involved toes. On the plantar surface, callosities often affect the metatarsal heads and the tips of the toes, particularly the second toe, due to excessive amounts of weight bearing and a more plantar position of one or more bones. Hyperextension of both the MTPJs and distal IPJs is associated with proximal IPJ flexion and is termed swan neck deformity. Flexion of the proximal IPJ produces a hammer-toe deformity. This malformation usually involves the second toes and is denoted by a proximal IPJ callosity due to shoe friction.

The shafts of the metatarsal should be palpated for localized trigger points and swelling. There are a number of soft tissue structures that should be noted. Resisted dorsiflexion and inversion of the foot makes palpation of the tibialis anterior tendon easy, as it courses between the malleoli most medially. With opposed extension of the big toe at the distal phalanx, the extensor hallucis longus tendon, lateral to the tibialis anterior tendon, becomes evident. If the pressure is applied before the IPJ, then the extensor hallucis brevis also is tested.

Resisted extension of the toes facilitates palpation of the extensor digitorum longus tendon, which lies lateral to the extensor hallucis longus. It is most easily felt where it crosses the ankle joint before it divides into its four tendinous insertions at the dorsal bases of the distal phalanges of the four lesser toes. Muscle formation should be grossly tested by having the patient invert and evert, abduct and adduct, and dorsiflex and plantarflex against resistance. Toes also should be flexed and extended against resistance. Muscle strength usually is graded on a 0 (no movement) to 5 (normal) scale.

The Athlete

Athletic examination should include treadmill evaluation, ideally with video, or watching the patient walk and/or run. Check running movements such as cutting and figure-of-eights. If the athlete is a cyclist, use a stationary trainer to see, dynamically, what actually is occurring during this activity. Evaluate the patient in shorts from the posterior—barefooted, in athletic shoe gear, without devices, and with devices if appropriate. In addition to watching the patient participate in his or her athletic endeavor, it is important to examine the athlete's foot gear.

Footwear Considerations
Evaluation

Shoe-gear evaluation is essential in the investigation of a foot problem. The investigation should include not only the presumed culprit but also a cross sampling of all footwear regularly used by the patient. Does the footwear accurately fit the feet? Are the shoes loose, tight, shallow, or deep? Carefully inspect the shoe for defects (Fig. 10). Excessive in-toeing causes pronounced amounts of wear of the lateral border of the sole and heel of the shoes. Hallux rigidus often causes a markedly oblique crease of the forepart of the shoe due to toe-off on the lateral side of the foot. The prominence of the talar head in individuals with flat feet tends to produce broken medial counters, whereas individuals with foot drop tend to scuff the shoes during the swing phase of ambulation.

Not just the outside of the shoe but the inside as well should be carefully examined for protruding seams, nails, rivets, or wrinkled lining. Very often a visible external convexity will have a concomitant internal concavity corre-

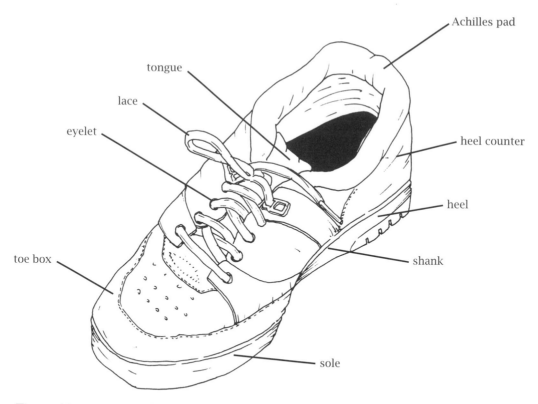

Figure 10. Anatomy of a shoe. (Drawn by Alan K. Whitney, DPM, Cherry Hill, New Jersey)

sponding to the hallux or the distal IPJs of the toes. Look for wear areas posteriorly, medially, and laterally. Such deformities are often associated with callus or corn formation. Look at the shoe from the rear and inspect the cant to the heel cup area. Does the shoe fit perpendicular to the sole, or is it inverted or averted? This gives evidence about the type of abnormal biomechanics. If the shoe is severely averted, pronation is compensatory; if the shoe is very inverted, a rearfoot varus position exists.

Next, look at the soles of the shoes and the wear pattern. If the patient is not propulsing off, there is no wear in the toe area. The type of material from which the shoe is constructed should be noted. Leather is more resilient and flexible than synthetic materials, which also tend to be allergenic. The height of the heel and dimensions of the last (the form that the shoe is made over) should be recorded.

Footwear Prescription

The foot tends to increase in size after the age of 20, although most individuals (75%), particularly women, have not had their feet measured in more than 5 years. In 60–70% of individuals one foot is larger than the other.

Forefoot abnormalities and incorrect shoe sizes are relatively common. Fashion has a significant role in the design of shoes and is the predominant cause of foot problems, particularly in women.

Over the years, comfort and protection in the design of shoes, particularly women's shoes, have been abandoned. Currently, most shoes are manufactured outside of the United States as "narrow," "medium," or "wide." Most of these shoe styles are copied from styles intended for the Italian and French, whose feet are shaped differently than those of most Americans. The tapered toe constricts the toes of a woman with a long foot, resulting eventually in a deformity. The high-heeled shoe does the same since it slides the foot forward. Lastly, shoes in numerous widths and styles and shoes with a combination last are prohibitively expensive to produce, and retailers cannot stock a large inventory.

The incidence of forefoot deformities in men is lower than 4% because the design of men's shoes does not lead to constriction or compression. As shoe heel height increases, forefoot pressure increases: 22% for a 3-inch heel, 57% for a 2-inch heel, and 76% for a 3 1/4-inch heel. The scaling process employed by shoe manufacturers to produce shoes of varying size enlarges or reduces all key internal dimensions of the shoe in a fixed proportion. As a result, it is difficult to procure a shoe with a disproportionate forefoot and hindfoot width available as a combination rack.

The lifetime mileage of a running shoe has been used to determine the longevity of its shock absorbency. The usual range is 500–1000 miles, after which a shoe offers little or no protection.

The following guidelines are suggested:

1. Educate patients about correct sizing of footwear and the ill effects of wearing inappropriate shoes.

2. The patient needs to consider the width of *both* feet as well as the width of the shoes and should fit the shoes to the widest foot. Sizing should occur at the end of the day, when the foot is the widest. For the most accurate measurement, the patient should stand and should measure the widest part of the foot from the outer aspects of the first metatarsal to the outer aspects of the fifth metatarsal. Alternatively, the foot outline can be drawn on a piece of cardboard. The patient then will have some idea of the discrepancy between foot width and shoe width, noting that the labeled shoe width correlates poorly with the actual fit of the shoe and the patient's foot.

3. Bear in mind that the width of shoes varies significantly between styles, lasts, and manufacturers. Shoes that are no more than 1/4 inch narrower than the foot, such as sports shoes, produce few problems. As the difference increases to 1/2 inch, 3/4 inch, and even 1 inch, the risk of compression, pain, and eventual deformity exponentially increases.

4. Because the forefoot tends to spread with age, it is important to inform the patient that he or she will not be wearing the same shoe later in life that was worn at 20 years of age.

5. Make certain that the shoe does not bulge over the welt (the strip of leather or other material that joins the upper with the outer sole).

6. The shoe upper should not wrinkle when the foot is flexed.

7. The toes should have room to extend and the toe box should be ample. The end of the longest toe of the biggest foot should be within 1/2 inch (a fingerbreadth) of the end of the toe box.

8. The forefoot should not feel tight in the shoe, and the counter should grip the heel relatively snugly.

9. Women who have a large discrepancy between forefoot width and heel width require a combination last to insure accurate fit. Other options include a lace-up sling-back or t-strap style.

10. All shoes should fit comfortably at the time of purchase and should not be bought with the expectation that they will stretch to fit. A "break-in" period for shoes should not be necessary.

11. Whenever possible the patient should purchase shoes made of soft leather or suede and should avoid shoes made of patent leather or synthetic materials that have no "give."

12. The heel counter should be stiff and compressible.

13. If necessary, discrepancies between shoe fit and foot size can be corrected with shoe inserts provided by a trained shoe technician or pedorthist.

14. Encourage the patient to try several shoes in the same style and size, even though from the same manufacturer, because some may fit better than others. This is particularly true for foreign-made shoes which tend to vary greatly in size.

15. It is essential to avoid seams over prominences of the forefoot since these may cause abrasion and lead to blisters and calluses. Women may want to consider men's or boys' shoes since these often are cut wider in the forefoot than women's shoes and generally run a size or two smaller.

16. For women who wish to wear fashion shoes with a high heel, styles with a rounder toe box are roomier and more comfortable. Limiting the heel height and the length of time these shoes are worn decreases exposure to deforming forces and probably the incidence of problems as well.

17. Wearing running shoes while walking to and from work should be encouraged.

Educate yourself, and encourage your patients to purchase shoes according to the fit and based on the measurements of their own feet, not the size stamped on the shoe. Flat soles are best. The "emancipation of feet," particularly of women's feet, will take time. The manufacture of healthy and fashionable shoewear and the education of consumers can help men and women look smart while they protect their feet.

References

1. American Academy of Orthopedic Surgeons: If the Shoe Fits, Wear It: Steps to Proper Shoe Fit. Rosemont, IL, AAOS, 1996. (Order by calling 1-800-824-2663.)
2. Bates B: A Guide to Physical Examination, 3rd ed. Philadelphia, J. B. Lippincott Co., 1983, pp 345–347, 498–503.
3. Coughlin MJ, Frey C: Cruel shoes. Biomechanics 1:34–39, 1994.
4. Czerniecki JM: Foot and ankle biomechanics in walking and running: A review. Am J Phys Med Rehabil 67(6):246–252, 1988.
5. Donatelli R: Normal biomechanics of the foot and ankle. J Orthop Sports Phys Ther 7:91, 1985.
6. Frey C: Pain and deformity in women's feet. J Musculoskel Med 12(9):27–32, 1995.
7. Hoppenfeld S: Physical Examination of the Spine and Extremities. New York, Appleton-Century Crofts, Inc., 1976, pp 197–236.
8. Nuber GW: Biomechanics of the foot and ankle during gait. Clin Sports Med 7(1):1–14, 1988.

3

Diagnostic Evaluation

Steven Garner, MD, Michael P. DellaCorte, DPM,
and Richard B. Birrer, MD

The Laboratory Examination

As with all areas of clinical medicine, laboratory tests in evaluating and managing podiatric problems are supplementary in nature. With few exceptions, laboratory data should not be routinely ordered. A complete blood count should not be ordered for screening purposes unless it is part of a preoperative evaluation. However, a urinalysis is appropriate if there is suspicion of underlying diabetic or renal disease. The hematocrit should be checked if the feet are cold or cyanotic or if an anemia or polycythemia is suspected. A hemoglobin level can confirm these findings as well as other diverse conditions such as pernicious anemia, leukemia, and dietary and hereditary anemias.

If an underlying infection is suspected, a white cell count with differential is appropriate. Rarely, a leukemia patient can be discovered by noting undifferentiated cells in the white cell count. Consider working with a venereal disease research laboratory when the differential diagnosis includes syphilitic-appearing dermopathy and unexplained ulcers and neuropathies. The erythrocyte sedimentation rate is of limited usefulness except in following the progress of patients with rheumatoid arthritis and in differentiating psychogenic from organic foot pain.

The physician must be selective in choosing from the numerous tests available—especially if there is clinical suspicion of underlying disease. For example, serum glucose is useful for following a diabetic's progress; serum urate is warranted in a gout patient. A clinical diagnosis of xanthoma should prompt a determination of the patient's lipid profile (cholesterol, triglycerides, lipoprotein electrophoresis). The physician should consider thyroid function tests if there is evidence of pretibial myxedema and hyperhidrosis (hyperthyroidism) or coarse nails, dry skin, and excess hair of the foot (hypothyroidism).

Doppler studies of the feet and legs are recommended whenever there is suspicion of blood supply impairment. Electromyography is reserved for suspected neuromuscular or neurologic disorders; it is useful in the diagnosis of compartment syndromes. Lastly, scrapings, culture, and biopsy techniques may be necessary for diagnosing a wide variety of infectious and noninfectious conditions.

The Radiologic Examination

Routine anteroposterior films of the foot do not demonstrate all areas satisfactorily due to nonconformity in thickness between the rearfoot and forefoot. Similarly, lateral x-rays are not informative at the level of the digits and metatarsals due to overlap. If the ankle is to be visualized also, then it should be x-rayed separately, because ankle films do not visualize the foot well. Therefore, x-ray evaluation of the foot and ankle should be undertaken *after* a clinical impression or differential diagnosis is established and should follow the high-yield criteria established by the Ottawa Study (Table 1).

Routine films of the foot usually are unwarranted, although they occasionally reveal an unexpected, asymptomatic, patho-

Table 1. High-Yield Criteria for Ankle and Foot X-Rays

Ankle	Foot
Pain in malleolar zone	Pain in midfoot zone
And	And
Bone tenderness at posterior edge or tip of lateral malleolus	Bone tenderness at base of 5th metatarsal
Or	Or
Bone tenderness at posterior edge or tip of medial malleolus-	Bone tenderness at navicular
Or	Or
Inability to bear weight both immediately and in emergency department	Inability to bear weight both immediately and in emergency department

logic problem. In general, views should focus on specific areas, and it is advisable for the purpose of diagnostic accuracy that radiographs be taken of the normal side for comparison.

Foot Projections

The following x-ray views are the ones most commonly used in standard x-ray evaluation. Each shows different aspects of the bony anatomy.

Dorsoplantar (Anteroposterior) Projection

The dorsoplantar projection allows for evaluation and examination of transverse plane deformities of the foot involving the phalanges, metatarsals, and tarsometatarsal joints, as well as the navicular, cuboid, and cuneiforms. Normal values of the angles between the metatarsals and the phalanges have been established.

Technique: The patient is asked to place the foot/feet on the x-ray plate (Fig. 1). (It is essential that the patient bear weight for a standard orthopedic evaluation of the foot. Weight bearing is not necessary in traumatic conditions.) The x-ray beam is angled 15° from the vertical to place the beam perpendicular to the metatarsals. The center of the beam is aimed at the lateral portion of the navicular. Both feet may be taken at one time, provided the plate is large enough, to decrease x-ray exposure.

Weight-Bearing Lateral Projection

This lateral view is important in evaluating flat foot and cavus foot deformities, dorsal and plantar exostosis, heel spurs, and the location of a foreign body, and in assessing the talus, calcaneus, and subtalar joint. The navicular, cuneiforms, metatarsals, and digits are views with overlap. Numerous angles have been de-

veloped to assist in surgical management of foot deformities.

Technique: The weight-bearing lateral view is taken with the aid of an orthoposer—a stand that holds the x-ray cassette vertical (Fig. 2). The patient stands on the orthoposer and places the medial aspect of the affected foot against the cassette. The central beam of the x-ray is aimed at the cuboid bone. Nonweight-bearing laterals are used in trauma.

Lateral Oblique Projection

The lateral oblique view is a nonweight-bearing supinated view of the foot. Supination

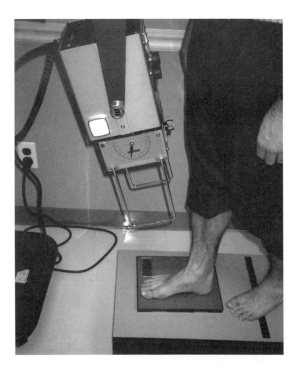

Figure 1. Dorsoplantar foot.

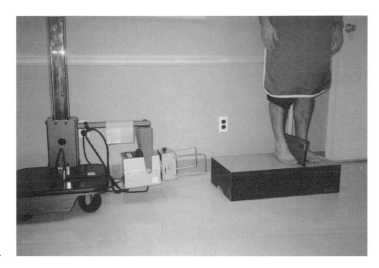

Figure 2. Lateral foot.

of the foot causes overlap of bony structures, allowing evaluation of the dorsolateral and plan.ar medial aspects of the foot only. It is used in trauma evaluation and as part of a complete foot x-ray series (dorsoplantar, lateral, medial oblique, lateral oblique).

Technique: There are two methods of taking this film. In one, the foot is placed flat on the plate and the x-ray beam is angled 45° on the medial side of the foot and aimed at the cuboid bone. The second method places the x-ray beam in front of the foot at 15° to the vertical (Fig. 3). The foot is then rolled on the lateral side, bringing the medial aspect 45° from the plate. The central beam is aimed at the cuboid bone.

Medial Oblique Projection

This nonweight-bearing view opens up the joints of the foot by pronation, allowing for in-

tra-articular evaluation. It often is used for evaluating forefoot trauma.

Technique: There are two methods of taking this view. In the first, the foot is placed flat on the plate, as for the dorsoplantar projection. The x-ray beam is angled 45,° aimed at the navicular bone, and positioned on the lateral aspect of the foot. The second method places the x-ray unit in exactly the same position as for a dorsoplantar view (angled at 15° to vertical directly in front of the foot). The foot is placed on the plate and the patient is asked to roll it on the medial side so that the lateral aspect is lifted 45° from the plate (Fig. 4).

Specific anterior/posterior (AP) films are recommended for toes and metatarsophalangeal joints (MTPJs). A sesamoid view of the sesamoid and metatarsal heads should be ordered. This view is best achieved by the patient passively dorsiflexing a toe or foot using an

Figure 3. Lateral oblique foot.

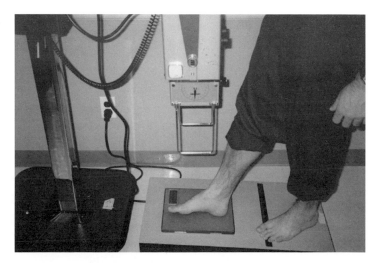

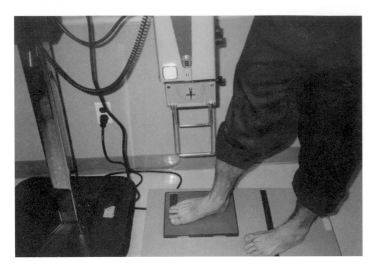

Figure 4. Medial oblique foot.

elastic bandage or piece of muslin to pull up the appendage.

The medial oblique view is best for determining pathology of the lateral talus and the calcaneonavicular and for fractures of the anterosuperior tubercle of the os calcis. Lateral and tangential radiographs (Harris view) are recommended for visualization of the os calcis. They should be slightly overexposed, and a lead marker should be placed for accurate localization of any underlying bony pathology or bony landmark.

Sesamoid-Axial Projection

The sesamoid-axial projection is used to evaluate sesamoid position during simulated propulsive phase of gait. This view is important in evaluating the patient with a painful bunion deformity. It also can assist in evaluating sesamoid fractures as well as plantarflexion of lesser metatarsals.

Technique: The sesamoid-axial view is taken with the aid of the orthoposer (Fig. 5). The cassette is placed upright in the orthoposer, and the patient places his or her toes in a dorsiflexed position against the plate with the ball of the foot on the ground. The heel is elevated from the weight-bearing surface. The central beam of the x-ray is aimed directly at the plantar aspect of the first metatarsal area at the sesamoids.

Calcaneal-Axial Projection

The calcaneal-axial projection is used to evaluate the intrinsic calcaneal position and fractures of the calcaneus, and to do a post-

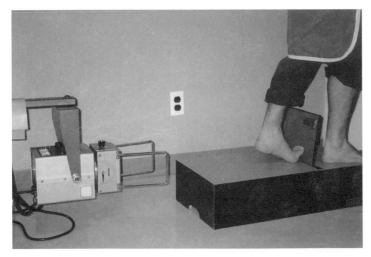

Figure 5. Sesamoid-axial projection.

operative check in arthrodesis procedures of the hindfoot.

Technique: The cassette is placed flat on the weight-bearing surface (Fig. 6). The patient stands on the plate in angle and base of gait, if possible, with the ankle at 90°. The x-ray beam is aimed centrally at the distal plantar aspect of the calcaneus at a 45° angle from the vertical. Nonweight-bearing films are used in trauma.

Ankle Projections

Routine ankle x-rays include AP, lateral, and oblique mortise films. Routine films should be supplemented by passive stress test radiographs when appropriate. Depending on the associated amount of spasm and pain, it may be necessary to use a local regional (i.e., peroneal) or general anesthesia. If the stress films are positive, further evaluation is unnecessary. If stress films are inconclusive and there is strong clinical suspicion of a complete tear, then an arthrogram should be ordered.

After sterile preparation and drape, the arthrogram is performed on the anterior portion of the joint opposite the area of suspected injury. Following initial aspiration, a 10 ml solution consisting of 1 ml lidocaine and 9 ml contrast material (e.g., 25% opaque solution) is slowly injected; then AP, lateral, and oblique films are obtained. Although the dye may enter tendon sheaths surrounding the an-

kle and may even flow to the subtalar joint, dye appearing outside the joint capsule or the surrounding tendon sheath is abnormal. The incidence of false negative examinations rises significantly 1 week after injury due to healing.

Another modality, arthroscopy, also can help detect tears and debris.

Anteroposterior Projection

The AP ankle projection is useful to evaluate the ankle joint complex and to evaluate ankle sprains and fractures.

Technique: The cassette is placed upright in the orthoposer (Fig. 7). The patient places his or her foot in front of the orthoposer at a 90° angle, with the posterior aspect of the heel against the cassette. The x-ray beam is aimed perpendicular to the cassette, centrally to the ankle joint between the malleoli.

Mortise Projection

The mortise ankle projection opens up the ankle joint, removing overlap of the fibula behind the tibia. This view reveals the entire superior aspect of the talar dome, which is useful to evaluate osteochondral fractures of the talus.

Technique: The foot is positioned as in the AP projection, with the foot internally rotated

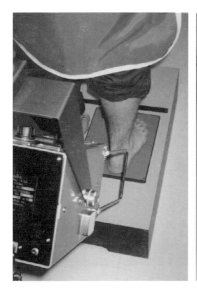 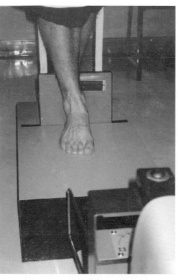 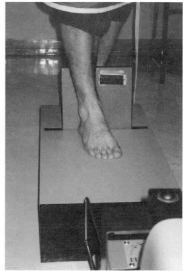

Figure 6. Calcaneal-axial projection.

Figure 7. Anteroposterior ankle.

Figure 8. Mortise view ankle.

until the high points of the malleoli are parallel (Fig. 8). The x-ray beam is aimed centrally, as in the AP projection.

Lateral Projection

The lateral ankle projection is useful to view the trochlear surface of the talus and to evaluate posterior malleolar fractures and posterior displacement of fibular fractures.

Technique: As in the lateral foot projection (see Fig. 2), the medial aspect of the foot and ankle is placed against the cassette. When isolating the ankle, there is no need to position the forefoot against the x-ray cassette. Conversely, more of the ankle and leg should be shown. The beam is aimed perpendicular to the cassette and directed at the malleolus.

Podiatric Imaging Modalities

There has been dramatic change and growth in the field of podiatric radiologic examination during the previous 5 years. Expanded use of ultrasound, digital subtraction angiography, duplex Doppler sonography, magnetic reso-

nance imaging (MRI), spiral computed tomography (CT), and nuclear imaging has enabled improved diagnostic capability in a more expeditious manner with less patient risk.

This section reviews recent advances and summarizes currently available radiographic modalities for work-up of the podiatric patient.

Radiography

A careful clinical examination of both the foot and ankle must be performed prior to ordering a radiograph. A careful history may help uncover the etiology of the patient's complaints. In evaluating foot and ankle complaints, consider the following categories:

- Traumatic
- Metabolic
- Infectious
- Neoplastic
- Congenital or developmental
- Arthritic.

Ankle and foot x-rays should not be included on the same film, as the technique for obtaining each area differs. Standard views of the foot include AP, weight-bearing lateral, and

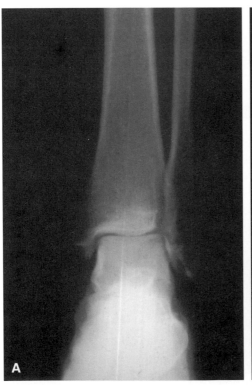 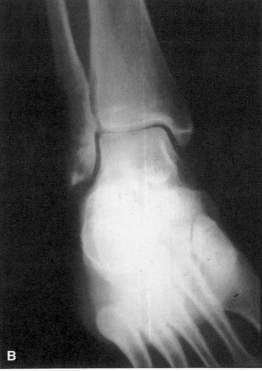

Figure 9. *A,* Anteroposterior view of the ankle—lateral aspect of distal tibia and talus obscured by overlying fibula. *B,* Mortise view—by 15° internal rotation, the lateral ankle is well visualized.

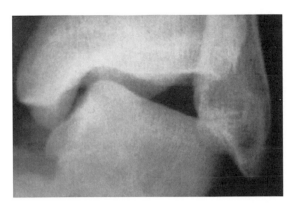

Figure 10. Stress view—excessive mobility at tibiofibular joint due to ligamentous tear.

one or both oblique views. As the digits and metatarsals overlap, all views must be obtained to adequately evaluate the foot.

Standard views of the ankle include AP, lateral, and oblique mortise. On the AP film, the lateral ankle joint is obscured by the fibula. Using 5–15° of internal rotation (mortise view), this area is well demonstrated (Fig. 9). Routine films should be supplemented by stress radiographs when appropriate, such as when there is considerable soft tissue swelling or pain in the absence of fractures. Stress radiographs, performed by adducting or abducting the heel, are useful in identifying ligamentous tears (Fig. 10). MRI and sonography have largely supplanted arthrography as the methods of choice in evaluating ligamentous and tendon injuries of the ankle.

In evaluating foot and ankle x-rays in trauma, accessory bones are a common problem. An accessory bone represents a supernumerary ossicle not ordinarily found in the skeleton, a bony process, or a secondary center for the tip of a process that has failed to fuse and remains as a separate bony structure. An accessory bone has smooth borders with a thin cortex. A fracture has an irregular border as well as a defect in the corresponding adjacent bone, which corresponds exactly in appearance to the fracture fragment. In addition, fresh fractures always are accompanied by swelling of the surrounding soft tissues. Further, accessory bones and anomalous bones commonly are bilateral, and, when in doubt, a view of the corresponding part in the opposite extremity can be obtained (Fig. 11). By understanding the appearance and distribution of accessory bones, diagnostic problems can be easily resolved.

When evaluating pediatric x-rays, most clinicians encounter diagnostic difficulty because the immature epiphyseal plates are not calcified. Consequently, there are numerous lucent areas noted about the joints. By obtaining comparison views and doing a careful clinical evaluation, the diagnosis of a fracture most times can be readily made (Fig. 12). It is extremely important to correctly identify fractures that involve the epiphyseal plate to prevent the occurrence of arthritic change and growth deformity. Therefore, it may be necessary to obtain additional studies, such as CT scans, when a diagnosis of a fracture is suspected.

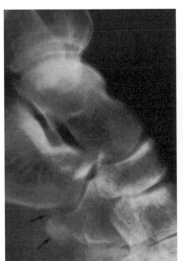
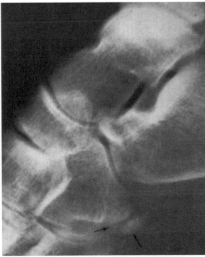

Figure 11. Comparison of large multicentric os peroneum in a patient's corresponding extremities.

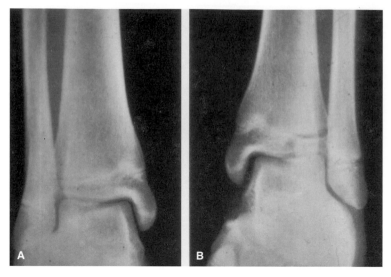

Figure 12.   Pediatric x-ray. *A,* Salter-Harris type 1 fractures of distal tibia and distal fibula. *B,* These fractures are best appreciated when compared to uninvolved opposite side.

Systemic diseases such as Cushing's syndrome, malnutrition, scurvy, and hyperparathyroidism manifest with characteristic bony changes in the foot and ankle. While the radiograph of the foot and ankle may not be specific for a disease entity, the clinician should realize that there is an abnormal appearance and should consider systemic etiology.

Arthritides such as psoriasis, Reiter's syndrome, and rheumatoid arthritis often present with characteristic changes. The plain film appearance of arthritides is characterized by distribution and symmetry, degree of osteoporosis, joint space narrowing, and associated soft tissue changes. In gouty arthritis, the joint most commonly affected is the first MTPJ (Fig. 13). In addition to typical erosive changes, there is a relative lack of osteoporosis.

The appearance of bone tumors in the foot and ankle is similar to that in other parts of the body. When a lesion is present, the zone of transition must be evaluated to determine how well-defined the abnormal bone is from normal bone. Benign tumors have a narrow zone of transition; malignant tumors have an ill-defined margin (Fig. 14). The matrix or the internal portion of the lesion also must be evaluated to determine the tissue of origin. If there are stippled areas of calcification noted within a lesion, then this is most often of cartilaginous origin. In the foot, a typical example is an en-

chondroma. Finally, any periosteal reaction should be examined. Malignant tumors can irritate the periosteal lining of bone, causing disruption of the regular periosteum. A benign

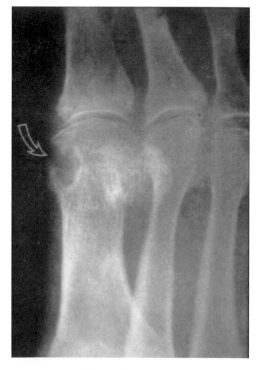

Figure 13.   Gout.

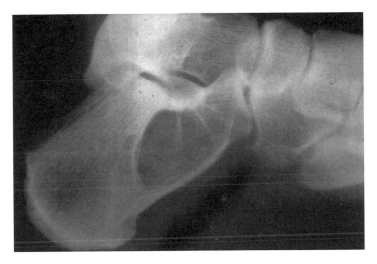

Figure 14. Solitary bone cyst—typically benign radiographic features.

process usually does not interfere with the periosteal lining, unless there is a fracture present.

While new imaging modalities have arisen for evaluation of podiatric disease, plain film radiography continues to be the mainstay in everyday practice.

Sonography

Evaluation of the soft tissues of the foot and ankle became possible with the advent of high-frequency, small part transducers. The small size of the "hockey stick" transducer allows easy access to small parts (Fig. 15). The ultrasound exam provides a dynamic means to observe tissues in full motion or while under stress. As is commonly the case, radiographs of painful feet are negative. The sonogram becomes extremely useful in evaluating soft tissue injury, abnormal fluid collection, or soft tissue masses not demonstrated radiographically. It also provides a more objective approach, in that soft tissue swelling and abnormality can be better characterized than on plain film radiography.

Almost all tendinous injuries of the foot and ankle can be evaluated by ultrasound. For example, tendon edema and true tears can be differentiated. In tendonitis, the tendon appears swollen and has fewer echoes, appearing darker than normal (Fig. 16). A torn tendon appears interrupted with the swollen ends easily visualized. The extent of bunions can be easily evaluated. Soft tissue masses such as hematomas, abscesses, or ganglia also can be diagnosed with sonography.

Sonography is useful in detecting nonradiopaque foreign bodies. It is extremely difficult to identify glass or wood on plain radiography, and extensive surgical exploration generally is necessary. Sonography can be used to guide surgical exploration in removal of nonradiopaque foreign bodies.

Ultrasound has become the modality of choice for detection of Morton's neuroma, which appears as a hypoechoic mass (darker than the surrounding tissue), most often in the

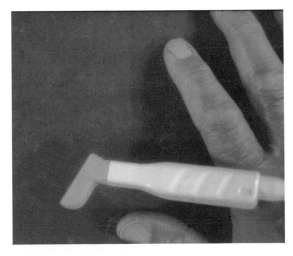

Figure 15. "Hockey stick" transducer used in sonography for access to small areas.

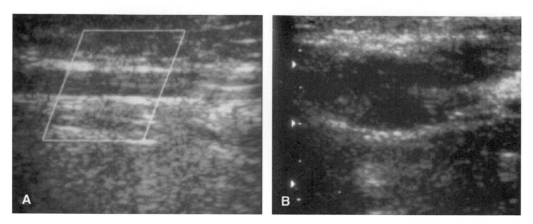

Figure 16. Ultrasound. *A*, Normal posterior tibial tendon. *B*, Swollen, hypoechoic inflamed tendon.

region of the second and third intermetatarsal spaces (Fig. 17). Treated patients can be followed sonographically. In the authors' experience of more than 100 examinations performed for evaluation of Morton's neuroma, there has been a 98% true positive correlation. This exceeds sensitivity of MRI evaluation. The examination is much easier for patients to endure, and the expense is dramatically less.

Ultrasound is of value in evaluating plantar fasciitis. The insertion point of the plantar fascia on the calcaneus may show thickening and edema. Inflammation of the periosteum of the calcaneus can be demonstrated as well.

With a doppler signal and real time sono-

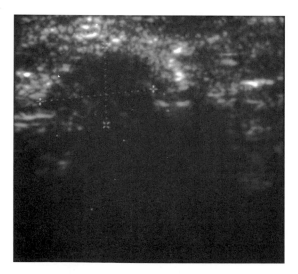

Figure 17. Morton's neuroma—hypoechoic mass in 2nd intermetatarsal space.

graphic imaging, the arteries of the lower extremity, including digital arteries, can be well evaluated. Based upon the waveform and velocity measured, stenosis as well as patency of small arteries can be predicted (Fig. 18). The doppler examination can be used to evaluate venous pathology such as deep venous thrombosis, for which it is considered the procedure of choice.

Digital Subtraction Angiography

The digital subtraction technique is performed with a small gauge catheter. As this technique allows for exquisite resolution, the amount of iodinated contrast injected can be reduced by 90% (Fig. 19). Thus, it is possible to evaluate the arterial system of the lower extremity in a safe outpatient setting. High-risk patients, including those who have renal dysfunction, often are able to undergo this examination.

Nuclear Radiology

Nuclear radiology provides a physiologic evaluation of pathologic bone. The radionuclide material is incorporated by osteoblasts which produce new bone. Stimulation of osteoblast activity occurs as a response to destructive processes such as infection and neoplasm. This new bone formation results in a "hot spot."

Nuclear radiology is valuable in evaluation of osteomyelitis. While plain radiographs do not disclose osteomyelitis at an early stage, bone scanning allows positive identification of infection within a few days of onset. A three-

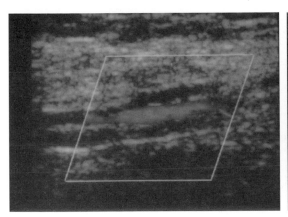 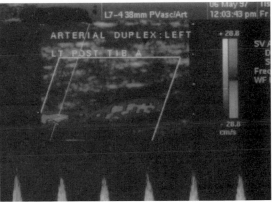

Figure 18. Normal duplex doppler of posterior tibial artery.

phase technique is performed: immediately after injection of radionuclide, images are obtained. Areas of infection or soft tissue abnormality display increased uptake due to increased blood flow. Approximately 3 minutes after the initial flow, a second evaluation is performed, known as the blood pool phase. In conditions of osteomyelitis and cellulitis, there is increased uptake in this phase as well, representing hyperemia that often occurs in the adjacent soft tissues. Finally, a three-hour delayed film is obtained, which demonstrates increased activity in bone (Fig. 20). Gallium scans can be informative in cases in which new bone formation (abnormal bone scan) may not be related to infection (i.e., diabetic neuropathy of chronic osteomyelitis).

Another common use for nuclear medicine in the podiatric setting is in detection of fractures not seen by other methods. A stress fracture often is difficult to identify on plain films but is easily demonstrated by nuclear radiology (Fig. 21).

Many patients are worried about risk from exposure to nuclear medicine agents. Patients should be reassured that the total dose to the body is extremely low and is less than a barium enema or a gastrointestinal series.

Computed Tomography

CT is of assistance in evaluating various foot disorders as often there is extensive overlap of the foot bones on standard views. CT scans are excellent for assessing cortical bone.

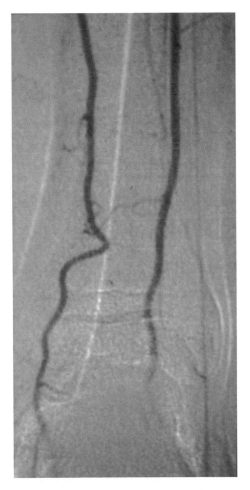

Figure 19. Digital subtraction angiogram—runoff provided via anterior and posterior tibial arteries. Only 8 cc of contrast was injected for this outpatient procedure.

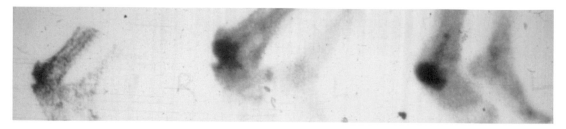

Figure 20. Three-phase nuclear bone scan—increased uptake noted in all phases consistent with osteomyelitis. The plain film was negative.

In addition, podiatric soft tissue tumors and infectious processes are well evaluated. With the capability of multiplanar reconstruction, CT generally is more sensitive than linear tomography and more specific than nuclear radiology in evaluating complex bone and joint cases.

In particular, CT scans are valuable in disorders such as trauma, arthritides, neoplasm, and congenital or acquired deformities. For example, the CT scan is the modality of choice in evaluating both tarsal coalition and complex fractures (Fig. 22). It also is useful in evaluating bone tumors (Fig. 23). The extent of the tumor and the periosteal reaction, the character of the matrix, or the presence of a pathologic fracture can be determined.

Magnetic Resonance Imaging

Most clinical indications for MRI examination of the ankle and foot are related to trauma. The purpose of the examination is to assess any damage to cartilage, ligaments, or tendons.

By altering the magnetic field, T1-weighted and T2-weighted images can be obtained. On a T1-weighted image, fat appears bright and fluid dark. On a T2-weighted image, fluid becomes bright and fat decreases in signal. By understanding the normal appearance of tendons, cortex, and marrow, the physician can detect areas of abnormality and propose an etiology for the abnormal appearance (Fig. 24). Normal tendons of the ankle and foot appear as low signal intensity (dark appearance) on all sequences.

In a tear, there is increased signal noted within the normally dark Achilles tendon. The ligaments of the ankle and foot exhibit a homogeneous low signal or alternating bands of low and intermediate signal intensity. The cortex is low-signal on all imaging sequences. By understanding the normal appearance, it becomes easy to evaluate pathologic structures.

Avascular necrosis represents the death of bone and marrow components due to vascular compromise. In the early stages of avascular necrosis, conventional radiographs usually are normal. The MRI, however, initially shows an area of increased signal noted centrally within the bone. As the lesion becomes chronic, the signal appears hypointense or dark on both T1- and T2-weighted images (Fig. 25).

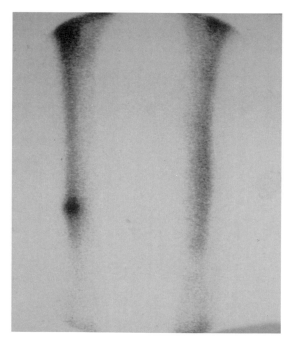

Figure 21. Nuclear image of stress fracture, which is demonstrated by increased uptake.

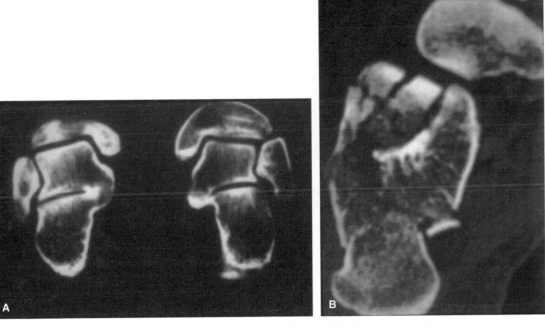

Figure 22. Computed tomography. *A*, Bilateral tarsal coalition in a female presenting with pain. X-rays were not diagnostic. Incidentally noted is a left calcaneal spur. *B*, Comminuted fracture of calcaneus involving the talocalcaneal joint.

MRI also may be an early indicator of osteomyelitis and can determine the extent, origin, and character of soft tissue tumors (Fig. 26).

Some Notes on Photography

The primary care practitioner may want to photograph podiatric pathology for medical, legal, research, or teaching purposes. The following guidelines are recommended:

1. In general, photograph only the area involved unless the etiology (e.g., pes planus, tight shoe) is obvious and can be easily included.
2. Take different views of the pathologic area.
3. If surgery is contemplated, take preoperative and postoperative clinical pictures.
4. A 35 mm camera with a behind-the-lens meter is practical and sufficient.
5. A close-up lens (1+ to 10+ diopters) or macro lens (50–90 mm), though not necessary, allows close, detailed photos without contamination of a surgical field.

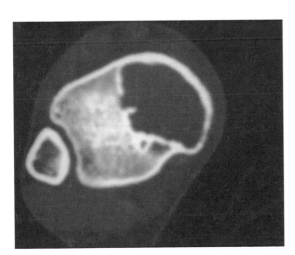

Figure 23. Computed tomography reveals a well-defined lytic lesion in the distal tibia without evidence of an associated fracture. At surgery, this lesion was found to be a benign giant-cell tumor.

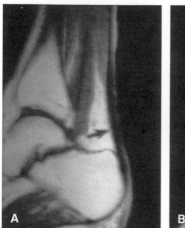
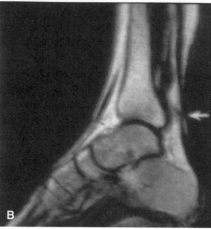

Figure 24. Magnetic resonance imaging of the ankle. *A,* Normal Achilles tendon. Note homogeneous low signal intensity and dark appearance (*arrow*). *B,* Increased signal and bright appearance within the normally dark Achilles tendon indicates a tear (*arrow*).

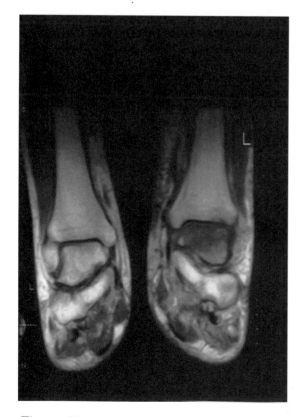

Figure 25. Avascular necrosis. T1-weighted image showing low signal in the left talus consistent with avascular necrosis.

6. Color film (ASA 100–400) is recommended for most office work. Speeds less than 100 often require additional lighting, but the color is better and grain finer.
7. Black and white film (ASA 100–400) is suitable for many deformities. Use a matte white for dark-skinned patients and a matte black for light-skinned individuals. Note that the speed needs to be decreased by 1 to 2 stops with matte white and increased 1 stop with matte black.

Summary

There is a wide array of radiographic options available for evaluating common podiatric problems. It is hoped that this chapter enables the clinician to understand the selections on the radiographic menu.

In all radiographic examinations, it is important for the radiologist to have access to the clinical picture, so that a close correlation may be made. While a brief history or indication can be included on the request, there is no substitute for direct verbal communication. Teamwork is the key to proper and successful management of the patient.

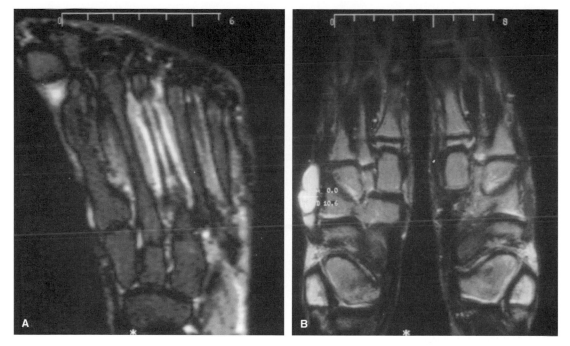

Figure 26. Magnetic resonance imaging. *A*, Osteomyelitis of 3rd metatarsal with extensive bone marrow edema and soft tissue inflammation. *B*, A bright, round density with septations on this T2-weighted image is consistent with a ganglion cyst.

References

1. Beltran J: Magnetic resonance imaging. Radiol Clin N Am 32(2):337–352, 1994.
2. Chhem R: Ultrasonography of the musculoskeletal system. Radiol Clin N Am 32(2):275–290, 1994.
3. Erickson S, Johnson J: MR imaging of the ankle and foot. Radiol Clin N Am 35(1):163–192, 1997.
4. Resnick D: Bone and Joint Imaging. Philadelphia, W. B. Saunders Company, 1989.
5. Stiell IG, McKnight D, Greenberg GH, et al: Implementation of the Ottawa Ankle Rules. JAMA 271(11):827–832, 1994.
6. Thrall James: Nuclear Medicine: The Requisites. St. Louis, Mosby-Year Book, Inc., 1995.

Skin

Richard B. Birrer, MD and Harrison Donnelly, MD

Anatomy

The skin of the sole and the skin of the dorsum of the foot are anatomically distinct, which is an important fact in differentiating features of their respective pathologies. The skin of the dorsum has a normal stratum corneum, while the skin of the sole is very thick. The next layer, the stratum lucidum, is present on the sole but is absent on the dorsal aspect of the foot. There are no hair follicles or sebaceous glands on the sole of the foot, but both are present in normal distribution on the dorsum. However, the eccrine glands are numerous on the sole, with a normal complement on the instep.

Examination

In addition to the routine skin exam (see Chapter 2), a Wood's light and biopsy may be useful. A Wood's, or black, light consists of ultraviolet long-wave light from a high-pressure mercury lamp fitted with a special nickel oxide and silica filter. All web spaces should be examined with light for fluorescein, particularly the coral-red color characteristic of the diphtheroid-causing erythrasma. However, it should be noted that a variety of dyes, ointments, and debris may fluoresce various colors and lead to false diagnoses.

Biopsy technique of the dorsum of the foot is similar to other areas of the body. A 1% lidocaine solution is used as a local anesthetic, and then an appropriate-sized cylindrical punch, ranging from 2–10 mm, is chosen. A rhythmic, alternating, clockwise-counterclockwise motion is made rapidly, and small surgical scissors are used to clip the biopsy plug from the underlying fat of the deep dermis. Bleeding can be easily controlled by the application of basic ferric sulfate or subsulfate solution (Monsel's). A smaller punch is used when cosmesis is important, whereas a scalpel with an elliptical biopsy may be more appropriate if a larger specimen is needed. Biopsies of the sole of the foot, especially weight-bearing areas, must be done with the utmost caution to avoid the development of painful scar tissue. The recommended size is 2–3 mm, with 4–5 mm considered the maximum.

Contact Dermatitis

Contact dermatitis is classified as either allergic or secondary to irritating chemicals (Fig. 1). Pathologically, both types are characterized by a nonspecific, eczematous reaction with variable amounts of edema, erythema, vesicles, and occasionally bullae, and both types can resemble the eczema seen in atopics. Exposure to the Rhus family (poision ivy, oak, or sumac) is a common cause of contact dermatitis, and the lesions tend to be linear and geographic in distribution, corresponding to the area of contact. Another common cause of contact dermatitis is shoe wear. The dorsal aspects of the foot, particularly the hallux and distal portions, usually are involved. The reaction is due to rubber found in the toe box of most shoes or to the cement used to bind together the shoe components. Leather usually is nonallergenic. In rare cases, the sole of the foot and other portions of the body may become involved in an id reaction. Pruritis is common.

Examples of primary irritants in contact

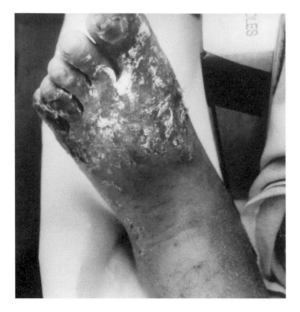

Figure 1. Contact dermatitis caused by new, synthetic shoes.

dermatitis include inadequately prepared chemical solutions such as permanganate and Burow's, irritating creams, hot water, and highly-concentrated chemical solutions. Individuals who have underlying systemic diseases, such as vasculitis, diabetes, or peripheral vascular disease, can develop a severe contact dermatitis using over-the-counter callus and corn remedies. Occasionally, the dermatitis may be iatrogenically induced from a prescribed orthotic or similar device.

Diagnosis of contact dermatitis is made by obtaining a careful history and an appropriate series of patch tests. The patch test is easily administered by serial dilution of the suspected agent(s) and application via Band-Aids or similar device to the upper back for 48–72 hours. A control also should be applied and the area examined every 24 hours with the results carefully documented. It is important to dilute and prepare the topical agents adequately according to a number of readily available tablets for patch tests and preparations. Inadequately diluted agents produce edema, erythema, and vesicles of an irritant nature in the majority of healthy individuals. A well-demarcated, unnatural outline to a patch test suggests contact sensitivity.

The treatment of choice is twofold. First, the offending agent must be removed. In the case of shoes, the substitution of a leather upper usually is sufficient, although in some individuals the substitution of a thermoplastic or Silastic toe box for a rubber one is necessary. The additional prescription of a regularly applied drying powder together with cotton or woolen socks rather than synthetic ones increases aeration and thus reduces the solvent effect of perspiration on allergens in the shoes. Second, in mild to moderate cases, a topical steroid such as hydrocortisone or triamcinolone is sufficient. Efficacy is enhanced by removing keratin with a keratolytic agent, soaking in water pre-application, and applying plastic film (Saran Wrap) post-application. In severe cases, a more potent topical steroid (e.g., betamethasone) in combination with a systemic steroid regimen for several days may be required.

Eccrine Gland Disorders
Hyperhidrosis

Hyperhidrosis is an annoying condition that typically affects the palms and soles, particularly when the patient's level of tension and excitement is high. It may be worse when accompanied by an offending odor (i.e., bromhidrosis). Hyperhidrosis usually is idiopathic, though it is important to rule out certain diseases that can aggravate or cause the condition: thyrotoxicosis, palmar and plantar keratoses, cholinergic medications, and fever from any cause, particularly the night sweats of lymphoma and tuberculosis, pheochromocytoma, gout, and the carcinoid syndrome. Because of the warm, moist environment usually associated with plantar hyperhidrosis, warts and tinea pedis often develop.

Treatment of the condition often is frustrating. Locally, a diluted formalin or glutaraldehyde solution (3–10%) may be useful, although there may be some discoloration and allergic sensitization in the susceptible individual. The glutaraldehyde should be applied to the bottom of the foot daily for 5 days and then as often as necessary (usually two to three times a week). Topically, aluminum chloride hexahydrate–based drying powders (Zea Sorb) applied at bedtime and occluded with a thin plastic film (Saran Wrap) are helpful, though far from curative. The combination of equal amounts of baking soda and talc applied twice daily also may be beneficial. Finally, the wearing of nonocclusive, nonsynthetic socks and leather footwear is essential for maximal aeration of the feet. In rare cases, systemic agents such as an anticholinergic drugs or anxiolytic tranquilizers can be used with some benefits.

Bromhidrosis

Although neither life threatening nor incapacitating, foot odor is upsetting to patients and to their families and friends. Hyperhidrosis, faulty foot hygiene, and improper footwear are factors. The following are suggestions for patient management:

1. Change socks twice a day, since wet socks defeat all therapies for foot odor.

2. Apply talcum powder directly to the bottom of the foot, where it is more effective than in the shoe or sock.

3. Purchase porous shoes rather than those made of hard leather, which tend to retain water.

4. Wear absorbent liners if using nylon stockings, since nylon tends to retain perspiration.

5. Avoid or reduce intake of spicy condiments such as onions and garlic.

While white socks are ideal from the viewpoint of absorbency, they often are aesthetically unacceptable. Gray or other light colored socks can be substituted, but the darker the sock the more moisture retention occurs. For resistant cases, consider prescribing propantheline bromide, which has a side effect of sweat reduction. Regular soaking of the foot in a diluted (1–2%) solution of formaldehyde or potassium permanganate or the application of a topical antibiotic such as erythromycin has been shown to decrease bacteria (*Corynebacterium minutissima*) that are associated with the degradation of perspiration.

Dyshidrosis

Dyshidrosis, an eczematous disease of the epidermis, is characterized by numerous, yellow, deep-seated vesicles affecting the soles and palms in the acute stage. Also termed pompholyx, the condition often is accompanied by hyperhidrosis and pruritus. Scaling and erythematous macules and papules denote the healing phase. The differential diagnosis should consider pustular psoriasis, tinea pedis of the plantar vesicular type, epidermolysis bullosa, and keratolysis exfoliative. The recommended management consists of wet soaks with saline or Burow's solution (i.e., aluminum acetate) followed by the application of a topical steroid and a keratolytic agent. Nightly occlusion is a good idea. Severe or refractory cases might benefit from the administration of a systemic steroid. Recurrences are common.

Fungal Infections

Tinea pedis (i.e., athlete's foot) is the most common dermatophytosis in the United States. It may be a relatively minor chronic infection, or it may cause a disabling dermatitis characterized by large blisters, fissures, thickening of the sole, and secondary infection—particularly of the fourth and fifth toes. The most common cause is *Trichophyton rubrum* and *Trichophyton mentagrophytes,* although the clinical presentation varies:

1. Dry type (moccasin type), usually in the fourth and fifth toe web spaces or on the sole and heel of the foot, is associated with varying amounts of scaling, erythremia, pruritus, and fissuring.

2. Wet type occurs on the sole of the foot or in the web spaces (Fig. 2).

3. A dermatophytic or vesicular variety typically involves the palms and fingers and is marked by a profound amount of inflammation.

The differential diagnosis should include erythrasma (Wood's light), soft corn, psoriasis, keratoses, contact dermatitis–dry form, epidermolysis bullosa, pustular psoriasis, dyshidrosis–wet form, or the vesicular form of tinea pedis.

A fungal infection of the foot is diagnosed by microscopic examination of the suspected material, which is scraped from the margin of the diseased area or from a vesicle wall (not its

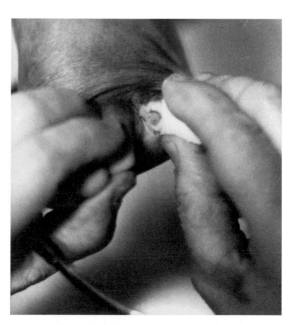

Figure 2. Fungal infection of the web space.

contents) with a No. 15 scalpel blade. The material is then gently heated with a few drops of 10% potassium hydroxide solution, and a cover slip is applied. Branching hyphae and myceliae are diagnostic of superficial dermatophytes. Budding cells and pseudohyphae are suggestive of yeast, particularly monilia. When the test is negative or nonconfirmatory, some of the suspected material should be planted on a suitable culture medium such as Sabouraud's agar or dermatophyte test medium (DTM). The top of the bottles should be loose to provide sufficient aeration, and at least 2 weeks in a dark, warm environment should be allowed for full growth to occur. The diagnostic accuracy of DTM for identification of dermatophytes (red color change) is over 95% within 14 days. If fluffy white colonies also are present, the diagnostic accuracy of DTM exceeds 97%.

The dry forms of tinea pedis usually respond well to antifungal solutions and creams applied at bedtime and in the morning (Table 1). Older topicals offer cure rates of 70–80% with newer ones achieving rates 5–10% higher. Lotions are more drying, less messy, and more useful for daytime application between toes. Creams have better penetration but can cause maceration if applied too thickly or if the site is occluded; they are better to use at night. The extra expense of using two formulations, however, usually is not warranted.

The most common side effect to the topical agents is irritation, but it is infrequent. The agents rarely cause hypersensitivity, are poorly absorbed systemically, and are unlikely to cause harm during pregnancy and lactation when used short term. However, they are not approved for the latter use.

Chronic infections, especially those associated with hyperkeratotic infections (usually caused by *T. rubrum*) and immunocompromised states, should be treated with oral therapy. Prolonged and/or intermittent topical or oral therapy may be needed to treat chronic infections. A mild keratolytic agent such as salicylic acid (Winfield's ointment) or a coal tar preparation (Pragmatar) is a useful supplement for the dry, diffuse plantar type associated with variable degrees of keratosis. Griseofulvin ultramicrosize (Fulvicin P/G, Grisactin Ultra, Gris-PEG, or Grifulvin V [children] 500–1000 mg daily for a month) may be useful for the refractory dry, interdigital type or the diffuse plantar form. The agent is well tolerated and side effects are minimal. Many experts do not consider hematologic and hepatic monitoring necessary.

Recalcitrant infections can be treated with oral ketoconazole 200 mg/day. However, liver functions must be monitored due to the risk of hepatotoxicity. Vesicular and dermatophytidic forms of tinea pedis respond well to the application of wet soaks (potassium permanganate 1:10,000, silver nitrate 1:200, or Burow's solution 1:20) initially until the skin returns to normal; then they should be discontinued. Prolonged application of these wet soaks can result in extreme desiccation, cracking, and fissuring, particularly of the surrounding normal skin.

A systemic antibiotic such as erythromycin or tetracycline may be required if there is a secondary bacterial infection. If the inflammation and vesiculation are severe, 40–60 mg of prednisone daily followed by 5 mg reductions every 2–3 days depending on response is quite helpful. Once the acute inflammatory response has subsided, griseofulvin by mouth or a topical antifungal agent in combination with a steroid cream completes the therapy. If the palmar surface of the hand also is involved, it need not be actively treated other than with the application of wet dressings, because the skin will return to normal after resolution of the pedal disease.

The patient should be carefully educated about adequate aeration of the feet through the use of nonocclusive, nonsynthetic socks and footwear and the use of open shoes (e.g., sandals). A mild antifungal powder can be applied in the morning, particularly in the web spaces, as a precaution. This is especially recommended in the more humid and warm months of the year and before exercising. The patient should be reminded that recurrences are common, particularly in susceptible individuals.

Viral Warts

Warts, or verrucae, are benign tumors of the skin. They are induced by papilloma viruses, which are ds DNA viruses, and are commonly caused by human papilloma virus (HPV) 1, 2, 4:

HPV 1—single, solitary, painful plantar lesions
HPV 2—mosaic plantar lesions
HPV 4—smaller, multiple lesions

Different types of verrucae are: verrucae vulgaris (common warts), verrucae plantaris (plantar warts, Fig. 3), verrucae plana (flat warts), and condyloma acuminata (genital warts).

Table 1. Topical Antifungal Medications

Drug	Dosage	Efficacy*	Cost*	Comments
Undecylenic acid and derivatives 2–10%	1–2 times daily as needed	+	+	Antibacterial and antifungal equivalent to tolnaftate for mild infections. May cause irritation if inflammation present
Tolnaftate 1%	Twice daily up to 4 weeks	+	+	Mild infections and prophylaxis
Gentian violet 1%	2–4 daily	+	+	Stains and tattoos skin; antibacterial and antifungal. Contraindicated for ulcerative lesions
Iodochlor-hydroxyquin 3%	2–3 daily for 1 week	+	+	Stains; interferes with thyroid function
Triacetin	Twice daily	+	+	Broad spectrum
Haloprogin 1%	Twice daily	+++	++	Broad spectrum
Nystatin 100,000 u/g	2–3 daily	+++	++	Mainly for Candida sp.
Amphotericin 3%	2–4 daily	++	++	Mainly for Candida sp.
Sulconazole nitrate 1% (Exelderm)	Twice daily for 4 weeks	++++	++	Comparable with nuconazole and clotrimyole
Econazole nitrate 1% (Spectazole)	Once daily for 4 weeks	++++	+++	Broad spectrum
Clotrimazole 1%	Twice daily for up to 4 weeks	++++	++	Broad spectrum OTC
Miconazole nitrate 2% (Monistat, MicaTin)	Twice daily for up to 1 month	++++	+++	Prescription and OTC broad spectrum, contraindicated in children < 2 years old
Oxiconazole nitrate 1% (Oxistat)	1–2 daily for up to 1 month	++++	+++	Broad spectrum
Ketoconazole 2% (Nizoral)	Once daily for up to 6 weeks	++++	+++	Broad spectrum
Naftifine HCL 1% (Naftin)	1–2 daily for up to 4 weeks	++++	++++	Broad spectrum
Terebinafine HCL 1% (Lamisil)	Twice daily for 1–4 weeks	++++	++++	Possibly more potent than naftifine, superior to gusefuloin

* + = low, ++++ = high
OTC = over the counter, HCL = hydrochloride

The average life expectancy of a clone of virions is 4–9 months; spontaneous regression is common. A number of small warty masses may coalesce, forming larger mosaic warts. Usually, patients who develop warts do not have a history of trauma, though they may have a history of warts elsewhere on the body. Warts may be asymptomatic or may cause severe pain and disability if present over sensitive weight-bearing areas of the foot.

The first step in treatment is to confirm the diagnosis (Table 2). Pinpoint bleeding on paring of the lesion is suggestive of verrucae from lesions, as is pain on compression; however, biopsy remains the definitive procedure for confirmation. Verrucae therapy is varied and not always effective. The large number of treatment plans shows that no single approach is always successful and alternative methods should be investigated for recalcitrant lesions.

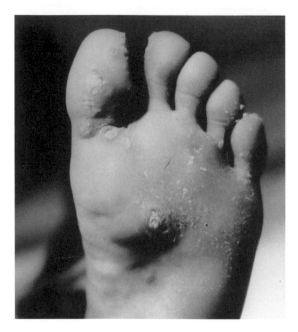

Figure 3. Multiple plantar warts.

Treatment is tailored to the type and location of the wart. Large plantar warts, particularly the asymptomatic mosaic variety, should be treated conservatively with weekly paring and the application of a keratolytic agent such as 40% salicylic acid plaster, 50% trichloroacetic acid, or lactic acid. Such treatment modalities suffice for the majority of asymptomatic plantar warts. More invasive techniques (e.g., electrosurgery, cryotherapy, excisional surgery, laser) should be reserved for painful lesions. After a local lidocaine (1%) anesthetic block with 1:200,000 epinephrine

Table 2. Differential Diagnosis for Verrucae

Eccrine poroma
Heloma durum
Heloma milliare
Heloma neurofibrosum
Heloma vasculare
Porokeratosis plantaris discreta
Squamous cell carcinoma
Basal cell carcinoma
Arsenical keratosis
Epidermoid keratosis
Fibrosarcoma
Molluscum contagiosum
Nevi
Pyogenic granuloma
Verrucous carcinoma

(avoiding epinephrine in the digits), the lesion is carefully pared to define its borders. Thereafter, an electrocautery needle is placed in the central superficial portion and the unit activated for a few seconds until the wart "boils." A small curette then can be used to remove the necrotic tissue; attempts to remove deeper tissue should be avoided, because scarring will result. Since verrucal growth is superficial, more effort should be spent on its lateral margins, because that is the area where recurrence is most likely. Hand pressure with a gauze pad after application of ferric subchloride (Monsel's solution) is sufficient to stop most bleeding. The wound should be packed with an antibiotic ointment (e.g., Ilotycin, Neosporin, Bacitracin) and a horseshoe-shaped, adhesive felt pad applied to disperse weight-bearing pressure (Fig. 4). The same techniques can be used if excisional therapy with a No. 15 scalpel blade is chosen. Once again, it is imperative not to invade the deeper tissue of the dermis, but rather to use light electrocautery and curettage to remove any remaining tissue.

Biweekly application of liquid nitrogen usually is received more favorably by patients. Although this technique is not as effective as excisional surgery or electrosurgery, it is far less painful. The more radical modalities should be reserved for the removal of a large "mother" wart, which will then cause regression of "baby" satellite warts. Rarely, radiotherapy can be employed for recalcitrant plantar warts, but only in consultation with an experienced operator.

Periungual or subungual warts are not uncommon. They often deform the nail plate and may, if deep enough, erode the underlying bony tuft. These lesions are best managed by conservative surgical removal following anesthetic nerve block. Blunt dissection or curettage is preferred over electrosurgery or the scalpel. Electrodesiccation or laser can be used to remove any remaining warty tissue, and Monsel's solution is preferred to electrosurgery for control of bleeding.

Calluses/Tylomata

A callus is a hyperkeratotic lesion which, like a corn, develops in response to pressure irritation and friction (Fig. 5). Remember, the keratin layer of the sole is up to 25 times thicker than anywhere else on the body; in hyperkeratotic conditions it may be five to ten times thicker still. Usually the sites of tylomata are the ball of the foot, a protuberant bony en-

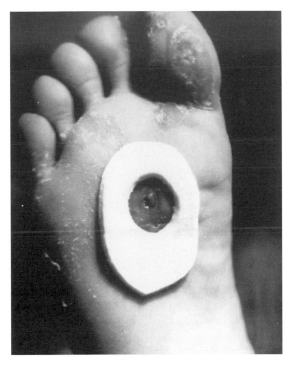

Figure 4. Plantar warts following two liquid nitrogen applications, with protective donut.

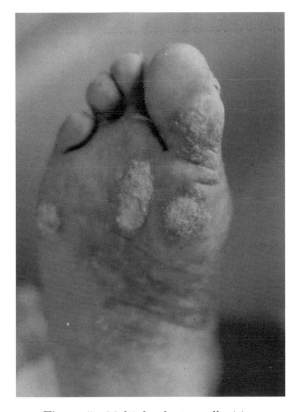

Figure 5. Multiple plantar callosities.

largement, or an area of abnormal weight distribution (i.e., lateral border of the foot and the fifth toe, below the metatarsal heads, or the perimeter of the heel, particularly the medial portion). Less common sites include the talar head, the prominent navicular tuberosity, the dorsal surface of the first metatarsal cuneiform joint, the medial portion of the first metatarsophalangeal joint over a hallux abducto valgus, and certain unusual areas in association with such congenital anomalies as clubfoot or clawfoot.

The lesion is diffuse and, therefore, does not have clearly demonstrated margins such as helomata. Initially the area is erythematous, but in time a yellowish-gray, slightly raised hyperkeratotic region forms. This region, often diffusely tender when direct pressure is applied, preserves the papillary skin lines. Conservative treatment includes periodic paring with a scalpel blade (weekly to monthly) and the application of an adhesive felt, latex, or foam rubber protective donut or horseshoe (see Chapter 20). Keratolytic agents such as 20–40% salicylic acid and plaster can be applied for several days every week over several weeks. Keralyt, a mixture of salicylic acid in propylene glycol, is one of the best keratolytic agents. A potent corticosteroid should be considered to suppress inflammation and give adequate lubrication and moisture retention. The patient is instructed to soak the callus in warm water and then abrade the area with a pumice stone for 1 or 2 minutes. A callus razor, in addition to or instead of the pumice stone, can be used to trim the dead, thickened skin. Great care is taken to avoid injury to the underlying healthy skin, which can be recognized by its softer texture.

As with corns, it is essential to treat the underlying etiology (deformity, disease, or biomechanical dysfunction) responsible for the stress. In the female, high-heeled shoes are often responsible for placing increased amounts of pressure on the metatarsal heads or the bases of the phalanges. A tight toe box forces the toes backward as well as together, particularly at the metatarsophalangeal joints. For athletes involved in stop-and-go sports, a full sole orthosis incorporating a metatarsal pad may better maintain the foot's position in the shoe. In the malfunctioning foot, a flexible sole aggravates abnormal stress. Shoes that are too narrow or that place frictional forces on the medial and lateral borders, particularly where the seams meet at the upper and insole, must be modified. Even elastic stockings can increase frictional forces on the ball of the foot, pulling the toes backward. Abnormal gait due to hyperpronated feet or genu valgus or varus deformity of the knees also causes pronounced stress on certain areas of the feet. Finally, local pedal conditions such as bursitis, tenosynovitis, tumors, spurs, exostosis, and osteophytes often can lead to or aggravate existing calluses. Therefore, effective management of the patient with a tylomata consists of treating the underlying etiology.

Corns/Helomata

Helomata, or clavus, have been classified into two types: dura (hard) and molle (soft) (Fig. 6). A corn is a focal hyperkeratotic lesion secondary to pressure or irritation from an external (e.g., shoe) or internal (e.g., exostosis, unreduced dislocation, hypertrophic phalangeal condyle) source. The most common sites for hard corns are the dorsal aspects of the lesser toes of the proximal or interphalangeal level and the lateral region of the fifth toe. If there is a flexion or mallet toe deformity, the terminal end of the small toes may develop an end corn. Over time, due to repeated microirritation, an inflammatory reaction occurs with a buildup of cellular debris and compensatory epidermal hyperplasia.

There is no age limit to corns; children have developed them. Corns may or may not be painful, though direct pressure over the lesion usually produces variable amounts of discomfort. Unlike warts, corns do not bleed when pared by a scalpel blade. They appear as a thickened epidermal area with a conical center or core that is lighter in color than the overlying epidermis. The epidermal lines are interrupted, unlike a callus, which preserves the lines. The porokeratotic corn is a distinctive species of wart that is very painful and has a white peripheral rim on paring, but no pinpoint bleeding. There is no central core, but the rubbery hard center is concave.

The differential diagnosis of hard corns should include verrucae—distinguished by their disruption of the papillary skin lines, capillary bleeding on surgical paring, and pain on lateral compression—and foreign bodies and fibromas.

Soft corns typically appear between the toes and result from irritative pressure of one condyle rubbing against its neighbor due to the differential lengths of the toes and metatarsals. Macerated skin, usually associated with soft corns in a toe web space, often

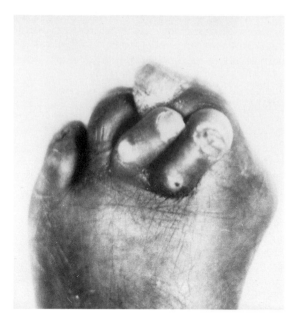

Figure 6. Helomata of the dorsal second and third toes in association with overlap and hallux valgus.

resembles a fungal infection. The treatment of a misdiagnosed soft corn with ointments, creams, and other chemical substances can aggravate the lesion and produce such complications as fissuring, further skin irritation, and fibrosis.

The treatment of corns is twofold: conservative and surgical. The conservative method of treatment consists of periodic, weekly to monthly paring of the hyperkeratotic area with a No. 15 scalpel blade. The paring procedure is done in short, rhythmical, crescentic movements until the overlying epidermis is removed and the softer portions of the underlying corn are visible. Specially tailored, adhesive-backed felt pads in the shape of a horseshoe or donut are then fitted to the area to allow pressure dispersion to nonaffected areas. Specially fitted foam or latex pads also can be used, depending on the preference of the practitioner. For soft corns, lamb's wool pads can be placed between the affected toes.

Shoewear should be carefully examined and modified to reduce frictional pressures. If the shoe is leather, a special device called a shoemaker's swan can be used to stretch the area causing the irritation. The prescription of an alternative shoe may be necessary for the healing phase. Generally, the shoe should have a wide, deep toe box, as low a heel as possible, laces or straps, a felt pad attached to the inside of the shoe tongue, and a space-occupying insole to lock the foot in place. Surgical excision of these lesions should be reserved for the most refractory cases after a 6-month trial of conservative therapy and should be conducted with the utmost caution in the foot at risk (e.g., in the patient with diabetes or peripheral vascular disease).

Surgical therapy should be handled in consultation with a podiatrist or orthopedic surgeon. The local excision of hard and soft corns without the simultaneous removal of the irritative focus (e.g., poorly fitted shoe, protuberant condyle, dislocated phalangeal joint) is not recommended because recurrence will follow, and complications such as fibrotic scarring and sinus tract development may result. The procedure can be performed under a local anesthetic nerve block and in the outpatient department. After a hemiphalangectomy or condylectomy, the wound is closed with sutures, and a dry sterile dressing is applied. Children and the elderly are best managed conservatively.

An end corn is managed similarly to corns in other areas; the treatment of choice is conservative and palliative. Moleskin, foam rubber, or latex is applied to the toe so that the distal end of the toe is protected, and the nail is trimmed to reduce impingement. If there is an abnormal flexion posture of the distal interphalangeal joint, with or without fixed skeletal deformity (e.g., mallet or claw toe deformity), it should be corrected (see Chapters 7 and 20).

Miscellaneous Keratoses

A number of other keratotic lesions that are not caused by friction and are frequently hereditary afflict the foot. Keratoses on the soles of the feet usually afflict the palms of the hands simultaneously. From the perspective of the primary care doctor, these conditions should form part of the routine differential diagnosis of plantar keratotic lesions. Examples of punctate keratoses include those inherited dominantly and recessively. Secondary syphilis, arsenic poisoning, Darier's disease, and the basal cell nevus syndrome may be associated with this form of keratosis. The differential diagnosis also should include guttate psoriasis. More diffuse forms of keratosis may be genetic, as in the dominant form of Unna-Thost disease, or may be inherited and associated with skin diseases such as psoriasis, pityriasis, rosacea, lichen planus, syphilis, or pityriasis rubra pilaris. Furthermore, noninherited diffuse keratosis may, in a small number of cases, be a harbinger of internal malignancy.

The treatment of these lesions is frustrating due to the rapid regrowth of skin. Frequent paring and the use of keratolytic agents (e.g., salicylic acid) and retinoic acid preparations have met with some success.

Infectious Diseases

Scabies

The web spaces of the toes often are affected by the itch mite, *Sarcoptes scabiei,* though less commonly than the hands. The patient usually complains of itching that is especially bad at night. The diagnosis of scabies is made by a suggestive history, observation of papulovesicles (nondescript papules), and identification of the characteristic burrow, which is a very thin, narrow, serpiginous track in which the egg-laying female mite resides. The identification of the mite in the skin scrapings, or more rarely, in a biopsy, is confirmatory. It is important to check the patient's torso, particularly in the bathing suit area, and genitalia. The differential diagnosis should include tinea pedis, contact dermatitis, and dyshidrosis.

Therapy consists of treating the patient and his contacts with one or two applications of 1% lindane (Kwell) or crotamiton solution (Eurax). It is important to advise the patient that it may be several weeks to months for the pruritus, probably an immunologic phenomenon, to subside.

Bacterial Infections

The elaboration of a keratolytic enzyme by a diphtheroid bacteria produces multiple, small, superficial pits that are rapidly filled with debris. The condition, termed pitted keratolysis, may produce a small amount of discomfort, slight pruritus, and characteristic dark punctate lesions of the heel. Diagnosis is confirmed by bacterial culture, although clinical observation usually is sufficient. Treatment is the application of erythromycin ointment or systemic erythromycin 400 mg twice daily for 2 weeks.

Streptococcus can follow fungal infections, especially if cracks and fissures develop between the web spaces of the toes. If early cellulitis and localized infection are not aggressively treated, recurrent bouts of lymphangitis and erysipelas can present variable degrees of elephantiasis. The treatment of choice is systemic penicillin given orally.

Impetigo contagiosa, secondary to staphylococci or streptococci, can also affect the feet, particularly if the epidermal barrier has been violated by previous fungal or vesicular disease. Papules with honey-colored crusts are characteristic. Penicillin or erythromycin by mouth are curative.

Gram-negative bacteria also can superinfect previously inflamed and injured areas of the foot, especially in the immunocompromised host. Characteristically, the erosions may suggest tinea pedis, but cultures and scrapings are negative. Diagnosis is made by smear and bacterial culture, and treatment consists of an astringent soak (e.g., silver nitrate 0.5% Burow's solution) and an effective systemic antibiotic. See Chapter 17 for additional information on infectious diseases.

Foreign Body

Foreign bodies in the plantar surface of the foot are not infrequent, particularly in shoeless individuals. They often enter the foot without the patient being aware of it. Splinters are the most common foreign objects, though hairs, needles, pebbles, glass, metallic slivers, plastic, and gun-shot pellets also are found. Foreign bodies in the foot sometimes are difficult to localize; if suspected, an x-ray should be taken. Multiview radiographs, xeroradiographs, radiopaque grid systems, surgical magnets, computed tomography, sonography, and/or fluoroscopy may be necessary. Most types of glass are radiopaque. Ultrasonography (10 MHz) is probably the most reliable method for detection of nonradiopaque superficial foreign bodies composed of wood or plastic. Magnetic resonance imaging is not recommended due to cost and low specificity.

The differential diagnosis should include corns, verrucae, granulomas, soft tissue masses, and miscellaneous conditions such as pyogenicum granuloma and fibroma. For superficial foreign bodies, the lesions should be gently pared and a curette and splinter forceps used to remove the object. Such management usually is curative, though wet dressings and a topical antibiotic may be useful. A foreign body may be left in place if it is asymptomatic, inert, not within a joint, or not a threat to function. Removal is advisable for reactive foreign bodies (near tendons, vessels, or nerves), large objects, and any item of concern to the patient. Rarely, if there is a secondary cellulitis or lymphangitis, a systemic antibiotic should be used. For deeper foreign bodies, surgery may

be necessary (see Chapter 13). Excisional biopsy for soft-tissue masses can establish the diagnosis and prevent unnecessary anxiety for the patient.

Atopic Dermatitis

The feet can be nonspecifically involved in atopic dermatitis or eczema. Look for lichenification in the nuchal, antecubital, or popliteal areas; a family or personal history of infantile eczema, hay fever, or asthma; and negative patch tests to shoe components. The acute pedal manifestations of the dermatoses include erythema, edema, warmth, and pain. Chronically, there is scaling and lichenification, and there may be fissuring and maceration of the toe web spaces following secondary infection. The differential diagnosis should be contact dermatitis and tinea pedis. Patch testing is confirmatory in the former condition, while scrapings and culture are confirmatory in the latter. Furthermore, atopic dermatitis typically does not involve the web spaces.

Treatment consists of the application of a steroid cream once or twice daily. Mild cases and those requiring long-term treatment are best handled by applying 0.5, 1, or 2.5% hydrocortisone. More severe, acute cases are handled with one of the newer fluorinated steroids (e.g., betamethasone). If the skin is dry and scaly, an ointment is preferred; however, a normally hydrated skin cream is useful. Lotions are more suitable for macerated, eczematous lesions. Use of a thin plastic film (Saran Wrap) at night improves the penetrating effect of the topical ointment. In severe cases, systemic prednisone with a several-week taper is necessary. Antipruritic agents such as cyproheptadine or diphenhydramine may be required to break the itch-inflammation cycle. Soaps, detergents, and other drying agents are best avoided during the acute phase, and nonsynthetic, loose stockings and socks should be worn.

Psoriasis

This condition is a dominantly-inherited disorder characterized by reddish-pink papules and plaques of silver-gray scales. Areas commonly affected are the scalp, knees, lumbosacral area, elbows, and penis, although there are more generalized forms of the eruption over the whole body. There may be variable degrees of pruritus and associated pitting of the nails, as well as an erosive, deforming arthritis. Psoriasis of the feet presents as random, scaly papules or plaques on the dorsal or plantar aspects of the foot; hyperkeratotic plaques that are fissured in the area of the heel and weight-bearing surfaces; pustular lesions of the sole; or macerated "white psoriasis" of the interdigital areas.

The differential diagnosis should include lichen planus, atopic dermatitis, lupus erythematosus, and, in the macerated area, tinea pedis, soft corns, and moniliasis. A diagnosis of psoriasis is made by careful history and clinical exam, although appropriate fungal cultures may be necessary to rule out tinea pedis.

Lesions usually respond well to application of steroid cream or ointment in conjunction with a keratolytic agent or with a tar and occlusive dressing such as a thin, plastic film that will increase the absorption and effectiveness of these agents. Interdigital psoriasis is difficult to treat but usually responds well to intralesional steroid therapy (weekly injections of 0.1 ml of triamcinolone 10 mg/ml). No more than 1 mg of triamcinolone should be injected in any one area, because atrophy may result. Pustular psoriasis does not respond well to most therapeutic regimens; it should be handled in consultation with a specialist. It may be necessary to administer periodic injections of triamcinolone (40 mg/ml) intramuscularly and incise and drain the pustules. Further, antimetabolites and ultraviolet-A (PUVA) treatments may be necessary.

Granuloma Annulare

This lesion is a symptomatic, idiopathic disease typically involving the dorsal surface of the feet. Children are more commonly affected than adults, and females twice as often as males. Diabetes mellitus should be suspected in the generalized form of the disease. The characteristic lesion is a donut-shaped ring of discrete, pink papules. In time, these papules coalesce into annular plaques.

The differential diagnosis should include lichen planus, erythema multiforme, larva migrans, and tinea pedis. Biopsy, usually unnecessary, is confirmatory. The natural history of granuloma annulare is spontaneous resolution in almost all cases; for those that are refractory or recurrent, intralesional injections of a steroid (e.g., triamcinolone) are useful.

Ulcers

There are three basic ulcer types: neurotrophic/neuropathic, vascular/ischemic, and stasis/pressure. Etiologies include diabetes, vascular disease, leprosy, cerebral palsy, alcoholism, and cord lesions such as spina bifida and syringomyelia. Ulcer presentations and treatments are discussed in Chapters 11, 16, and 18.

Miscellaneous Conditions

The erythematous bull's-eye lesions of erythema multiforme may affect the feet. Diagnosis is made by noting the presence of the lesion in other areas of the body, including mucous membranes, and identifying the underlying predisposing conditions. The differential diagnosis should include tinea pedis, which can be documented by fungal culture and microscopic examination of the scrapings, and granuloma annulare. The pedal manifestations of erythema multiforme improve when the systemic disease is treated.

Epidermolysis bullosa is a vesiculobullous disease. Its presentation depends on a variety of hereditary factors, the presence or absence of fibrotic scarring, and the location of the split in the skin. Depending on the type, there are variable amounts of vesicles and bullae in association with erythema and hyperkeratosis. Diagnosis is made by a careful history and clinical exam and a biopsy. Immunofluorescent tests usually are negative. The differential diagnosis should include pustular psoriasis and dyshidrotic eczema. Of note is the fact that the noninherited, acquired form of epidermolysis bullosa, which begins later in life, may be associated with underlying multiple myeloma, diabetes mellitus, or colitis. All forms of this disease respond to systemic steroids. Trauma should be avoided. Wet dressings and topical steroid creams are helpful. Chronic foot and toe contractions may develop, requiring correctional surgery and rehabilitation.

A number of autoimmune diseases can cause pedal dermopathy. In rare cases the atrophic, erythematous, irregular plaques of discoid lupus erythematosus can involve the sole of the foot. Diagnosis is established by biopsy and by immunofluorescent and serologic tests. The differential should include psoriasis and tinea pedis. Intralesional steroids plus topical applications are helpful in resolving the plaques. Systemic lupus erythematosus may cause distal periungual redness of the toes. Gottron's sign—the appearance of glazed, purplish-red, coalescent papules forming plaques over the ankles and large toe—may be seen in patients with dermatomyositis. The usual skin changes associated with systemic scleroderma can be seen in the foot. When palpated, the skin typically is hard and blanched; chronically there may be ulceration and calcinosis of the heel.

Finally, syphilis, the "great mimicker," always should be considered in any dermatologic condition involving the foot. The skin lesions of secondary syphilis generally produce bilaterally symmetric, dry, reddish-brown macules, papules, pustules, or papulosquamous lesions. These syphilids are seldom pruritic and occasionally may involve the interdigital area and escape notice. A careful history and exam, accompanied by the appropriate serologic tests, confirms the diagnosis. The differential diagnosis should include psoriasis, lichen planus, drug eruptions, pityriasis rosacea, and other acute exanthemata.

═══

References

1. Gooding GA: Foreign bodies. Clin Diagn Ultrasound 30:99–111, 1995.
2. Lammers RL: Soft tissue foreign bodies. Ann Emerg Med 17(12):1336–1347, 1988.
3. Monu JUV, McManus CM, Ward WG, et al: Soft tissue masses caused by longstanding foreign bodies in the extremities: MR imaging findings. Am J Roentgen 165:395–397, 1995.
4. Oikarinen KS, Nieminen TM, Makarainen H, et al: Visibility of foreign bodies in soft tissue in plain radiography computed-tomography, magnetic resonance imaging, and ultrasound: An in vitro study. Int J Oral Maxillofac Surg 22: 119–124, 1993.
5. Parieser DM: Superficial fungal infections. Postgrad Med 87(5):205–214, 1990.

5

Nails

Richard B. Birrer, MD

Anatomy

The nail, or unguis, is a horny, elastic plate covering the dorsal surface of the distal half of the terminal phalanx. Histologically, the nail consists of three layers: ventral, intermediate, and dorsal. The distal exposed portion, termed the nail body, is derived from the proximal hidden part, called the root. The nail wall, which is a fold of skin, surrounds the nail bed on each side. The nail groove is a slit between the wall and the bed. The eponychium is a proximal skin fold covering about 25% of the nail and its root. The lunula is a white, semicircular area just distal to the eponychium. The nail plate grows longitudinally from the nail matrix. Finally, the paronychium represents the soft tissue surrounding the nail border.

It takes 4–6 months for a toenail to grow from its matrix to the free edge. Growth of the nail is continuous throughout life and averages 0.2–0.4 mm per week.

Nail Disorders

Dystrophic Nails

Dystrophic nail (onychodystrophy) is a general term representing the end-stage degenerative changes of the nail bed and plate (Fig. 1). The etiology may include poor hygiene, the aging process, trauma, or a variety of chronic diseases (e.g., hypothyroidism, diabetes). The nails are brownish-black in color and tend to be thickened by cellular detritus, which fragments easily and has a waxy consistency. It is not clinically possible to distinguish dystrophic nails from fungal infections, although the former tend to involve all the toes, whereas the latter involve only one or two adjacent ones. Culture and microscopic exams are essential. Treatment consists of careful paring of the nails with a clipper on a monthly basis and a review of nail hygiene. It is important to inform the patient that the nails will never return to their previous state.

Onychomycosis

Fungal infections of the toenails (tinea unguium) occur in at least 2% of the population. They are particularly frustrating because of their chronic relapsing nature (Fig. 2). The infection occurs under or within the nail plate and causes a proliferation of keratinized debris under the nail. The nail thickens and crumbles when the plate is infected. Onychomycosis must be differentiated from nail dystrophy through microscopic examination and culture of the scrapings. Bacteria and candida, not dermatophytes, typically infect paronychial tissue. The differential diagnosis should include psoriasis.

Treatment is twofold. Conservatively, the nail should be periodically trimmed both in length and depth. Shoe gear should be adequately sized, particularly the toe box, and the socks should be nonsynthetic and loose. Topical antifungal agents are, for the most part, ineffective. The current treatment of choice is micropulverized or microcrystalline griseofulvin in doses of 500–1000 mg daily. Therapy must be continued for 1–2 years for a favorable response. The patient should be warned of such common side effects as headache, gastrointestinal discomfort, and, occasionally, photosensitivity and liver dysfunction. Terbinafine

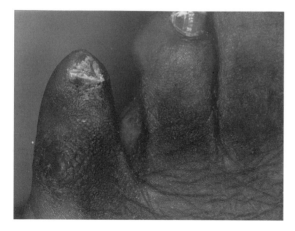

Figure 1. Dystrophic nails.

(250 mg) and itraconazole (200 mg) also are effective and well tolerated, although the latter is significantly more successful in eradication of fungal pathogens. Neither drug is associated with significant hepatotoxicity, and duration of therapy is a short 12 weeks. Itraconazole is contraindicated with co-administration of astemizole, cisapride, cyclosporine, and terfenadine. Procedures such as laser waffling and surgical removal of the nail with matricectomy are reserved for refractory cases that serve as a nidus for infection in the diabetic or vascular disease patient (see Chapter 20).

Subungual Hematoma

A traumatic blow to the nail can lead to a subungual hematoma. The individual often is immobilized due to throbbing pain as the blood tries to expand in the closed space. The severity of pain is proportional to the amount of trauma and pressure caused by the expanding hematoma. Ice should be applied immedi-

ately and the nail plate punctured to release the blood. Several methods are available. In the office, a dentist drill (or a laser in the pulse mode) is the fastest and least painful. A soldering gun with a fine point also is useful, although considerable expense can be saved by heating a paper clip or safety pin. In the field, a hand-held, battery-operated cautery gun can be used, as can a heated paper clip. Perhaps the best all-around modality in terms of expense and ease is an 18-gauge needle gently rotated through the plate. No anesthesia is necessary.

Once released, cold water soaks with gentle pressure removes the blood. A small absorbent bandage is supplied, and nonsteroidal anti-inflammatory drugs or analgesics are prescribed for pain. The patient should be advised that the nail plate will be discolored by the hemoglobin pigments as it grows distally. If the blow was severe and the hematoma large, then the nail may be lost entirely, although a new one will grow from the matrix in several months. Occasionally, the matrix is damaged during the trauma, resulting in a permanently deformed nail. X-rays should be taken to assess bone integrity.

Ingrown Toenail

Although jokes about ingrown toenails (unguis incarnatus/onychocryptosis) abound, for the patient who has one it is far from being a laughing matter. Ingrown toenails constitute 3–5% of all foot problems. A tight toe box or a congenital variation of tubular nails causes the nail plate to become curved rather than flat. The lateral (fibular) and medial (tibial) edges of the nail tend to become vertical, resembling an inverted "C," and impact on the horizontal bed

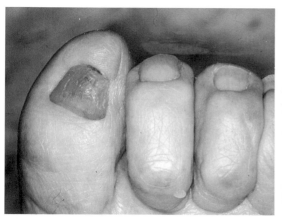

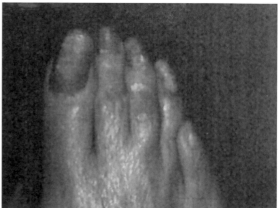

Figure 2. Onychomycosis.

of the nail. Usually the first toe is involved, although in some individuals any of the other toes may become similarly affected.

In time, the leading edge of the curled toenail acts like a sharp foreign body, causing local inflammation and fungal or bacterial infection. A localized abscess with swelling and purulent discharge can occur. The abscess typically is located on the lateral (fibular) side, perhaps due to pressure against the second toe. With recurrent formation of small abscesses and inflammation, exuberant granulation tissue can form, thus creating a vicious cycle of inflammation, inadequate drainage, and enlargement of granulation tissue followed by fibrosis and further inhibition of drainage. The differential should include paronychia, tumor, and foreign body.

Treatment of the infection and inflammation response consists of saucerization and removal of the ingrowing nail edge. If the lesion is mildly infected and has a minimal amount of granulation tissue, saucerization may be sufficient. A small amount of cotton is packed under the ingrown nail edge so that the skin is separated from the nail, thus allowing better drainage as well as preventing any further cutting action of the nail. The cotton, soaked in 40% salicylic acid, and application of anhydrous lanolin for 7–10 days are helpful. If possible, without local anesthesia, trim away the ingrown part of the nail and instruct the patient to soak the toe three times a day in a solution of 1 tbsp Epsom salt and 1 tbsp povidone-iodine solution per pan of water. This conservative management suffices in the majority of mild to moderate lesions. If the lesion is exceptionally painful, a local anesthetic block is necessary (see Chapter 20).

Recurrence may be prevented by teaching the patient to regularly file the central portion of the nail to keep it thin and cause it to grow centralward to compensate for loss of thickness. Trimming nails flat, wearing shoes with wide toe-boxes, and correcting over-pronation if present also are helpful.

Individuals who have chronically recurrent infections of ingrown toenails should be considered for complete and permanent removal of the nail. Consultation should be sought if the practitioner is unfamiliar or uncomfortable with the technique, because it is essential that the nail bed and matrix be removed completely since small islands of nail tissue can reappear. A phenol, laser, or surgical matricectomy may be employed.

Removal of the nail matrix can follow partial or complete nail avulsion and may be chemical, surgical, or laser. The procedure usually is reserved for recurrent or refractory cases of ingrown toenails. There should be no infection present (see Chapter 20).

Common Nail Deformities

The three most common nail deformities are tubular nails, hypertrophic thickening (onychophosis), and onychogryposis. The Ram's horn deformity of onychogryposis most commonly involves the first toe, but may also affect the small toes. Usually the nail plate is separated from the nail bed and is relatively brittle. Onychogryposis typically is seen in the elderly individual who is unable to trim his or her toenails. Treatment is conservative: trimming the nails. In the younger individuals, excision of the matrix and entire nail may be warranted.

Tubular nail deformity usually is congenital, though it may be exacerbated by a tight toebox. The inverted "C" becomes exaggerated and sometimes almost forms a complete circle ("O"). Treatment is identical to that for an ingrown toenail. Subungal exostosis, diagnosed by radiography, should be surgically removed.

More commonly seen in middle-aged and geriatric groups, hypertrophic nail thickening is marked by considerable deformity and the deposition of discolored subungual detritus. Treatment is conservative and consists of periodically trimming the nail, although in the more refractory cases excision of the nail and matrix may be necessary. Koilonychia, or spoon-shaped nails, are seen in cases of iron deficiency anemia. Onychorrhexis consists of marked longitudinal striations in the nail and is associated with nutritional disorders or rheumatoid arthritis.

Finally, trauma to the nail matrix can lead to a number of deformities, such as splits, ridges, and pits. These usually are asymptomatic.

Miscellaneous Subungual/Paraungual Lesions
Osteoid Osteoma

A benign bone lesion, common in children and young adults, osteoid osteoma produces recurrent pain attacks that usually are relieved by aspirin. There is focal tenderness on pressure to the involved nail plate, but due to the paucity of symptoms, the lesion frequently is not diagnosed. X-rays usually are diagnostic and show a central, round, radiopaque nidus surrounded by a thin, rarefied zone. Treatment consists of surgical excision under local anesthesia. Consultation is recommended. Subungual osteomas, also an uncommon tumor seen mostly in children or young adults, produce few long-term symptoms other than separation and deformity of the nail. X-rays are confirmatory, and the treatment of choice is surgical excision under local anesthesia with preservation of the nail, if possible. The differential diagnosis should include exostosis, which is reactive bone formation from repetitive microtrauma.

A number of rare lesions also may be visible through the nail plate. For instance, a small, round, bluish-red lesion that is paroxysmally painful, especially on exposure to cold, suggests a subungual glomus. Treatment consists of surgical removal of the distal nail plate and curettage of the tumor. Warts also may be located subungually and in this position can erode the adjacent tuft. Treatment is surgical excision. A subungual abscess often is first noted by the presence of a small, whitish area, which represents pus collection, underneath the nail bed. Decompression by removal of the overlying nail or perforation with a dental drill or 18-gauge needle is curative. Rarely, a melanoma may present as a discolored (black, purple, or red) nail bed; this sign should prompt a biopsy.

Periungual lesions include fibromas, warts, corns, and granuloma pyogenicum. The former three conditions are discussed in Chapter 4. A granuloma pyogenicum consists of an exuberant mass of granulation tissue overlying an ingrown toenail. Treatment is excisional biopsy of the pseudotumor and removal of the nail edge and its underlying matrix.

Paronychia

Paronychias are one of the most common problems encountered by healthcare professionals treating the foot. A paronychia is an inflammation of the nail fold, due to fungi or bacteria, that results in separation of the skin from the proximal portion of the nail (Fig. 3). Potential etiologies are ill-fitting shoes, foreign bodies, poorly administered self-care, and trauma. Systemic conditions such as diabetes mellitus, alcohol abuse, collagen vascular diseases, peripheral vascular diseases, and immunosuppressive states may predispose the patient to paronychias.

Paronychias can be acute or chronic. Acute paronychias are associated with red, hot,

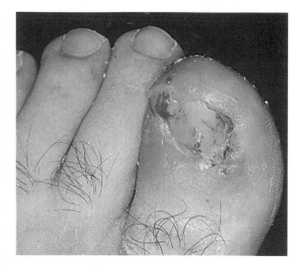

Figure 3. Paronychia.

swollen, and painful digits, especially in the distal periungual fold. The nail may be discolored, loosened from the bed, and fragmented. Often a pyogenic granuloma is present, which may cover a large portion of the nail plate. The most common organism causing the infection is *Staphylococcus aureus.* Chronic paronychia is similar, but severe tenderness and gross infection are not present. Candida species are often etiologic.

In treating acute or chronic paronychia, it is important to remember that the offending nail border must be removed (see Chapter 20). Once this is accomplished, local care consisting of dilute povidone-iodine (10%) soaks four times a day for 2–3 days usually resolves the infection. A topical antibiotic preparation also can be applied. Systemic antibiotics should be reserved for cellulitis extending to the metatarsophalangeal joint.

Pigmentation Changes

Toenails, like fingernails, are affected by systemic disease. A blue or azure lunula occurs in argyria. Diffuse melanosis suggests Addison's disease, neoplasia, hemochromatosis, or the adverse effects of chemotherapy (using quinacrine, antimalarials, etc.). Single or multiple white lines across the nail (Mee's lines) are found in arsenic and other heavy metal poisoning. White discloration (leukonychia) has many causes, including autosomal dominant inheritance; hypoalbuminemia (Muehrcke's lines) is one well-known acquired cause. Others include cirrhosis, rheumatoid arthritis, and diabetes. A sudden interruption in matrix vascularity as a result of myocardial disease produces one or more white lines across the nail (Beau's lines).

Gray discoloration occurs with chronic mercury poisoning. Yellow nails are associated with lymphatic edema from neoplasia or hypoplasia. Blackish discoloration of a nail may represent a melanotic whitlow or subungual hematoma if trauma has occurred. Half and half nails (Lindsay nails) are characterized by a deep reddish color distally and a white proximal portion. They are seen in renal and liver failure. Terry's nails (deep red distal one-quarter and white proximal three-quarters) are seen in chronic liver disorders or connective tissue disorders.

══

References

1. Stone O, Mullins JF: Chronic paronychia—Clinical aspects and therapy. Clin Med 73:30–34, 1996.
2. Yale JR: Yale's Podiatric Medicine, 3rd ed. Baltimore, Williams and Wilkins, 1987, pp 131–246.

6

The Big Toe

Richard B. Birrer, MD

Hallux Abducto Valgus

The term hallux abducto valgus denotes lateral (fibular) deviation of the great toe in association with prominence of the medial portion of the first metatarsal head, both of which tend to be constant features of the disorder (Fig. 1). The complex deformity of hallux valgus needs to be distinguished from a bunion, which refers to the acute swelling or chronic tumefaction of the bursa overlying the first metatarsophalangeal joint (MTPJ). A bunion may or may not accompany hallux valgus. Though the condition may be associated in up to 30% of cases with a number of inherited problems such as hypermobile joints, Ehlers-Danlos disease, splaying of the forefoot (excessive foot width—size B in females and size D in males), Achilles tendon contraction secondary to cerebral palsy, or metatarsus primus varus, it is almost exclusively a consequence of short, narrow shoes with pointed toes, high heels, or tight-fitting stockings or socks. Trauma leading to subluxation, dislocation, or rupture of the medial capsule (turf toe) of the first toe also can be causative. The complex is far more common in females than males (15:1) due to the types of shoes worn by females. Over time, there are accommodative changes seen in the cartilage, articular ligaments, sesamoids, tendons, and joint capsule forming the first MTPJ. Normally both feet are affected, but one side has a more marked degree of deformity and symptoms.

The pathogenesis of hallux valgus consists of gradual lateral inclination of the great toe, pushing on the second, third, and fourth toes so that there is gradual fibular drift of these toes (Table 1). The first, second, and third metatarsals tend to adduct, while the fourth and fifth abduct. Atrophy of the exposed condylar cartilage of the metatarsal and phalanx is present. The sesamoids are displaced laterally into the first intermetatarsal space. This migration causes the sesamoids to undergo chondromalacia as well as erode the cristae under the first metatarsal head, leading to denudation and ulceration. There is valgus rotation of the phalanx as it slips over or under its immediate fibular fellow. Subluxation of the first MTPJ causes the great toe to slide toward the axis of the foot and the metatarsal head to slip toward the mid axis of the body. Usually less than 50% of the metatarsal articulates with its proximal phalanx. The soft tissues of the great toe undergo progressive accommodative shortening and lengthening of the lateral and medial sides, respectively. With degeneration of the joint's cartilaginous surface as well as recurrent microtrauma due to abnormal joint biomechanics, greater surface incongruity occurs, and exostosis, osteophytes, and early degenerative joint disease develop.

Shoe friction and irritative tension of the medial collateral ligament of the first MTPJ lead to chronic inflammation of the overlying bursa and further proliferation of fibrotic and osteoblastic activity. Once the resistance of normal bone structure and function has been partially removed, the unbalanced pulls of the flexor, extensor, adductor, and abductor hallucis muscles complete the process through their unopposed contractions. It is not uncommon to see the great toe in marked lateral deviation, held in extension away from the

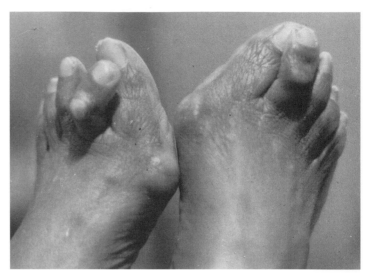

Figure 1. Bilateral hallux valgus with overlap of the second toe.

ground due to the "bowstring" effect of the extensor hallucis longus.

The symptoms of hallux valgus are not related solely to the degree of deformity, but also to complications. Repeated pressure and irritation from constricting shoewear usually leads to pain and inflammation. Pressure over the sensory nerves occasionally may cause paresthesias on the medial aspect of the toe. In time, there is development of bunions, corns, calluses, tight heel cord, ingrown toenails, septic bursitis, and occasionally septic arthritis due to the occurrence of a sinus or fistula tract. Pain typically arises in the region of the sesamoids, secondary to lateral displacement and degenerative changes.

Radiographs are confirmatory. The intermetatarsal angle is greater than 8° and the MTP angle greater than 15°. The head of the first metatarsal usually is irregular, flat, and broad, and osteophytic spurs may be seen at the joint margins. There may be trabecular hypertrophy, joint effusion, and an irregular, dense, subarticular sclerotic line under the base of the proximal phalanx. Soft tissue swelling may overlie the deformed joint, which may represent bursal inflammation. Occasionally, degeneration and calcification along the medial aspect are noted. The sesamoids are displaced, and degenerative changes such as spurs and osteophytes occur. The differential diagnosis should include forms of arthritis

Table 1. Hallux Valgus—Stages and Treatments

Stage	Description	Treatment
1	Little toe deviation but large medial prominence of MTP joint	NSAIDs, contrast soaks, OTC pads, wide and soft-soled shoes
2	Mild deformity with deviation (<20° MTP angle and <10° intermetatarsal angle); no subluxation of sesamoids	As above plus night splints, bunion posts
3	Moderate deformity with 20–40° MTP angle and 75% subluxation of sesamoids	As above plus custom orthosis
4	Severe deformity (>40° MTP angle, pronation of the first toe, marked lateral deviation and overlapping of the second toe); 100% subluxation of the sesamoids	Surgery

NSAIDs = nonsteroidal anti-inflammatory drugs, OTC = over the counter, MTP = metatarsophalangeal such as rheumatoid, gout, gonorrhea, and bursitis, as well as osteonecrosis, osteochondritis, stress fracture, and turf toe.

Therapeutic management of hallux valgus depends on the symptomatology, degree of deformity, extent of pathology, and presence of complicating factors. The majority of mild to moderate cases can be conservatively treated with good results. A bunion shield can be fashioned from tube foam, latex, or adhesive felt in such a manner that the pressure forces on the medial aspect of the first MTPJ are displaced circumferentially to noninvolved areas (Fig. 2). If adhesive felt is used, it is important to bevel the edge so that transition from felt to normal skin tissue is smooth and does not provide a focus for further hyperkeratotic reaction.

Anti-inflammatory agents (e.g., aspirin, nonsteroidal anti-inflammatory drugs) also are useful during the acute phase. Overlying hyperkeratotic tissue should be carefully pared down with a No. 15 scalpel blade. If there is a high degree of suspicion of an underlying bursitis, the injection of a long-acting steroid (e.g., methyl prednisolone acetate) is acceptable. A night splint and spacers between the first and second toe also should be prescribed, as well as regular active and passive rehabilitative exercises, perhaps in conjunction with low voltage stimulation.

Finally, the patient's footwear should be carefully examined and modified where appropriate: the toe box and width should be adequate, the heel low, and socks and stockings loose. Shoes should be leather so that they can be modified by stretching to relieve pressure points. Without attention to footwear, the therapeutic regimen will fail.

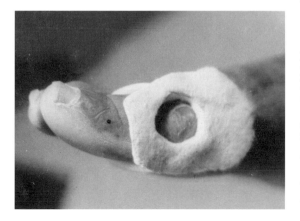

Figure 2. Adhesive felt bunion shield for hallux valgus.

Surgical therapy is reserved for individuals who have severely symptomatic deformities and those who have failed an adequate (6–12 months) trial of conservative management. Because there are over 100 surgical operations for hallux valgus and its attendant complications, the choice should be handled in association with a specialist. Preferred techniques include the Silver, Chevron, McBride, Akin, Lapidus, McKeever, Mitchell, Keller, Mayo-Stone, and Hoffman procedures. Surgical complications are not infrequent—metatarsalgia, floppy great toe, stress fracture of the lesser metatarsal rays, recurrence, development of hallux varus, adhesive neuritis and tendonitis, infection, dehiscence, and hemorrhage can occur. Once again, rational footwear must be presented postoperatively in order to minimize recurrence.

Hallux Rigidus

Limited range of motion of the first MTPJ due to previous trauma has been termed hallux rigidus, hallux limitus, hallux flexus, hallux nonextensus, metatarsus primus elevatus, and dorsal bunion. It is the second most common disabling deformity of the first toe. In addition to trauma, other etiologies are rheumatoid arthritis, gout, hallux valgus, and hereditary factors. The condition typically is unilateral and is more common in young adult males than females. There may be a single episode of severe trauma (e.g., stubbing of toe, kicking a hard object, falling from a height), though more commonly recurrent microtrauma is at fault (e.g., low-cut shoes with a tight toe-box).

Predisposing factors include a long, dorsally-tilted first metatarsal ray, pes valgus planus, a forward projecting big toe, and obesity. The patient usually complains of pain around the joint, especially upon tiptoeing or during the push-off phase of ambulation. The physical examination notes painful limitation, particularly of extension (<60°) and also flexion. Pain and tenderness are usually located dorsolaterally and may be associated with small amounts of erythema and edema. The patient may walk with an abducted gait or with the distal phalanx dorsiflexed to provide an accommodative fulcrum during gait.

Pathologically there is periarticular fibrosis with associated changes of ligaments and tendons as well as accommodative muscular spasms. Radiographic clues are narrowing of the MTPJ space and the development of spurs, lipping, and osteophytes at the articular margins, particularly the dorsal aspect of the first metatarsal head. Adolescents generally have articular cartilage changes, whereas adults develop degenerative joint pathology. The family doctor also may discover a thickened hallucis longus tendon as it crosses the dorsal spur of the first metatarsal head or a fluctuant swelling on the plantar aspect of the joint, which is most likely a subcutaneous adventitial cyst secondary to constant friction. In rare cases, there may be complete ankylosis of the articulation. The differential diagnosis should include gout and rheumatoid arthritis.

The injection of 1–2 ml of anesthetic (e.g., lidocaine, bupivacaine hydrochloride) and 0.25–0.5 ml of long-acting steroid (e.g., methyl prednisolone acetate) allows for immediate pain relief, relaxation of periarticular tissues, and long-term improvement of joint function. Traction with some basic range-of-motion exercises should be started. A foot appliance can be fashioned from rigid metal or an acrylic polymer, with the ultimate goal of shifting the weight to the lateral aspect of the foot. A Thomas or Denver heel, Jones bar, rigid shank, and extended counter accomplish the same goals. Complete splinting of the joint through the use of a steel insole or an inlay appliance with a longitudinal portion extending just behind the sesamoids (Morton's extension orthosis) also is quite effective. Surgical intervention is reserved for a joint with no function or for cases of failed conservative therapy (see Chapter 20).

References

1. American College of Foot and Ankle Surgeons: Preferred practice guidelines: Hallux valgus in the healthy adult. Park Ridge, IL, ACFAS, 1991.
2. Hawkins BJ, Haddad RJ: Hallux rigidus. Clin Sports Med 7(1):37–50, 1988.
3. Mann RA: The great toe. Orthop Clin North Am 20(4):519–534, 1989.

7

The Small Toes

Richard B. Birrer, MD

Disorders of the Small Toes

Corns

The dorsal aspect of the smaller toes at the proximal interphalangeal (PIP) and distal interphalangeal (DIP) level and the lateral border of the fifth toe (i.e., tailor's bunion) are common sites for hard corns. Corns also can occur on the terminal end of the toes, especially if there is an associated flexion or mallet toe deformity. Corns may occur at other areas due to frictional irritation of the shoe against a phalangeal condyle, bony prominence, unreduced dislocation, or exostosis. Differences in toe length (e.g., fifth toe) can lead to the formation of soft corns in the interdigital web spaces secondary to the pressure of a proximal phalangeal base and the head of a metatarsal against a condyle of a contiguous toe or vice versa. Diagnosis and treatment of corns are detailed elsewhere (see Chapters 4 and 20).

Mallet Toe Deformity

Contracture of the DIP toe joint in plantar flexion has been termed a mallet toe (Fig. 1). The deformity may be fixed or dynamically flexible and usually is limited to the lesser digits of the foot (the second, third, or fourth toes), although the condition may be bilateral. High-heeled, pointed-toe shoes aggravate the deformity. The clinical exam reveals PIP joint flexion and one or more complications, such as nail deformity or end or dorsal corn formation. The latter conditions are due to abnormal frictional irritation against the shoe or walking surface.

Treatment of mallet toe can be conservative or surgical. The secret to successful management is to detect it early while the deformity is flexible. At a minimum, the shoe should be roomy and well-fitted, with a high, wide toe box and crepe soles, to avoid pressure on the toes. A metatarsal bar or an insole (Plastazote) may be added to distribute pressure on the plantar aspect of the foot. Protective pads of moleskin, adhesive, or felt foam can be custom designed to protect the distal tuft or the dorsal aspect of the toe. An elastic sling made from similar materials can be used to reduce the flexion deformity.

A program of daily manipulation and stretching of the toes by the patient helps flexibility and delays a fixed deformity. A specialist should be consulted for surgical correction (e.g., flexor tenotomy, fusion, arthrotomy) of a fixed deformity.

Hammer Toes

Hyperextension of the DIP joint in combination with a rigid flexion deformity of the PIP defines this deformity, also termed digiti flexus. Malposition of the proximal phalanx on the metatarsal head joint and contraction of the metatarsophalangeal capsule in dorsiflexion (claw toe) are commonly associated. Hammer toes may be fixed, semiflexible, or flexible. Characteristically the second toe is involved; its length makes it susceptible to trauma by short or extremely pointed shoes or short stockings. The condition often is associated with hallux abducto valgus, rheumatoid arthritis, and osteoarthritis.

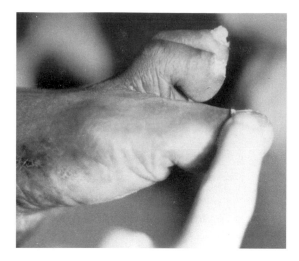

Figure 1. Mallet toes.

Incidence of hammer toes among persons 30–60 years old is one in 15 among Caucasians and one in five among African-Americans, with a female to male ratio of 2.5:1. Complications include the development of corns, calluses, and bursitis over the PIP joint. Claw toes generally are neurologic in origin, also may be fixed or flexible, and frequently are complicated by the development of corns on the dorsum over the PIP joint or at the tuft of the involved toe.

Hammer toes may be either congenital or acquired. The acquired condition primarily is associated with abnormal biomechanics (e.g., excessive pronation and supination). The deformity may occur in the transverse, sagittal, and frontal planes. A short first metatarsal ray, as seen in a cavus foot, results in the increased transfer of weight to the second toe with eventual formation of the deformity. In addition, in cavus foot there is decreased motor strength of the extensor digitorum brevis which causes weakening of normal extensor power, aggravating hammer toe formation. Finally, neurologic conditions that weaken the anterior tibialis muscle and lead to extensor substitution (i.e., poliomyelitis) also may produce the classic hammer toe posture.

In time, contracture of the flexor and extensor tendons, fascia, and collateral ligaments develops, and the skin of the plantar surface wrinkles and fissures. Painful hyperkeratotic lesions overlying or adjacent to the interphalangeal joints or on the distal tips of the digits are common. The joints become enlarged, deformed, and, occasionally, ankylosed. X-ray examination may reveal calcification of the overlying bursa or a calcified sinus tract. Se-

questration and local bone necrosis may occur, as well as osteophytic spurring and lipping.

Successful management of hammer toe may be conservative or surgical, depending on the degree of deformity, the number of joints involved, whether the deformity is fixed or flexible, the presence of complications, and the age and health of the patient. Palliative treatment, when the condition is recognized early and is still flexible, consists of custom-fitting the appropriate adhesive felt, foam rubber, or similar device to protect pressure areas from the development of hyperkeratosis. Forced extension of the toes can be assured by the fitting of a toe crest pad on the plantar surface (Fig. 2). A plantar splint with a dorsal elastic sling also may be used for considerable improvement.

It is important that the footwear be carefully examined and an extra-depth toe box be prescribed. Inlaid depth shoes may allow suf-

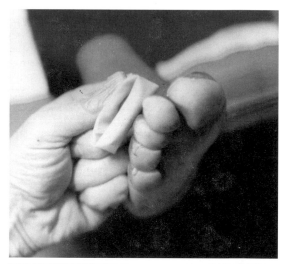

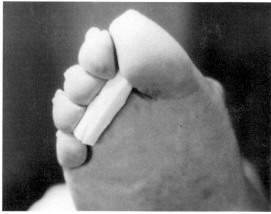

Figure 2. Toe crest pads for treatment of hammer toes.

ficient freedom and relief of pressure in the forefoot. Moldable plastic materials and silicone products can be used along with tube gauze to produce an accommodative appliance for the palliative management of hammer toes (e.g., Budin splints and the double-ring hammer-toe device of Polokoff).

A number of surgical techniques can correct hammer and claw toes; these approaches should be handled by consultation. Some examples include proximal hemiphalangectomy (DuVries and Mann method), Kelikian syndactylation, distal hemiphalangectomy, forced straightening, metatarsal head resection, diaphysectomy or waist resection of the proximal phalanx, and osteotomy (Tierny's method) (see Chapter 20).

Trigger Toes

Tenosynovitis of the flexor hallucis longus tendon with resultant triggering due to rupture of its central fibers has been noted in ballet dancers and joggers. The athlete usually complains of tenderness, perhaps swelling, and painful clicking, snapping, or popping during the exacerbating activity. Careful, controlled injection of a long-acting steroid may be useful (see Chapter 20), although surgical lysis of adhesions and removal of the entrapment often is necessary.

Underlapping Toes

This deformity, also referred to as curled undertoes, must be distinguished from mallet and claw toes. Overriding and underriding toes usually are acquired and frequently are associated with the development of a hallux abducto valgus deformity (Fig. 3). If the hallux underrides the second toe, there typically is atrophy and discoloration of the toenail due to the prolonged forces of weight bearing. Overriding of the second toe by the hallux causes severe contraction of the adductor hallucis, joint capsule, and articular ligaments. The third, fourth, and fifth toes also may overlap or underride, particularly if there is hypermobility of the foot.

Most of the deformities occur at the interphalangeal joint with abnormal metatarsophalangeal joints. The third and fourth toes tend to underlap one another and the second toe, whereas the fifth toe often overlaps the fourth, though underlapping is not uncommon. There is associated contracture of the skin, joint capsule, and extensor tendon. Complications in-

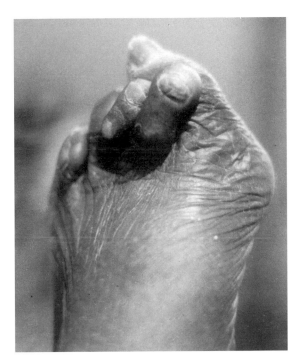

Figure 3. Overlapping toes.

clude the development of soft and hard corns and dystrophic changes of nails due to repeated trauma.

Treatment depends on the degree and type of deformity, as well as the age and overall health status of the patient. For instance, overlapping of the second toe due to hallux abducto valgus usually requires treatment of the hallux in order for the second toe to resume its neutral position. Regardless of severity, if the deformity is flexible, then a trial of conservative therapy still is warranted. Adequacy of footwear, particularly a sufficient toe box, is paramount. Tailored splints, removable crests, or similar appliances located on functional insoles also help to improve the condition (e.g., transverse Budin splint).

Surgery should be reserved for the most refractory cases and should be handled in consultation. Surgical options include metatarsal head resection, diaphysectomy, hemiphalangectomy of the proximal portion of the proximal phalanx, tenectomy, tenotomy, capsulotomy, syndactyly, arthroplasty, and a variety of method combinations.

Paraungual Lesions

The most common paraungual lesions of the small toes are nail groove corns. Gentle curetting with a 1-2 mm curette usually is sufficient, although lesions associated with the fibular side of the fifth toe may be more troublesome. The lesion typically is due to frictional shoe pressure secondary to tight-fitting shoegear that "squares off" the toes. Gentle, periodic paring and the wearing of a liberal, open-toed shoe or a deeper toe box are mostly curative, although removal of the entire nail and matrix (Syme procedure) may be required. The most common subungual lesion is an end corn adjacent to the free nail edge due to a complicating, fixed, hammer toe deformity. Correction of the hammer toe is usually all that is required.

Miscellaneous Conditions

Repetitive microtrauma, common in long-distance runners and joggers, may be seen in the small toes as an asymptomatic, subungual, brownish-black lesion due to micro hemorrhage (see Chapter 13). The condition has been termed "runner's toe." The differential must include malignant melanoma and pigment-producing fungal and bacterial infections. Ulcerations in the toe web spaces and on the tips of the toes should suggest a peripheral neuropathy or microvascular impairment.

The small toes are involved in rheumatoid arthritis more frequently than the big toe , but are affected less frequently in gout and arthritis. There may be an associated interphalangeal joint flexion contracture or fixation in extension. The initial presentation of psoriasis and rheumatoid arthritis may involve the isolated swelling of the small toe in the form of linear periostitis. A relatively rare condition primarily seen in African-Americans is the spontaneous auto-amputation of the small toes, termed ainhum. The fourth and fifth toes are most commonly involved, though the second and third ones can be affected, as well as the fingers. Over a period of several years, a narrow, band-like constriction develops, normally at the base of the fourth or fifth toe. It starts medially and spreads progressively plantarward and dorsolaterally. The condition may be bilateral; it affects both men and women around the age of 45 and tends to be symptomless. Treatment is expectant.

References

1. American College of Foot and Ankle Surgeons: Preferred Practice Guidelines: Hammer Toe Syndrome. Park Ridge, IL, ACFAS, 1991.
2. Coughlin MJ: Lesser toe abnormalities. *In* Chapman M (ed): Operative Orthopedics. Philadelphia, J. B. Lippincott, 1988, pp 1765–1776.
3. Coughlin MJ: Subluxation and dislocation of the second metatarsophalangeal joint. Orthro Clin N Am 20(4):535–551, 1989.
4. Dale SJ, David DJ, Sykes TF: Effective approaches to common foot complaints. Patient Care 30(3):158–180, 1997.

8

Metatarsals

Richard B. Birrer, MD

Anatomy

The many anatomic relations among the metatarsals are important for understanding pertinent pathophysiology. Even though the fifth metatarsal usually is the longest in the foot, the most important relation is between the first and second. Twenty-five to 30% of individuals have an "index plus/minus" type of foot in which the first and second metatarsals are approximately equal in length, and the forward ends of the other three metatarsals progressively diminish in length. Fifty-five to 60% of people exhibit the "index minus" prototype in which the first metatarsal is shorter than the second. Finally, in the "index plus" conformation, the first metatarsal is longer, and the forward ends of the others decrease progressively.

Physiology

Under normal physiologic conditions, the heads of all metatarsals should rest evenly on the floor in the standing position, particularly in the tiptoe position, regardless of the type of forefoot. In one study of 100 normal people, a podoscope demonstrated that 30% use all of the metatarsals, 28.5% the first three metatarsals, 28.5% the lateral metatarsals, and 13% the central rays. These static findings are preserved during the dynamic aspects of gait, and it is the biomechanical alteration of the metatarsal area that is the most frequent cause of pain in the forefoot (e.g., metatarsalgia). Remember that the center of weight-bearing pressure in over 50% of the stance phase of gait remains on the metatarsal heads. The pathomechanics of metatarsal pain can be classified according to anatomic location and the distribution of weight—diffuse or local—on the metatarsal supports. Diffuse overload occurs in anterior support problems; focal overload follows first ray overload and insufficiency syndrome, as well as central ray overload and insufficiency syndrome.

Metatarsal Disorders

The term "metatarsalgia" has been used loosely to describe painful conditions that affect the plantar surface of the forefoot. As a generic term that allows us to localize pain to the forefoot, it has absolutely no relevance to underlying pathology, specific diagnosis, or appropriate management. The most common causes of metatarsalgia are either metatarsophalangeal (MTP) joint disorders or plantar keratoses that develop under bony prominences (Table 1).

Anterior Support Overload

Anterior support overload occurs in the equinus foot, the cavus foot, and the foot in a high-heeled shoe. Eight-five to 90% of metatarsalgia occurs in females. Shoes with elevated heels greatly increase the force exerted against the metatarsal heads. In addition, a cramped, pointed toe box crowds the toes together in dorsiflexion so that the metatarsal condyles lose the normal anterior support from the toes. These changes can be readily demonstrated with a Harris foot mat. The success of all therapy in this situation depends on wearing a low-heeled shoe with an adequate toe box.

Table 1. Common Causes of Metatarsalgia

MTP joint problems	Keratotic disorders
Systemic arthritis	Long metatarsal
Lyme disease	Rigid first ray
Degenerative arthritis	Hypermobile first ray
Synovial cyst	Varus or valgus forefoot
Interdigital neuroma	Prominent fibular condyle
Freiberg's infraction	on metatarsal head
Capsular degeneration	Flatfoot or cavus foot

MTP = metatarsophalangeal

Equinus foot deformity caused by contracture of the Achilles tendon from congenital as well as inherited disorders (e.g., cerebral vascular accidents, poliomyelitis) results in limited dorsiflexion and the consequent overload of the anterior support on the metatarsal heads. Abnormal increases of the plantar arch in the form of a cavus foot results in the maldistribution of weight at the heel as well as at the metatarsal heads. The associated subluxation and occasional dislocation of the toes also aggravate the metatarsalgia by removing normal toe support of the metatarsals. Finally, in equinus, the metatarsal heads generally are the first point of contact with the floor, again increasing the symptoms of metatarsalgia. Because the gait malfunction—dynamic cavus foot—appears before the pathologic manifestation—structured cavus foot—early diagnosis and treatment can prevent many of the principal biomechanic disturbances of the deformity. The differential diagnosis should include systemic causes such as gout and rheumatoid arthritis (i.e., degenerative, rheumatoid, psoriatic disorders).

Treatment

The therapeutic approach to anterior support overload may be conservative or surgical. If there is no underlying foot deformity, the recommendation is to prepare a metatarsal bar or pontoon fashioned out of adhesive felt or foam rubber (Fig. 1). The device is placed behind or adjacent to the metatarsal heads to diffuse the frictional pressure. A low-heeled shoe and stretching of the Achilles tendon are imperative to reduce frictional irritation.

In the child with a dynamic cavus foot, normal gait through regular rehabilitative exercises must be established, particularly walking barefoot on a smooth floor. The emphasis here is to impact the floor with the heel rather than the ball of the foot. Supplementary arch

supports as well as a metatarsal bar and pontoon are useful. Physical therapy can be supplemented by diathermy, ultrasound, hydrotherapy, and massage to minimize fibrotic contraction (see Chapter 20).

Once there is structural deformity present in the soft tissue or bones, a qualified specialist should be consulted to determine the appropriate course. Examples of soft tissue operations include the method of Steindler and Camera; operations for skeletal deformities consist of arthrodesis and the metatarsectomy method of Lelievre.

First Ray Overload

Overload of the first ray occurs under two circumstances. The first involves an overly long big toe that is joined to a strong metatarsal. With repetitive microtrauma to the MTP joint, enhanced by an insufficient toe box and metatarsus elevatus, osteoarthritis of the joint develops, leading to hallux rigidus. The second pathogenetic mechanism of first ray overload involves frontal load imbalance of the head of the metatarsal and the sesamoids. Acute overload can follow a fall on the tiptoes

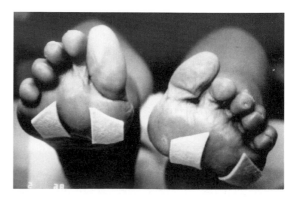

Figure 1. Metatarsal pontoons made of adhesive felt.

or the sudden application of brake pressure, as in a traffic accident. Repetitive microtrauma resulting from dancing, particularly ballet, can lead to front load imbalance. A chronic syndrome can result when the angle that the first metatarsal forms with the floor is greater than 25°. The most common causes are high heels and the presence of a cavus foot.

The patient usually complains of chronic pain, particularly a dull ache. The clinical exam also discloses pain at the level of the head of the first metatarsal; there may be some indurated edema and limitation of motion noted. The internal arch usually is increased, the condyles of the first metatarsal are prominent, and the big toe is held in hyperextension. Hyperkeratosis, in the form of tylomata and helomata, are characteristic in the region of the overload zone. In more advanced cases, the bursitis may be noted by crepitus, a small ulcer, or a sinus tract. Radiologically, there is hypertrophy of the margins of the first MTP joint; narrowing of the joint space; and lipping, exostosis, and osteophytic spurs of the articular surfaces. Soft tissue swelling may be noted in longer term cases, and the bursa may be fibrotic and calcified.

Treatment

Palliative treatment consists of custom fitting an orthotic, pontoon, or cushion in the form of a half-moon that protects the overload zone or designing an insole that has a retrocapital support. Diathermy can be applied in selected cases and, especially with complicating bursitis, a long-acting steroid-anesthetic combination can be beneficial (see Chapter 20). Anti-inflammatory agents are useful supplements. A dancer's pad can be prescribed. If the underlying etiology is repetitive microtrauma, well-fitted, firm-soled footwear with an anterior heel or Jones bar is helpful. Surgery should be reserved for the most refractory cases after several months of conservative therapy. Standard surgical interventions include the Jones operation, metatarsal base osteotomy, and sesamoidectomy.

First Ray Insufficiency

Insufficiency of the first ray—due to relatively long second and short first metatarsal bones—causes dysfunction of the foot by overloading the other rays, particularly the second and third metatarsals. The condition is variably described as open foot, splay foot, metatarsus varus, transverse or anterior flat-foot, or Dudley J. Morton's syndrome or foot. The mechanics of gait are disturbed, resulting in march fractures (Deutschlander's disease) and trigger points in the gluteal muscles, especially the gluteus medius.

A long-term effect of first ray insufficiency is overlapping of the toes. The prominent head of the second metatarsal acts as a leading "knife-edge" that extends through the heel. This makes the foot unstable and prone to rock during the push-off phase of the gait cycle. The ankle pronates, the knee internally rotates, and the hip adducts and internally rotates. The glutei, vastus medialis, and peroneus longus muscles are strained. Referred pain to the buttock and sacrum is common, and sensory defects including foot drop may mimic nerve entrapment or intervertebral disc disease.

The causes of first ray insufficiency are congenital (e.g., posterior placement of the sesamoids, a shortened first metatarsal, or varus deviation of the first metatarsal); soft tissue dysfunction (e.g., laxity of the Lisfranc ligament); dislocation of the sesamoids; flattening of the longitudinal arch; and such iatrogenic causes as the Hueter-Mayo operation, in which the metatarsal head is removed and remodeled; metatarsal osteotomy, which usually shortens the first ray; and a variety of operations that diminish the strength of the big toe (e.g., Brandes-Keller operation). Regardless of etiology, insufficiency of the first ray must be borne by the adjacent rays.

Acutely, the insufficiency is manifested by sudden decompensation in the form of a march fracture. There is a sudden onset of intense pain in the second or third metatarsal due to a spontaneous fracture associated with long periods of walking or as a consequence of the type of marching performed by military personnel. The afflicted individual generally must stop walking, and swelling may occur over the dorsal aspect of the affected foot. The condition is unilateral and most commonly affects the second ray, though the third and fourth may be involved as well. Radiologically, except for an obviously shortened ray, there usually are no acute changes noted, although 2–3 weeks after the injury a periosteal reaction occurs around a clear line at the union of the distal and middle thirds of the bone.

Deutschlander, who originally described the condition in 1921, noted three phases: an acute phase, which lasts 2 months and is characterized by pain and usually negative radiographs; a periosteal reaction lasting about 3 months, during which time the radiographs are positive; and a reparative or healing phase of approximately 4 months, during which the bone structure returns to normal. The availability of bone scan techniques makes possible the earlier diagnosis of march fracture—even within the first week.

Progressive first ray insufficiency causes characteristic pathophysiologic changes. A thick, diffuse callus or hyperkeratotic area develops under the heads of the second, third, and fourth metatarsals in over 75% of patients. The hyperkeratosis often is associated with submetatarsal bursitis. Thickening of the cortex of the second metatarsal also may be seen radiographically, along with stress fractures. Finally, the abnormal biomechanics cause dorsal dislocation and subluxation of the second and third toe, resulting in claw deformity.

Treatment

The treatment of first ray insufficiency depends on the etiology as well as degree of deformity. The treatment of a lesser metatarsal stress fracture is best managed by the application of a posterior splint or soft cast (e.g., Unna boot) or surgical adhesive strapping in combination with rest, elevation, ice, and anti-inflammatory agents. The cast should remain in place for 2–3 weeks; thereafter, progressive ambulation with taping or a shoe with a rigid sole and supportive inlay is advised. Once healing has occurred, attention must be directed to the underlying etiology in order to prevent recurrence.

Treatment of the chronic form may be palliative or surgical. Analgesics and anti-inflammatories should be prescribed during the initial visit to relieve intense pain and discomfort. The hyperkeratotic area should be carefully trimmed. An elastic bandage 3–5 cm in width around the metatarsals, in an attempt to reduce their distal divergence and correct the varus of the first metatarsal or the valgus deformity of the fifth, is *not* useful. A number of orthotics are available to restore the normal tripod base. These include a metatarsal bar or anterior heel (an elevated transverse bar of the shoe sole situated behind the central metatarsal heads) that diffuses excess pressure causing the metatarsalgia. A Morton's device fashioned from two layers of Kiro felt provides an insole that has a prolongation beneath the first metatarsal of the big toe to the MTP joint crease to correct the insufficient first ray. The Martorell arch support consists of a metatarsal bar plus a toe crest placed in the digital plantar fold; the crest prevents foot slippage on the insole surface and provides for further pressure dissipation from the metatarsal heads. These supports can be supplemented by dorsal digital splints that force plantar toe flexion. Such adhesive felt or sponge rings are placed at the base of the toes so that, with normal pressure, the toe is forced downward.

These therapeutic modalities should be supplemented by an active physiotherapy program for the best functional result, regardless of whether there is surgical intervention or not. It is essential to develop the flexor muscles of the forefoot since a great tendency toward toe dorsiflexion exists in this syndrome. The exercise program consists of both active and passive components. Active exercises should begin in a tub of warm water and should feature a full range of motion emphasizing plantar flexion. The exercises can be performed on a small wooden platform placed inside the tub so that the metatarsal heads rest on the edge of the platform and the toes overhang. Thereafter, a number of mechanical exercises are routinely practiced for eight repetitions. Examples are towel grasps, pencil curls, and small ball pickups.

An exercise session should include a short period of barefoot ambulation on a smooth surface. During the push-off phase, all the toes must make surface contact, especially the big toe. A surface of wet sand is extremely valuable as it clearly demarcates the contact points of the five toes and reinforces the importance of plantar flexion. Passive exercises include manipulation and postural modifications. The ball of the foot and the MTP articulations of each toe should be gently, but progressively, squeezed to overcome the stiffness and inflammation of the metatarsal areas and the dorsal retractions of the musculotendinous units in the region. Postural treatments include bending the foot in strong plantar flexion when the patient is seated or adopting a knee attitude and producing the same plantar flexion.

A 6-month trial of this conservative treatment should be applied rigorously before surgical consultation is sought. Discussion of the surgical management of the first ray insufficiency syndrome is beyond the scope of this chapter. In general, the approach depends on the type of deformity and its attendant complications. Thus, depending on circumstances, the first metatarsal may be lengthened, realigned, or fused, or the remaining metatarsals shortened by resection or osteotomy.

Central Ray Overload

Overload of the central rays rarely involves a single metatarsal ray but rather affects several, in diminishing order from the second to the fourth metatarsal. The syndrome typically is seen in compensatory combination with insufficiency of the first ray. Overloads of a single central ray occur congenitally or when there is loss of proximal articulation dorsiflexion—a condition most commonly seen in the fourth ray.

The patient usually complains of pain in the area of the inflamed condyle, and the clinical exam reveals hyperkeratosis in the form of corns and calluses. In the chronic situation there may be a bursitis, which can become infected and progress to an ulceration if not treated early. Treatment for central ray overload syndrome is similar to first ray insufficiency. Surgery, usually osteotomy or condylectomy, should be reserved for failures of palliative modalities.

Central Ray Insufficiency

Insufficiency of the central rays is characterized by overload of the first and fifth metatarsals. The etiology may be congenital, neurologic, or iatrogenic. The most common congenital cause is aplasia of one or more metatarsal segments. The fourth metatarsal typically is involved with the deformity, becoming evident in early infancy or following cases of poliomyelitis. Clinically, the condition does not become symptomatic until later in childhood when the third and fifth toes deviate compensatorily, producing metatarsalgia. With few exceptions, the treatment of this syndrome is surgical removal of the entire ray and corresponding toe.

Interdigital Neuroma

An interdigital plantar neuroma is a common cause of metatarsal pain. The condition, variably referred to as Morton's disease, Morton's toe, Morton's metatarsalgia, Morton's digital neuralgia, interdigital perineural fibrosis, and anterior metatarsalgia, frequently is confused with first ray insufficiency syndrome. Classically, the condition affects adults 20–50 years of age, typically female (8:1 ratio), in the region of the fourth MTP articulation. Although most commonly unilateral, it may be bilateral.

The patient complains of sharp, lancinating pain in the second and third metatarsal interspaces, with radiation of the pain toward the second, third, and fourth toes. It may have a burning or electric shock sensation and occurs at rest following a period of prolonged walking or strenuous foot exertion. The pain is not directly under the plantar condyle of the metatarsal head. The patient often attempts to relieve the discomfort by removing the shoes and massaging the feet. Initially the pain crises are intermittent, but over time they may become chronic in nature.

The clinical exam tends to be unremarkable. Some pressure pain at the distal end of the second and third interspaces may be noted when the soft parts are compressed. Mediolateral compression of the adjacent bones may produce plantar pain, particularly if dorsoplantar web space squeezing is applied. Occasionally a "click" (Mulder's click) can be heard or felt as the swollen nerve is forced between the metatarsal heads. Rarely, a small tumor may be palpable in the affected areas.

Radiologic investigations also are unremarkable since there are no fixed concomitant bony alterations. An ultrasound exam usually shows a hypoechoic nodule. The differential diagnosis should include Deutschlander's disease (pain produced by pressure on the distal third metatarsal diaphysis), Morton's syndrome, bursitis, tumors, stress fractures, and other causes of metatarsalgia (pain in the head of the involved metatarsal).

Pathogenetically, there is external pressure and repetitive microtrauma to a branch of the lateral plantar nerve. Tight shoes, frequently noted in women, and certain professions such as ballet dancing are predisposing factors in the pathogenesis of the lesion. Strong evidence suggests that the particular branch of the lateral plantar nerve is congenitally enlarged, although other theories include neoplastic and vascular etiologies for the neuroma. The majority of interdigital neuromas respond to conservative therapy. A metatarsal pad and a progressive, stepped program is recommended (Table 2).

Shoes must have an adequate toe box and length. High heels are not advisable. A rigid insole, preferably of metal, is carefully fitted to immobilize the metatarsals as well as compensate for any biomechanical dysfunction that may exist (e.g., flat feet or first metatarsal insufficiency). A trial of anti-inflammatory agents may be helpful, and patient education—reinforced on a regular basis—is important.

Table 2. A Progressive, Stepped Program for Interdigital Neuroma

Stage	Treatment Methods	Duration	Expected Outcomes*
1	Properly-fitted, wide shoe Metatarsal pad Patient education and reinforcement	3 months	40–45% improve
2	Injection therapy: 　Lidocaine (1%) 2 cc 　Trimanotone hexacetomide 　Triamcinolone Patient education and reinforcement	3 months	45–50% improve 12% no improvement
3	Surgery		96% improve

*Overall improvement rate is 85%.

Standing, walking and running activities often must be modified, shortened, or temporarily discontinued. Alternating hot and cold compresses for several minutes each two or three times often relieves pain. If the patient does not respond to this initial form of palliation, injection of a combination anesthetic and corticosteroid (see Chapter 20) into the dorsal part of the foot at the point of pain is most beneficial and diagnostic. This treatment can be combined with short-wave diathermic applications. Several authors also have recommended large doses of vitamin B. For the refractory case, surgical extirpation of the pathologic area—as proximally as possible via a longitudinal dorsal approach—is curative. Consultation with a specialist is advised.

Note: For a discussion of **sesamoiditis,** see Chapter 13.

Periarthritis Synovitis

Periarthritis between the first two MTP joints, also called the second metatarsal interspace syndrome, manifests itself as sharp pain in the distal second metatarsal interspace. Occasionally the condition may involve the third metatarsal head. There may or may not be signs of local inflammation, swelling, and callus formation. The pain does not radiate, worsens with ambulation, and disappears at rest. Careful palpation reveals a trigger point at the metatarsal head and flexion increases the pain. Etiologically, repetitive microtrauma is typical, although there may be a short first ray. Intermittent forefoot dysfunction also is common and usually is secondary to poorly fitting or inappropriate footwear.

The differential diagnosis includes Morton's neuroma, stress fracture, arthritis, and Freiberg's disease. Symptoms of generalized synovitis in association with subluxation and dislocation of multiple MTP joints suggest a generalized disease process such as arthritis (see Chapter 14). Treatment includes removing stress (e.g., pads, medial longitudinal arch support for overpronators), controlling inflammation, and strengthening the toe flexors through toe curls (lifts the metatarsal heads). The injection of a combination local anesthetic and long-acting steroid is not only diagnostic but also curative (see Chapter 20).

Freiberg's Infraction

Osteochondrosis of the metatarsal head occurs most commonly at the second head, particularly in female adolescents who perform on their toes and in jumping and sprinting activities. Presumably, there is ischemic necrosis of the epiphysis or subchondral cancellous bone. Pain at the MTP joint is aggravated by increased activity, but improves with rest.

On exam, range of motion is variably decreased, and generalized thickening at the MTP joint is noted. Osteosclerosis and head flattening occur early and are detectable on x-ray; osteolysis and collapse are late findings (1–2 months). Conservative therapy using a metatarsal pad, short leg weight-bearing cast, or stiff postoperative shoe until asymptomatic (6–12 weeks) is appropriate for painful cases without destruction. Individuals with increased bone formation and range-of-motion loss should have a surgical consultation.

Miscellaneous Causes of Metatarsalgia

A variety of neuropathic processes (e.g., cerebral palsy, poliomyelitis, Charcot-Marie-Tooth disease) increase the longitudinal and transverse arches of the foot so that the first and fifth metatarsals tend to lie more inferior in the horizontal plane than the central rays. Pathogenetically, there is an imbalance of the anterior tibial and peroneus longus muscles. Subcutaneous hygromata, hyperkeratotic zones, and incapacitating pain of the first and fifth metatarsals are characteristic; chronically, trophic ulcers may develop in the same region.

The underlying condition must be diagnosed and treated before podiatric manifestations can be addressed. Normally, palliative therapy in the form of orthotics produces beneficial results. Surgery should be reserved only for a failed trial of conservative therapy (several months) and the confirmation of a static lesion (e.g., nonprogressive).

References

1. Bennett GL, Graham CE, Mandlin DM, et al: Morton's interdigital neuroma: A comprehensive treatment protocol. Ankle 16:760–763, 1995.
2. Cracchiolo A: Morton's metatarsalgia: Clinicians' guide to diagnosis consultant. 26(5): 1034–1942, 1996.
3. Gould JS: Metatarsalgia. Orthop Clin North Am 20(4):553–562, 1989.
4. Scranton PE: Metatarsalgia: A clinical review of diagnosis and management. Foot Ankle Int 1:229, 1989.
5. Wyngarden TM: The painful foot. Part I: Common forefoot deformities. Am Fam Phys 55(5): 1866–1876, 1997.

9

The Heel, Subtalar Complex, and Ankle

Michael P. DellaCorte, DPM

The Heel

Plantar Fasciitis

Despite the mythical connotations of vulnerability (i.e., Achilles heel), the heel of the foot has efficiently carried humans through a long evolutionary process. The heel is not immune to injury, however, which usually presents as pain. Plantar pain may be due to plantar fasciitis (3 million cases per year in the United States) or the formation and inflammation of calcaneal spurs. Both conditions are the result of repeated microtrauma to the plantar aponeurosis, which causes straining of its posterior attachment to the medial tubercle on the plantar surface of the os calcis and of its adjacent short muscles. Excessive pronation also is a factor. This repetitive microtrauma occurs in a variety of running sports, such as football and soccer, and is especially detrimental in the unconditioned or obese individual. There may be secondary involvement of adjacent structures, such as the medial calcaneal nerve and the adductor digiti quinti.

Plantar fasciitis typically is unilateral, but it is bilateral in approximately 10% of cases (consider Reiter's syndrome, ankylosing spondylitis, and obesity-rheumatism diseases). The condition is associated with cavus and planus feet. Regular use of high-heeled shoes appears to be the culprit; 75% of patients are women. Pain is more pronounced on initial weight bearing in the morning or after prolonged periods of sitting, and five to ten steps are necessary before the patient feels comfortable walking. Forty to 50% of symptomatic individuals and 16–27% of asymptomatic individuals have a calcaneal or heel spur diagnosed on x-ray, although only 15% of these cases exhibit cause and effect. The clinical examination confirms diffuse tenderness in the region of the calcaneal tuberosity, particularly the medial side, but not over the area of the spur. Pain can be elicited by toe walking and passive dorsiflexion of the first toe. The differential diagnosis should include tarsal tunnel syndrome, heel pad atrophy, calcaneal stress fracture, spondyloarthropathies, and Achilles tendonitis (Table 1). A positive bone scan supports a stress fracture or fasciitis.

Treatment is conservative. Nonsteroidal anti-inflammatory drugs (NSAIDs) and local corticosteroid injection are useful in reducing the acute inflammation. Acutely, tincture of benzoin should be applied, and the lesion should be carefully strapped with surgical adhesive tape (see Chapter 20, Fig. 8). Barefoot walking and unsupported standing in the morning are contraindicated because the new, immature collagen may tear. Rather, the first step out of bed should be made with a supportive shoe or sandal. Thereafter, an inexpensive, off-the-shelf shoe insert or a custom-fitted medial arch support—both with heel dispersion and designed from adhesive felt, foam, Plastazote, or polypropylene—is used to hold the foot in inversion or, for recalcitrant cases, in adduction. These supports plus a stiff-soled shoe reduce medial longitudinal arch stretch. A simple 4-mm varus wedge may be effective, but in refractory cases a carefully fitted, transferable orthotic producing 10° of dorsiflexion is required, particularly at night.

Injection therapy (one to three steroid injections given medially 2–4 weeks apart) and physiotherapy may help. MH$_z$ ultrasound and iontophoresis soften the collagen and loosen the fascia, allowing calf and Achilles tendon stretching to be beneficial. Self-stretching is accomplished with a towel drag, which is done by sitting with the leg straight out, looping a towel or belt around the forefoot, and applying tension to the medial band of the fascia. A weighted towel drag should be prescribed to improve the intrinsic strength of the fascia. An alternative is for the patient to place the palms on a wall and lean against it with the heels pressed to the ground. Stretching for 3–5 minutes three times daily throughout the duration of pain is recommended. A recent study by the American Orthopedic Foot and Ankle Society demonstrated evidence of 81–95% improvement using a simple home stretching program in conjunction with store-bought shoe inserts.

An ice massage should conclude the rehabilitation session, as it helps to soften the fascia, enabling it to elongate and better cope with the enormous, winding tensile strain that occurs during ambulation. Transverse friction massage and a night splint with 5% of ankle dorsiflexion are useful. Application of a short leg walking-cast for 4 weeks is reserved for recalcitrant cases.

While the average recovery time is 6–8 weeks, several years may be required for ultimate recovery. Conservative therapy is ineffective for 10% of patients. Endoscopic release surgery is recommended prior to open resection of heel spur. Up to 90% of such patients return to their former activity levels after surgery.

Heel Spur

The process of spur formation has been termed heel spur syndrome. Initially presenting as a periostitis, a calcaneal spur is an osseous extension of the medial process of the calcaneal tuberosity in a forward direction within the central plantar fascia. The etiology is presumed to be chronic traction of the plantar fascia and intrinsic muscles. Although the lesion may develop in a young athlete, it is more typically found in an older, obese adult in whom the plantar padding has thinned due to aging (see Chapter 11). The patient complains of an acutely painful heel, particularly on rising in the morning or following periods of rest (poststatic dyskinesia). Normally, the pain disappears after ambulation, but it does tend to reappear after prolonged walking and weight bearing.

Table 1. Differential Diagnosis of Plantar Heel Pain

Skin
　Hyperkeratosis
　Verruca

Nerve
　Plantar nerve entrapment
　Tarsal tunnel
　Neuritis
　Radiculopathy

Infection
　Acute osteomyelitis
　Plantar abscess
　Dermatophytoses

Miscellaneous
　Foreign body
　Nonunion of calcaneus
　Fractures and stress fractures
　Arthritis—seronegative, rheumatoid,
　　gout, sarcoidosis
　Psychogenic disturbance
　Benign or malignant bone tumors
　Atrophy of fat pad
　Fasciitis
　Bursitis

The pain is described as a nail or pin sticking in the foot and is located at the medial tubercle on the plantar surface. Palpation and the stress maneuver—stretching the plantar fascia at its insertion site by dorsiflexing the digits at the metatarsophalangeal (MTP) joints—are helpful. Tenderness is pin-point rather than diffuse, and the x-ray examination clearly demonstrates the spur formation emanating from the calcaneal tuberosity.

Absence of a spur suggests fasciitis. Spur size does not necessarily correlate with clinical findings. In fact mature, large heel spurs often are asymptomatic, and patients with early symptoms may have no visible spur. The differential should include an acute bursitis and plantar fasciitis, both of which may coexist with a spur. Gout and, rarely, bone tumors can cause heel pain. X-rays are useful—not so much to visualize a spur, but to rule out fracture or tumor.

Treatment in the majority of cases (90%) is conservative and follows the guidelines outlined for the treatment of plantar fasciitis. In addition, a custom-fitted orthotic from a suitable material can be used to displace pressure from the spur, add shock-absorbing materials, and reduce pronation. Injection of the trigger point should be reserved for severe pain or a chronically recurrent situation, but should be attempted before surgery (see Chapter 20). Surgical excision through a medial incision is indicated for refractory cases (minimum of 6 months of failed conservative therapy or intractable pain). Postoperatively, the patient is kept in a nonweight-bearing cast or splint for 3 weeks to prevent a calcaneal fracture. Gradual weight bearing is then initiated in conjunction with postoperative biomechanical control of pronation with orthotics.

A new, less debilitating procedure, called endoscopic plantar fasciectomy, is available to alleviate intractable heel pain. Via a stab incision, an endoscope and special blade are used to separate the medial slip of the plantar fascia from the calcaneal tubercle. Despite the fact that no bone is removed, heel pain is relieved by reducing the chronic traction of the fascia. The patient can walk immediately, and the success rate is high. Again, however, all conservative treatment must be exhausted before contemplating surgery.

Heel Pain

Posterior heel pain can be due to calcaneal exostosis, retrocalcaneal bursitis, a short Achilles tendon, Achilles tendonitis, and bursitis, as well as a variety of athletic injuries. Recurrent irritation and pressure to the posterior heel—from poorly fitting shoes as well as sling-backs; high-heeled pumps; shoes with stiff, tight counters; and athletic footwear typical of hockey and figure skating—is the most common etiology, particularly in the young patient. In the older patient, who is most frequently female, chilblains, frostbite, and rheumatoid arthritis can lead to heel pain. With long-term, repeated injury there may be formation of visible "pump bumps" which represent the generic end-state of a number of problems.

Athletic causes of posterior heel pain in the adult include rupture of the plantaris tendon and strains of the Achilles tendon. Apophysitis of the calcaneus occurs in the pediatric age group (see Chapter 10).

Lateral heel pain typically is due to pathology involving the peroneal tendons, particularly subluxation or frank dislocation of the peroneus longus (see Chapter 13). Other causes include irregularities of the calcaneus and fibula and static disorders.

Causes of **medial heel pain** include the tarsal tunnel syndrome, strains of the tibialis posterior, and neurodynia of the medial calcaneal nerve. Compression of the posterior tibial nerve by the laciniate ligament can produce debilitating hyperesthesias along the medial plantar surface of the foot. Initially, there is ill-defined discomfort and pain on the posterior aspect of the heel below the medial malleolus to the mid-tarsal zone during activity. Over time, the pain becomes more severe, aching in quality, and also present at rest. The pain can be a shooting, radiating, electrical type pain.

Reproduction of the pain and discomfort during palpation and percussion (Tinel's sign) in the region of the laciniate ligament, located about a finger's breadth below the medial malleolus, is highly suggestive. The disorder is confirmed by electromyography and nerve conduction velocity studies.

Conservative treatment consists of custom fitted orthotics, NSAIDs, steroid injections, and rest. Such palliative therapy usually is sufficient in the initial stages of the syndrome. Chronically, surgical neurolysis is necessary. Occasionally, posterior tibial nerve impingement is caused by a soft tissue growth in the area, which can be identified by magnetic resonance imaging. If a growth is symptomatic, then it must be surgically excised.

Retrocalcaneal Bursitis

Inflammation of the bursa lying between the Achilles tendon and the posterior border of the os calcis is termed retrocalcaneal bursitis, anterior Achilles bursitis, achillodynia, and Albert's disease. There often is enlargement of the superior tuberosity of the os calcis ("pump bump"). Trauma can cause acute bursitis; gout, rheumatoid arthritis, pes planus, and such infectious diseases as tuberculosis and gonorrhea can lead to chronic bursitis. Trauma can be direct, such as a blow or kick to the heel, or indirect, such as sudden jumps in gymnastics and running that strain the Achilles tendon.

Posterior heel pain is insidious and is aggravated by increasing activity and shoes with tight heel counters. The clinical exam discloses localized tenderness at the sides of the tendon at its insertion site. The patient holds the foot in eversion to avoid dorsiflexion, and there may be some swelling and erythema evident at the tendon's lateral borders.

Ice, aspirin, and NSAIDs are useful during the acute phase, as is a 1/4-inch, U-shaped heel wedge. Heel immobilization by adhesive strapping is helpful, and injection of a long-acting steroid and local anesthetic combination occasionally is beneficial (see Chapter 20).

Achilles Bursitis

Inflammation of the posterior Achilles or precalcaneal bursa also may occur from the predisposing factors already mentioned. The bursa between the skin and Achilles tendon may have bullae, fissures, and ulcerations associated with its chronic inflammation. The inflammation site typically is at the margin of the shoe counter, and chronic calcification as well as the formation of a calcaneal exostosis located at the attachment of the tendon may be noted on x-ray. Over time, there may be enlargement of the posterior superior surface of the calcaneus, termed Haglund's deformity. This lesion, in turn, aggravates the overlying bursitis. Pain usually is severe with any movement of the Achilles tendon, and although the conservative modalities already mentioned for retrocalcaneal bursitis should be attempted, surgical removal of the exostosis generally is necessary.

Haglund's Deformity

Haglund's deformity is sometimes called "pump bump" because of its frequency in women who wear pumps (high-heeled shoes). It is an osseous deformity of the posterior superior aspect of the calcaneus. The patient presents with pain over the osseous deformity. A subcutaneous bursa, a tyloma, or both may contribute to the patient's symptoms. Pain occurs on ambulation with the offending shoe gear.

The etiology of the condition is pronation associated with several biomechanical problems (e.g., partially or fully compensated rear foot varus, plantarflexed first ray, or rigid forefoot valgus). As the calcaneus everts during stance phase, friction between the calcaneus and the shoe counter leads to the formation of an exostosis and also may contribute to the formation of a tyloma. On x-ray, the lateral view reveals a prominence or ridge (1–2 cm) at the postcrosuperior aspect of the calcaneus. There is pain upon palpation of the exostosis, tyloma, or bursa, particularly just proximal and slightly lateral to the insertion of the Achilles tendon.

Conservative treatment of Haglund's deformity can be achieved with NSAIDs, padding (1/4- to 1/2-inch lift), rubber heel cup, change of shoe gear, control of pronation with orthotics, and steroid injections (see Chapter 20).

Sandals or shoes with a soft heel counter and no prominent seams or stitching over the ridge are recommended. A reduced training schedule is appropriate, as are a softer running surface, temporary cessation of interval training and hill workouts, and a stretching and strengthening program for the gastrocnemius-soleus complex.

If conservative treatment fails, surgical resection of the prominent posterosuperior aspect of the calcaneus is indicated. A linear incision is made over the prominence just lateral to the insertion of the Achilles tendon. Resection of the exostosis should be aggressive because of the high incidence of the deformity's recurrence. Postoperatively, the patient should be kept nonweight-bearing for several weeks to guard against possible rupture of the Achilles tendon. The patient also should be placed in orthotics to decrease the incidence of recurrence. Of affected patients, 70% are able to return to their previous level of activity following surgery.

Retrocalcaneal Exostosis and Tendocalcinosis of the Achilles Tendon

These two conditions can occur together or by themselves. The patient complains of pain, described as a dull ache, across the posterior aspect of the heel at the site of insertion of the Achilles tendon. A tender, palpable exostosis and/or hypertrophied Achilles tendon may be present, and pain usually can be elicited by range of motion. On the initial visit, a lateral x-ray of the heel is recommended. An exostosis emanating from the posterior central aspect of the calcaneus or calcifications within the Achilles tendon may be observed. Occasionally, the spur may fragment at the site of the insertion of the Achilles tendon. If these findings are not seen, then a retrocalcaneal bursitis or a hypertrophied Achilles tendon may be the etiology of the symptoms.

Conservative treatment of these conditions includes padding, heel lifts, orthotics, and NSAIDs. Steroid injections are not recommended because of close proximity of the Achilles tendon insertion; cortisone injections in this area have been known to cause weakening and rupture. If all conservative treatment fails, surgical removal of the exostosis and/or removal of calcific deposits within the Achilles tendon may be required. A significant portion of the Achilles tendon insertion on the calcaneus may have to be detached in order to gain exposure to the retrocalcaneal exostosis.

The exostosis can then be removed with an osteotome or power burr.

Postoperatively, the patient is kept 4–5 weeks nonweight-bearing in an above-knee cast or splint, with the knee flexed and the foot in plantarflexion. Immobilization is required to allow for tenodesis of the Achilles tendon to the calcaneus.

Notes: For a discussion of **tibialis posterior strain**, refer to Chapter 11. For a discussion of **Achilles tendonitis**, refer to Chapter 13.

The Subtalar Complex

Pathologic conditions involving the subtalar joint (STJ) can be due to abnormal biomechanics, fixed pathology, arthritides, and trauma (Table 2). This important articulation between the calcaneus and talus has been called the "torque converter" of the foot because of its important biomechanical influence on the other joints of the foot.

The STJ allows for the triplane motions pronation and supination, which permit adaptation of the foot to uneven terrain, shock absorption, locking of the midtarsal joint for stability and propulsion, and normal transverse plane knee motion in gait. The STJ, basically the hinge joint between the leg and the foot, is responsible for a smooth transition of forces as the leg moves over the foot in gait. Any pathology in the STJ leads to progressive problems in the foot and leg.

Os Trigonum Syndrome

The os trigonum is an accessory bone that forms when the ossification center for the lateral tubercle of the talus fails to fuse with the body of the talus. Usually this is an anomaly seen on routine lateral x-rays of the foot. However, this accessory bone may become pinched between the calcaneus and tibia leading to pain above the calcaneus at the posterior ankle joint. The condition typically is seen in ballet dancers.

A physical exam may reveal direct tenderness in the posterior ankle or pain with ankle joint range of motion. Pain can be reproduced by palpating medial and deep to the peroneal tendons. It is important to rule out fracture of the lateral tubercle by taking a lateral x-ray of the foot and ankle. Dorsiflexing the hallux can elicit this pain because the flexor hallucis longus tendon is close to the os trigonum.

Conservative treatment includes NSAIDs, strapping, and physical therapy. If these

Table 2. Pathology of the Subtalar Joint

Biomechanical (Chapter 12)
  Excessive STJ pronation leading to pes planus and its related foot pathology
  Excessive STJ supination leading to pes cavus and its related foot pathology

Fixed Pathology
  Tarsal coalition (Chapter 10)
  Varus valgus (Chapter 12)
  Congenital vertical talus (Chapter 10)
  Os trigonum syndrome

Arthritides
  Degenerative joint disease (Chapter 15)
  Gout (Chapter 14)
  Rheumatoid arthritis (Chapter 15)
  Sinus tarsi syndrome
  Posttraumatic syndrome

Trauma (Chapter 13)
  Calcaneal fractures
  Talar fractures

STJ = subtalar joint

fail, surgical excision of the accessory bone through a posterolateral incision is indicated.

Sinus Tarsi Syndrome

Grooves in the articulated talus and calcaneus form a bony canal called the sinus tarsi, which is occupied by a ligament and a small neurovascular bundle. Inflammation within the sinus tarsi secondary to trauma, marked pronation, or overuse can lead to a painful condition called sinus tarsi syndrome. Chronic inversion ankle sprains also are a common etiology.

Pain can be elicited by directly palpating the sinus tarsi on the lateral aspect of the rear foot. There also is pain during inversion and eversion of the STJ. The condition may be difficult to differentiate from a tear or sprain of the anterior talofibular ligament. A small injection of lidocaine into the sinus tarsi that alleviates the pain is diagnostic.

Treatment includes injection therapy, NSAIDs, orthotics, taping/strapping, and physical therapy. Oblique radiographs or a computed tomography scan should be taken to rule out fracture or arthritis of the STJ.

Arthritides

Degenerative joint disease, rheumatoid arthritis, and gout may affect the subtalar joint (see Chapter 15). Posttraumatic arthritis of the

STJ is common following calcaneal fractures, especially if they are intra-articular. Many of these patients require triple arthrodesis.

The Ankle

The ankle is a key focal point in the transmission of body weight during ambulation and bears more weight per unit area than any other joint in the body. It is capable of adjustments necessary for fine balance on a wide variety of terrain. Its integrity depends on the paradoxical functions of stability and mobility. Because the joint is subject to the concentrated stresses associated with standing as well as with movement, the ankle is involved in both static and dynamic deformities. In fact, injuries to the ankle joint are the most common athletic injuries seen in the primary care office. Various estimates place the prevalence of such injuries between 10 and 90%, with the highest rate occurring in basketball players. At least one study has estimated the incidence to be one significant ankle sprain per day per 10,000 individuals.

Ankle injuries are not always minor and may be associated with prolonged disability and recurrent instability. In 25–40% of patients, healing may require several months to years. Therefore, a casual approach (e.g., "it is only a sprain") to the diagnosis and management of these injuries is not tenable. It is the rare ankle sprain that requires only an Ace bandage and some ice. The ubiquitous and unpredictable nature of ankle injuries mandates a precise understanding of the mechanism of injury, a clear ability to assess the degree of damage, and a solid understanding of appropriate treatment modalities in the acute and rehabilitative phases.

General Pathogenic Mechanisms of Ankle Injury

Ankle trauma frequently involves both ligamentous and bony damage. There are a number of anatomic factors that contribute to such a combination injury. Ankle mortise asymmetry creates inherent instability during inversion. The longer lateral malleolus provides a mechanical barrier to eversion ligamentous injury due to its greater surface contact with the talus. In addition, the dome of the talus is appreciably wider anteriorly than posteriorly. During inversion and plantarflexion, the narrow posterior aspect of the talus occupies proportionately less space within the mortise. As a result there is increased ankle joint play which, together with the inherent block to eversion, results in predominantly lateral stress forces. Additional complicating factors include a tight heel cord and deficient proprioception. Many athletes, particularly females, have tight Achilles tendons that force heel inversion. Lack of sufficient flexibility greatly increases the risk of ankle sprain. Finally, the lateral ligaments of the ankle are smaller and weaker than the medial deltoid ligament.

Nonanatomic factors such as surface configuration and footwear often are responsible for injury. Irregular surfaces, particularly those with holes, can produce damage to the ankle. Less obvious circumstances such as banked tracks can lead to repetitive ankle trauma and long-term ankle disability. Finally, defective, old, or inappropriately fitted footwear can result in inversion or eversion stress.

Clinical Evaluation of the Ankle

The following items should be carefully investigated in all ankle injuries:

1. What were the position of the foot and the direction of stress when the injury occurred (e.g., eversion, inversion, flexion, extension, or a combination)?

2. Was there immediate disability or did symptoms occur at a later time?

3. At the time of injury, were any snaps, pops, or crunches noted?

4. When and to what degree were pain, swelling, and discoloration noted?

5. Were there any pre-existing problems associated with the joint (e.g., previous injury or systemic disease)?

6. Was medical care sought out? What did the evaluation show? Was treatment initiated? What were the results of any treatment?

7. Did the injury occur acutely or from overuse?

8. What is the functional capacity of the joint at present?

9. What were the surface conditions at the time of injury?

As a final comment, it should be understood that a careful history usually will identify the site of pathology and severity of tissue trauma. There are situations, however, when a misdiagnosis can result. For specific types of ankle trauma, consult Chapter 13.

References

1. Amis J, Jennings L, Graham D, et al: Painful heel syndrome: Radiographic and treatment assessment. Foot Ankle 9(2):91–95, 1988.
2. Baxter DE, Pfeffer GB, Thigpen M: Chronic heel pain: Treatment rationale. Orthop Clin North Am 20(4):563–570, 1989.
3. Kwong PK, Kay D, Voner RT, White MW: Plantar fasciitis: Mechanics and pathomechanics of treatment. Clin Sports Med 7(1):119–126, 1988.
4. Wyngarden TM: The painful foot. Part II: Common rearfoot deformities. Am Fam Phys 55(6): 2207–2212, 1997.

10

The Pediatric Foot

Stuart Plotkin, DPM

Limb Embryology

Foot pathology in the infant can be associated with an intrauterine position, a congenital anomaly, or a genetic predisposition. Because of this genetic component, a thorough family history of foot pathology including siblings, parents, and grandparents should be obtained. Bunions, tarsal coalition, and in-toe gait all have a genetic link. The genetics of limb patterning and development are rapidly being resolved. We now know that the *HOX* gene cluster gives anterior-posterior and proximo-distal limb patterning. Transforming growth factors such as TGF-β superfamily, fibroblast growth factor, and bone morphogenic protein have been isolated and shown to play an important role in limb development.

The lower limb bud starts to form at the end of the fourth week, following slightly behind the upper extremities. By day 57, all tarsal and digital elements are present and are chondrifying. During the eighth week, ossification begins and critical rotations take place: the upper extremity rotates 90° outward, placing the palms forward; the lower extremity rotates 90° inward, placing the soles posteriorly. A developmental over-rotation leads to an in-toe gait.

By the ninth week, the metatarsals are adducted, and the calcaneus, which has been adjacent to the talus, begins to migrate plantarly. The ankle joint develops its articulation with the talus. The foot is still parallel to the leg and inverted. During the next few weeks, the ankle dorsiflexes, and the inverted attitude of the foot decreases due to bony torsional changes in the calcaneus and talar neck. If this attitude does not fully resolve, a permanent rearfoot or forefoot varus may occur.

In utero, the leg can be visualized with B mode diagnostic ultrasound by week 10 and the foot by week 24 (Fig. 1). Many congenital deformities can be diagnosed at this time, including spina bifida, neural tube defects, clubfoot, amelia, phocomelia, achondroplasia, anencephaly, dwarfism, osteogenesis imperfecta, rocker-bottom feet, and polydactyly. Early diagnosis is important because some structural deformities have been linked to significant if not life-threatening medical disorders. Such is the link between clubfoot and renal agenesis.

Correct development requires a competent nervous system and muscle innervation. Movement allows for precise formation of joints and skeletal structures. Average milestones for gait include crawling at 9 months, cruising at 12 months, and independent walking at 15 months.

Lower Extremity Examination

As much as 70% of the adult population suffers from foot ailments as a result of untreated pediatric anomalies. These include disabling deformities such as bunions, hammer toes, heel spurs, degenerative arthritis, and knee, hip, and back pain. Many of these disabilities can be prevented if structural and functional biomechanical faults are detected and treated early. The importance of early diagnosis and intervention cannot be overemphasized. It is a common misconception that many pediatric

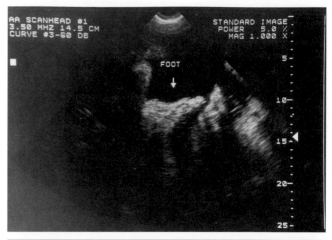

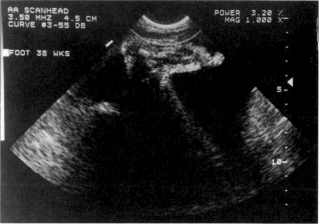

Figure 1. Ultrasound scans of a foot at 38 weeks of gestation.

gait abnormalities are outgrown. Another serious misconception is that lack of pain means there is no reason to intervene. Pediatric patients rarely complain of frank pain because their symptoms are much more subtle. More common complaints include tripping and falling, clumsiness, asking to be carried, refusing to walk any distance, and lack of interest in sports.

In examining a joint's range of motion, the examiner should take note of: (1) symmetry with respect to the contralateral mate, (2) quality of motion, (3) quantity and direction of motion as measured in degrees, and (4) structural (bony) or functional (soft tissue) deformities. Structural deformities tend to be more rigid and are difficult to treat conservatively. Functional or positional deformities, such as a tight hip joint capsule causing an in-toe gait, are easily reducible and more successfully treated. Because the entire lower extremity functions as a unit, all proximal joints ultimately affect foot function in gait.

Disorders in the Pediatric Patient

Ankle Problems

An infant's ankle can be dorsiflexed almost to the point at which the dorsal foot contacts the leg. Dorsiflexion in the adolescent is up to 15°; the normal value for plantarflexion is 20°. Limitation of dorsiflexion (i.e., equinus) is common and quite debilitating. It is important to rule out any neurologic causes of equinus, such as cerebral palsy.

A child with limited ankle joint dorsiflexion demonstrates a bouncy type of gait with a premature heel-off and flexed knees, an externally rotated gait, or severe flat foot. There are many ways a child can compensate for an equinus. In an older child, a growth spurt may produce a temporary equinus, as may muscle overdevelopment in an athletic child. Hamstring contractures frequently accompany an equinus, and they should be evaluated as well.

Treatment in the infant consists of passive

stretching. With the baby lying supine, the knees locked, and the foot slightly supinated, the parent can slowly dorsiflex the foot and hold it for 5 seconds. The exercise is repeated five times at each diaper change. The older child can stretch by leaning toward a wall (Fig. 2). There are devices that can assist the patient such as a Theraband rubber stretcher and a Prostretch rocker, both available from physical therapists.

Ankle sprains are common in youngsters and yet frequently are not taken seriously. Often, if a fracture is not visualized, the child is sent away with only an ace bandage and instructions to rest. Since childrens' bones are pliable and ligaments are not, injury to the lateral calcaneofibular ligament is common. Stability and muscle strength should be evaluated and compared to the contralateral mate, and

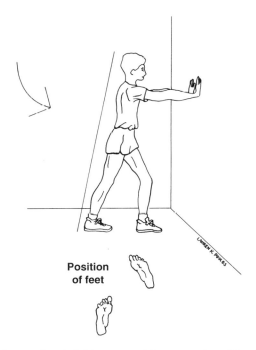

Position of feet

Figure 2. Achilles stretching exercise. Hands on wall, elbows locked, one leg back and one forward, toes turned inward. Front knee bends and elbows bend as patient leans into wall. Head, neck, back, and rear leg should be kept straight. When done correctly, patient feels a strong pulling at back of rear leg. If not felt, then position should be checked; patient may need to move slightly away from wall. Stretch is held for 5 seconds and repeated five times—no bouncing—then performed on other leg. With progress, patient gradually moves further from wall.

gait should be observed. If stability is questionable, then an Unna boot cast, aircast splint, or even a below-knee fiberglass cast should be applied. Rehabilitative physical therapy should be considered after immobilization. A common associated finding is a fracture of the base of the fifth metatarsal. Lack of proper treatment can lead to a chronically unstable ankle.

Subtalar Joint Problems

In neonates, the subtalar joint (STJ) is not completely matured; the calcaneus is still in varus. In the young walker, the STJ is markedly pronated—there is a wide base of gait, the legs appear bowed, and the angle of gait is high. If the angle of gait approaches 0° or becomes internal, then it is considered pathologic and a specialist should be consulted. It should not be left to chance to be outgrown. By age 3 years, the child's gait is approaching maturity; however, the foot may remain pronated. By age 7, the STJ should no longer be excessively pronated. At this point, treatment should be initiated even without symptoms.

Valgus Deformities

Planovalgus. Planovalgus (flat arch with an everted heel) is a congenital deformity easily identified at birth. All children walk with some degree of planovalgus, more appropriately termed pronation. The differential diagnosis consists of idiopathic flat foot, calcaneovalgus, vertical talus, tarsal coalition, ligamentous laxity, and biomechanical disorders (such as equinus). Vertical talus and tarsal coalition are rigid deformities; the others are flexible.

Calcaneovalgus. Calcaneovalgus is characterized by dorsiflexion and eversion of the entire foot and occurs in approximately 1 in 1000 births. It is 1.6 times more common among females and significantly more common in firstborns. It is believed to be caused by excessive intrauterine pressure. X-rays reveal a normal bony architecture and normal articulations. Calcaneovalgus is a positional, soft-tissue deformity caused by contractures of the anterior and lateral muscle groups and associated skin and joint capsule structures. When the deformity is significant and untreated, an unstable pronated foot frequently results.

In mild to moderate deformities, treatment consists of manipulation and stretching by the parent. This is best accomplished by inverting and plantarflexing (supinating) the foot to resistance for 5 seconds, repeated ten times at each diaper change. For severe deformities, stretching, manipulation, and serial casts changed weekly are recommended. After the deformity is reduced, a splint or shoe should be used to maintain the correction.

Congenital Vertical Talus

Vertical talus, also known as rocker-bottom foot or convex pes valgus, is a dorsolateral dislocation of the talocalcaneal navicular joint. The navicular articulates with the dorsal neck of the talus, locking it in a vertical plantarflexed position. Vertical talus is a rare deformity often associated with important neuromuscular diseases, including myelomeningocele and arthrogryposis multiplex. There are significant anomalies in the body of the calcaneus, talus, and navicular, in addition to secondary contractures of ligaments and tendons.

Clinically, the sole of the foot is convex, with the apex being the protrusion of the talar head plantarly. The forefoot is dorsiflexed and abducted, and the rearfoot is plantarflexed. The diagnosis can be made radiographically in the newborn despite the fact that the navicular has not yet ossified. The severely plantarflexed talus and the equinus position of the calcaneus are pathognomonic. Because it is a rigid deformity, it is not significantly improved by conservative means. Despite the fact that the young child may not complain of pain, undiagnosed vertical talus leads to significant soft tissue and arthritic pathology early in life. This deformity requires surgical intervention.

Flatfoot

Flatfoot, while not a diagnostic term, is used to indicate the absence of a normal arch. The incidence of flatfoot is approximately 30–40 per 100 children aged 1.5–3 years. This high incidence is due to the large plantar fat pad obscuring the arch in this age group. The rate decreases to about 4 per 100 in older children and adults. It is important to differentiate a flexible flatfoot (arch is present non-weight bearing, absent weight bearing) from a rigid flatfoot (arch is present weight bearing, absent non-weight bearing). Excessive pronation is the most common cause of flexible flatfoot. In patients less than 6 years old, it is treated only if symptomatic or severe. After age 6 it is considered abnormal, and treatment should be considered. Rigid flatfoot deformities are usu-

ally caused by muscle spasm, tarsal coalitions, or trauma.

Flexible Flat Foot

Biomechanical abnormalities leading to excessive pronation are the most common causes of flexible flatfoot. These include a rearfoot or forefoot varus, equinus, tibial varum, genu valgum, in-toed gait, scoliosis with limb length discrepancy, and others. A comprehensive biomechanical evaluation of the lower limb will identify the causative segment (see Chapter 12). The patient may be asymptomatic or complain of severe pain in the arch, heel, leg, knee, or back. Keep in mind that knee pain often is due to excessive pronation, as is shin splints (growing pains). Growing pains should not be thought of as part of "normal development," but should be addressed with stretching, shoe modifications, or functional orthotics.

Occasionally, a bony abnormality causes a flexible flatfoot. In approximately 2% of the population, an accessory bone—the os tibial externum—is found medial to the navicular. It is invested in the posterior tibial tendon, weakening its ability to support the medial arch in gait. Clinically, the non-weight bearing foot has a normal range of motion, but on weight bearing collapses and pronates maximally. A significant medial bulge can be seen near the navicular, which often is inflamed due to shoe irritation, causing a painful adventitious bursitis and posterior tibial tendonitis. This can be treated conservatively with functional orthotics, but severe cases must be dealt with surgically.

For children age 3 and under, an asymptomatic flexible flatfoot requires no treatment. In severe flatfoot deformities and mildly symptomatic patients, a medial Thomas Heel wedge can be added to the shoe. In symptomatic toddlers, a stabilizing orthotic that holds the heel vertical can be used to prevent severe eversion of the calcaneus.

For children age 3–7 years, severe flatfoot should be treated regardless of symptomatology because of the likely adult sequelae (e.g., bunions, hammer toes, heel spurs). Proper treatment is directed to the involved segment and may include Achilles tendon stretching, proper footwear, and functional orthotics with deep heel cup and no forefoot posting. Medial heel wedges can be used for a moderate flatfoot. A lateral heel wedge should *never*, under any circumstances, be used. An orthotic reduces symptoms caused by an overpronated foot by controlling heel eversion, talus adduction, and plantarflexion (see Chapter 12). A course of conservative therapy for acute pain—consisting of rest, ice, nonsteroidal anti-inflammatory drugs (NSAIDs), and immobilization—should be followed initially.

For children age 7 and up, treatment is similar to that for an adult, with functional orthotics and appropriate heel and forefoot posts. The earlier treatment is initiated, the better the long term prognosis. Children should be reassessed biannually.

It is important to note that arch integrity is determined by the shapes and articulations of the tarsal bones. They fit together like an interlocking puzzle, creating a foot that can be flexible to accommodate uneven terrain, yet rigid for a propulsive gait. Muscles are not significantly involved in maintaining arch height. It is therefore futile to attempt to increase arch height by various exercises. Picking up pencils or marbles with the toes and other "arch-strengthening" exercises should be abandoned. Additionally, the archaic technique of encasing the flatfoot in a rigid orthopedic shoe should be discarded.

Rigid Flatfoot

A rigid flatfoot usually is caused by a tarsal coalition, which is an osseous, cartilaginous, or fibrous bridge between two tarsal bones. The two most common coalitions involve the talocalcaneal medial and posterior facets (Fig. 3) and the calcaneonavicular joint (Fig. 4). The prevalence of tarsal coalitions has been estimated to be approximately 1%, and a genetic component has been identified.

Clinically, many coalitions are not symptomatic in the young child, but may present in the second decade of life as the coalition be-

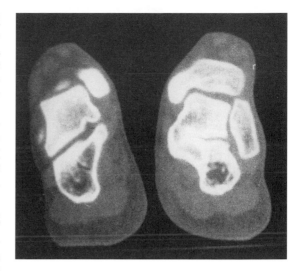

Figure 3. Computed tomography scan showing tarsal coalition of medial facet.

gins to limit joint motion. Complaints of leg pain exacerbated by activity are frequent. This pain is due to a peroneal spasm, caused by the body's attempt to splint the painful segment. The most common physical finding is limitation of STJ range of motion. Conventional x-rays may not demonstrate the coalition, but they are visible using magnetic resonance imaging. If diagnosis and treatment do not occur early, then degenerative arthritis in the surrounding joints often develops.

Treatment is geared to the severity of the symptoms. For mild discomfort, NSAIDs and rest may be all that is required. For moderate discomfort with peroneal spasm, a peroneal nerve block followed by a below-the-knee cast with the STJ held in neutral position may be required. After 6 weeks, a functional orthotic with a flat heel post to control STJ motion should be added. If conservative treatment fails, surgical excision of a calcaneonavicular

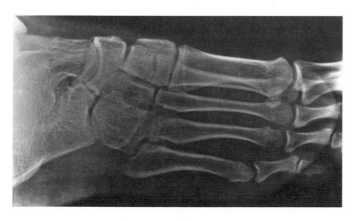

Figure 4. Tarsal coalition of calcaneonavicular joint.

coalition is required. Talocalcaneal coalitions are more difficult to treat, and surgical correction remains controversial. The differential diagnosis includes vertical talus and traumatic arthropathies.

In-Toe

In-toeing is defined as one or both feet pointing toward the midline of the body. Even the nonambulating infant can be identified as in-toed, allowing for early intervention. A family history, including any delivery complications or developmental changes, is important. Questions about older siblings can supply invaluable information concerning the likelihood of outgrowing this disorder. The level of the parents' concern also should be assessed and considered in the treatment plan.

A systematic, segmental, biomechanical examination can determine the level of the deformity (see Chapter 12). Multilevel deformities are quite common (Table 1). In the walking child, gait examination can direct the practitioner to diagnose the correct level of involvement. If the patella is deviated medially, then the femur or hip joint is involved. If the patella is in the frontal plane, then a tibial or STJ segment is involved. If only the distal foot is deviated, then a metatarsus adductus deformity is likely. Treatment must be directed to the specific level or levels of deformity. Positional in-toe deformities (soft tissue) are more easily and successfully treated than structural (bony) deformities.

The decision to treat can be difficult. Does one wait for physiologic correction to take place? How can one determine to what degree the deformity may spontaneously resolve? What symptoms are present, and what can be expected? What are the risk factors of the treatment plan? How concerned are the parents? What is the family history? The answers to all of these questions must be considered in formulating a treatment plan. If the treatment is easily tolerated and carries little iatrogenic

Table 1. In-Toe Gait

	Hip	Hip	Knee	Tibia	Foot
	Level of Involvement				
	Positional, tight hip capsule and ligaments	Structural, antetorsion in femoral head and shaft	Positional "pseudolack," high transverse plane knee motion	Structural, decreased tibial torsion in tibial shaft. >10% do not spontaneously resolve	Metatarsus adductus, mostly positional, becomes rigid with age
	Treatment				
Age < 1 year	Stretching, adjust sitting and sleeping positions, CRS	Same, but less successful due to bony pathology	None—usually resolves spontaneously	CRS, Wheaton brace	Stretching, Bebax shoe, Wheaton brace, serial casts
Age 1–4 years	Same	Same	None	Same, but less tolerated. Use as night splint	Same, plus straight last shoe with medial heel wedge
Age > 4 years	Same, plus gait plate orthotic and certain sports (ballet, skating)	Same, plus gait plate	None	Gait plate, functional orthotics	Same—*never* use reverse last or pronator shoe

CRS = Counter Rotational Splint

risk, then initiating treatment is reasonable. The consequences of waiting and watching may be worse than the consequences of treating a patient who would have undergone a spontaneous correction. The vast number of adults with disabling foot pathology is, in itself, confirmation that it is better to err on the side of hypervigilance.

The cornerstone of any treatment plan is mobilization of the affected part. In addition to stretching exercises and sitting/sleeping position changes, the Counter Rotational Splint (CRS) marketed by Langer Biomechanics is effective in treating a tibial and femoral component (Fig. 5). Its many advantages include attachability to any standard shoe, adjustability to precise angles, and acceptance by the child. The device protects the vulnerable STJ and midtarsal joints from excessive pronation and, most importantly, allows complete freedom of independent leg motion in all directions except internal rotation. Its dynamic motion and enhanced patient compliance result in a high success rate. The CRS is a non-weight bearing device indicated for children up to age 4 years. It is used as a night splint in walkers and allows for crawling in prewalkers. After age 4, orthotics are used to manage in-toed gait.

The CRS should replace the use of rigid bars between the feet (e.g., Denis Browne bar) to treat in-toe secondary to rotational disorders of the leg. Denis Browne bar–type devices must be fitted and worn correctly or damage to the distal joints can occur. Because of the obvious axiom that the effects of a treatment plan must not be worse than the disease itself, gentle guidance that assists normal development, rather than forced stress on the lower extremity joints, is recommended. Therefore, if the bar is used at all, it should be as a night splint to eliminate an in-toed sleeping position. The bar must be bent 5–10° to invert the feet and

protect the STJ from excessive pronatory forces. The foot angle should be increased gradually, and the connecting bar should be approximately equal to or slightly greater than the distance between the anterior superior iliac spines.

It is common today to see adults with significant pathology resulting from improper use of the Denis Browne bar. An iatrogenic flatfoot is an example of the outcome of a treatment plan being worse than the disease. It is essential not to discontinue treatment prematurely, which can lead to relapse. A general guideline is to continue treatment at least half again the time it took to correct the deformity. It is important to remove the device during the day in order to mobilize and stretch the joints. If a decision is made to treat the patient, initiating treatment as early as possible is imperative.

Internal Hip Position

If the in-toeing originates at the hip joint, the parent can be taught the following stretching exercise. The parent holds the femur firmly above the knee with one hand and gently holds the foot with the other. The femur is externally rotated and held firmly at its end range of motion for a count of five, repeated five times at each diaper change. It is important *not* to apply any force to the foot, as this will strain the STJ and knee.

The child's sitting pattern also must receive attention. When in-toeing originates at the hip, the child is most comfortable sitting with the legs underneath in a "W" position because this internally rotates the hip. Positions with the legs outstretched or "Indian style" should be encouraged. Following this reasoning, prone sleeping with the legs internally rotated should be discouraged. In older children, sports such as ice skating, roller blading, and ballet may be of help.

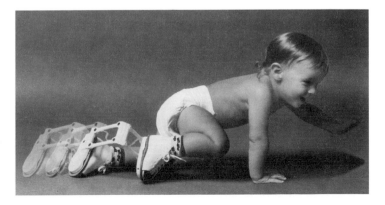

Figure 5. Counter Rotational Splint for treatment of in-toeing. (Courtesy of The Langer Biomechanics Group, Inc., Deer Park, New York, Tel. 800-233-2687.)

Tibial Torsion

There is a normal physiologic torque in the tibia/fibula that starts on the frontal plane by the knee joint and ends approximately 15° externally rotated at the malleoli. Malleolar position can be measured by placing the knee on the frontal plane and visualizing the two malleoli. A 13–18° external rotation should be noted. If this torque does not fully take place within the first 6 years of life (with some variability), an in-toed gait results. Although this deformity frequently is outgrown, a full 10% of cases do not resolve. A thorough family history helps decide when to treat.

Problems develop when the patient tries to compensate for the in-toe gait by actively pronating the foot. STJ pronation allows the forefoot to abduct, decreasing the appearance of an in-toe gait. This compensatory, pronated, unstable foot—and not one foot catching against the other in the swing phase of gait—often is the cause of tripping and falling.

When initiated early, the Wheaton tibial torsion brace or the Langer CRS are appropriate treatments. Since this is a bony pathology, muscle-stretching exercises have little effect. In an older child, treatment consists of functional orthotics—not to correct tibial torsion, but to prevent compensatory pronation. Despite the fact that the child initially may appear more in-toed, the symptoms eventually abate.

Metatarsus Adductus

Medial deviation of the tarsometatarsal joints also can cause in-toe gait. Metatarsus adductus is the adduction of metatarsals 1–5 at the tarsometatarsal joints. There also may be an associated varus deformity of the forefoot. The etiology may involve a delay in fetal maturation of the forefoot, intrauterine crowding, abnormal muscle activity, or genetics. The incidence of metatarsus adductus is 1 per 1000 births.

Clinically, there are forefoot adduction, separation between the hallux and the lesser toes, and a C-shaped foot. Other common findings are abnormal pulls of the abductor hallucis and the anterior and posterior tibial muscles, which may be due to abnormal innervation or insertion. Age permitting, the child should be examined sitting and weight bearing. It is important to determine the degree of flexibility, or reducibility, by stabilizing the rearfoot and abducting the forefoot on the rearfoot. Note that the rearfoot must *not* be allowed to

pronate during this exam or the results will be invalid. A readily reducible deformity is significantly easier to treat. A good indication of likely success is a straight or easily straightened lateral column of the foot (fifth metatarsal, cuboid articulation).

Although many foot bones have not completely ossified at birth, an x-ray can determine and document the severity of the deformity. On an anteroposterior view (see Chapter 3), a heel bisector line should pass through or near the second toe. If it passes lateral to the third toe, then a metatarsus adductus is present. Metatarsus adductus can be differentiated from talipes equinovarus clubfoot by the appearance of a normal rearfoot and a normal talocalcaneal angle on x-ray. If only the first metatarsal is affected, then the disorder is designated a metatarsus primus adductus. This foot is prone to developing a hallux abducto valgus deformity.

It is vital to initiate treatment as soon as possible, while the deformity is most flexible and easily reducible. If the child is merely watched until it is obvious that metatarsus adductus will not be outgrown, then successful treatment will be difficult, if not impossible, due to increasing rigidity and decreasing tolerance to treatment as the child ages.

Since the cause of this in-toe gait lies solely in the foot, treatment must be directed to this segment alone. A Denis Brown–type bar is ineffective and inappropriate for use in metatarsus adductus. For a mild-to-moderate, flexible deformity, the following stretching exercise is recommended. The parent is instructed to hold the heel firmly with one hand. The index finger of the other hand is placed medial to the first metatarsal (not the hallux), and lateral pressure is applied. The forefoot is maximally abducted for 5 seconds, repeated five times every diaper change. It is imperative that the STJ does not pronate while the forefoot is being abducted. The hand holding the heel must prevent heel eversion, which would injure the STJ and cause an iatrogenic flatfoot.

The treatment of choice in severe, flexible metatarsus adductus traditionally has been serial plaster cases. This remains an excellent treatment but has been replaced by cleaner and less psychologically disturbing (to the parents) techniques. The technique for using serial plaster casts requires several minutes of initial mobilization of the forefoot. The foot and leg are well padded with cast lining (e.g., Webril). A 2-inch, extra-fast-setting plaster roll is immersed in water and rolled onto the foot starting at the metatarsal heads to one inch below the fibular head. The toes are free. An assistant often is required to hold a baby. Most important, after the cast is applied, the rearfoot is held in neutral position and only the forefoot is abducted. Again, the STJ must not be allowed to pronate or an iatrogenic flatfoot may be produced. The cast is changed every 7–10 days and is removed by soaking in dilute vinegar. A cast cutter should be avoided because of its frightening noise. Generally, four to six casts are required to achieve correction; these should be followed with a night splint to prevent relapse. Again, the earlier the treatment is initiated, the faster the resolution.

There are two devices now marketed for treatment of metatarsus adductus, both equally effective, clean, and well tolerated. The Bebax shoe (Fig. 6), distributed by CAMP (Jackson, Michigan, Telephone 800–492–1088), has separate rearfoot and forefoot sections connected by two multidirectional swivel joints. It can be adjusted in all three body planes to correct for metatarsus adductus and varus deformities. The exact angle is set by the practitioner and is adjusted slowly over a few weeks. The Bebax shoe also is useful postoperatively and as a night splint after serial casting to maintain correction. It maintains the STJ in neutral position while applying abductory pressure to the forefoot.

The Wheaton brace (Figs. 7 and 8) is a thermoplastic, heat-adjustable splint also designed to maintain the STJ in neutral position while abducting the forefoot. In the past, splints have been ineffective in treating metatarsus adductus due to their inability to immobilize the rearfoot. The Wheaton brace, by extending above the ankle, does protect the rearfoot while correcting the forefoot.

Both devices are well tolerated and allow for frequent removal for range-of-motion manipulation by the parents. They are recommended for children age 2–8 months, are non-weight bearing, and require early intervention.

In the older child with flexible metatarsus adductus, the above treatments are poorly tolerated. A straight-last shoe with a medial heel wedge and stretching exercises may be helpful. Never use reverse-last or pronator shoes, and never reverse left and right shoes. These techniques unquestionably cause damage to the STJ, leading to iatrogenic flatfoot or skew foot. Again, a Denis Browne bar is completely ineffective for metatarsus adductus. For rigid deformities, serial casting should be applied

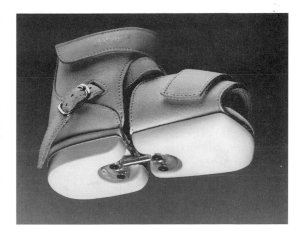

Figure 6. Bebax shoe for treatment of metatarsus adductus.

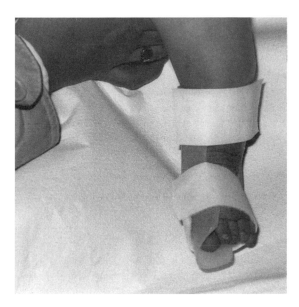

Figure 7. Wheaton brace. (Wheaton, Inc., Carol Stream, Illinois, Telephone 800–227–6769)

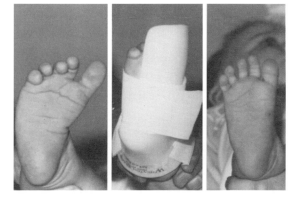

Figure 8. Metatarsus adductus before, during, and after treatment with Wheaton brace.

for 2–3 months, but surgical intervention may be necessary if the problem does not resolve.

Cavus Foot

The high-arched, or cavus, foot type in many ways is the mirror image of the flexible flatfoot. It is a rigid foot unable to adapt to uneven terrain and prone to ankle sprain, and it has diminished shock-absorbing capability. This lack of shock absorption can lead to knee, hip, and back pain. A cavus foot should elicit a high index of suspicion for neuromuscular disease (Table 2). A neurologic work-up and spine x-rays are recommended. While a small percentage of cases are simply idiopathic, up to 70% may be traced to underlying neuromuscular disease.

In appearance, the cavus foot demonstrates an excessively high arch, a forefoot equinus, and a fixed rearfoot varus. The deformity is progressive, leading to contractures of the digits, atrophy of the plantar fat pad, metatarsalgia, and heel pain. There is debate over the exact etiology, but most agree there is an imbalance in the intrinsic and extrinsic musculature of the foot, with weakness and spasticity. Treatment must be directed to the neurologic causes but may include soft orthotic devices, stretching exercises, soft tissue surgical releases, and bony procedures if the deformity is rigid.

Clubfoot

The characteristics of clubfoot, or talipes equinovarus (TEV), include an adducted forefoot, inverted rearfoot, equinus, and subluxation of the talocalcaneal navicular joints (Fig. 9). There is a medial rotation of the entire foot around the talus. The navicular is medial to the talus and almost abuts the medial malleolus. It is believed that the primary deformity is in the

Table 2. Neurologic Differential Diagnosis for Cavus Foot

Charcot-Marie-Tooth disease
Cerebral palsy
Dejerine-Sottas disease
Polio
Friedreich's ataxia
Spina bifida
Muscular dystrophy
Tumor
Trauma
Myelomeningocele

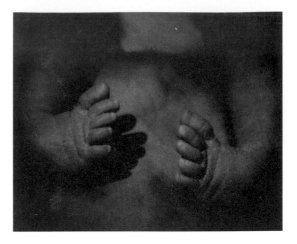

Figure 9. Talipes equinovarus, or clubfoot.

talar neck. Secondary changes include subluxation of the tarsal joints and soft tissue contractures in the triceps, posterior tibial, flexor digitorum longus, and flexor hallucis longus muscles. An acquired clubfoot may be associated with polio or cerebral palsy.

TEV can be clinically divided into two groups—rigid and flexible. The rigid deformity is more common and is characterized by a true anomaly in the talar neck, joint subluxations, leg atrophy, and a deep skin furrow across the medial ankle and heel. The skin is stretched so tight as to obliterate the normal skin lines on the dorsolateral aspect of the foot. Rigid TEV often is treated surgically, although conservative treatment should be initiated first. Flexible TEV probably is caused by intrauterine crowding and has no bony anomalies, no joint subluxations, no atrophy, and no skin furrow. It is relatively easy to correct this deformity with manipulation, casting, or splints.

Common radiographic findings include a reduced talocalcaneal angle almost to the point of superimposition of the talus on the calcaneus. An angle of less than 15° is significant. Serial x-rays are useful to monitor the progress of treatment and to check for indication of an iatrogenic rockerbottom foot.

Treatment should begin within the first few days of life, and manipulation is the key. For the pediatric patient, it is important to remember that ligaments and tendons may be stronger than osteocartilaginous structures, so manipulation pressure should be gentle. Each segment is manipulated and corrected separately in the following order: metatarsus adductus, calcaneal varus, and then equinus. The leg should be stabilized with one hand while the other hand is placed across the metatarsal plane with the thumb dorsal and lesser fingers plantar. The foot is distracted and gentle pressure applied to the talar head. The talus is pressured medially, the navicular and forefoot are pressured laterally (pronated), and the calcaneus is everted. This is performed for 10 minutes, after which an above-the-knee cast is applied.

The equinus is not addressed initially. Aggressive attempts to reduce the equinus can lead to an iatrogenic rockerbottom foot—a subluxation of the tarsometatarsal or midtarsal joint causing a rigid, painful flatfoot. After the adduction and varus components are addressed, the equinus deformity can be treated. With both thumbs, plantarly press on the distal calcaneus in a dorsiflexion direction. Gently manipulate the calcaneus in this manner for 10 minutes and then apply an above-the-knee cast. The eventual goal is a foot with 10° of ankle dorsiflexion, a calcaneus that can evert past perpendicular, a straight medial and lateral border, and aligned talonavicular and talocalcaneal joints as confirmed on x-ray. If no improvement is noted, it is better to address the problem surgically than forcibly damage the foot.

At this point, the risk of relapse is great. Retention casting must be continued for 2–3 months, followed by a splint such as the Wheaton brace or Bebax shoe.

Juvenile Bunions

This common adult deformity also is seen in adolescents. In both cases, it is more typical in females. For generations, bunions were blamed on tight shoes. The science of biomechanics has shown that hallux abducto valgus (HAV) deformity is caused by excessive STJ pronation. Since the condition may include internal gait disorders, equinus, limb length inequalities, varus or valgus foot, and leg deformities, a complete biomechanical evaluation is necessary. Most cases of symptomatic HAV present in the older adult population after decades of walking. The fact that some adolescents present with this deformity suggests that significant pronatory forces are acting on the foot. Although there may be a familial history of bunions, this should not be perceived as proof of a "bunion gene" but rather as evidence of an inherited foot structure that predisposes to excessive STJ pronation. Thus, it is imperative to identify the child with a significant flatfoot gait and treat with functional or-

thotics before HAV develops. After appearance of the disorder, it can be corrected only with surgery (see Chapter 20).

Kohler's Disease

Kohler's disease, or osteochondritis of the navicular, is common, particularly in 5- to 7-year-old boys. Clinically, it presents with pain over the navicular area. Kohler's disease may have a mechanical basis; the navicular is subject to great stress during locomotion and is one of the last bones to ossify. Radiographically, sclerosis and flattening of the navicular are diagnostic. This often is a self-limiting disorder with a good prognosis, but it may take up to 18 months until symptoms abate. Treatment consists of rest, ice, NSAIDs, and a below-knee cast if necessary. Functional orthotics also can help reduce symptoms by decreasing stress.

Sever's Disease

Sever's disease, also called calcaneal apophysitis or osteochondrosis of the calcaneal apophysis, is a common cause of heel pain, particularly in active, stocky, 7- to 12-year-old boys. It is caused by excessive traction on the calcaneal apophysis by the Achilles tendon, particularly during running and jumping sports. Pain is elicited on palpation of the Achilles tendon insertion on the posterior calcaneus. An equinus may predispose to this condition. X-rays are useful only in ruling out fracture or tumor, as the normal calcaneal apophysis ossification is very irregular and dense.

The differential diagnosis includes Achilles tendonitis and bursitis. Treatment again consists of rest, ice, NSAIDs, elimination of certain sports (e.g., basketball, soccer), shock-absorbing heel lifts (Sorbothane, Spenco, Poron), and Achilles stretching exercises. In severe cases, a below-knee cast may be used for 4–6 weeks. The prognosis is good, with resolution expected in the early teens.

Growth Plate Injuries

Epiphyseal or growth plate injuries are specific to the pediatric patient. Salter-Harris Classifications are:

Type 1—shearing of the epiphysis, no bony injury

Type 2—fracture through the epiphysis and proximal site

Type 3—fracture through the epiphysis and the distal joint

Type 4—combination of types 1, 2, and 3

Type 5—crush fracture.

Salter-Harris 1 and 2 have a good prognosis with 6-week immobilization. Types 3 and 4 have a poorer prognosis and surgical repair of the joint surface is recommended. Type 5 often produces a shortened limb or one with an angular deviation.

Shoe Gear

In the prewalker, shoes are not recommended except for protection from the environment. In the beginning walker, a shoe with a sturdy heel counter and a shank flexible enough to bend under the child's weight is advised. Such a shoe holds the heel vertical and counteracts the physiologic excess pronation that is due to lack of maturation. Running shoes made for toddlers are excellent in this regard. Do not encase the foot in a rigid, hard-leather shoe. For the older child, the same criteria hold. A running shoe offers good shock absorption and control and is excellent for accommodating a functional orthotic when needed.

References

1. Crawford AH, Gabriel KR: Foot and ankle problems. Orthop Clin North Am 18(4): 649–666, 1987.
2. Drvaric DM, Kuivila TE, Roberts JM: Congenital clubfoot: Etiology, pathoanatomy, pathogenesis and changing spectrum of early management. Orthop Clin North Am 29(4):641–648, 1989.
3. Ganley J (ed): Podopediatrics Clinics in Podiatry. Vols. 1 and 3. Philadelphia, W. B. Saunders Co., 1984.
4. Killam PE: Orthopedic assessment of young children: Developmental variations. Nurse Pract 14(7):27–30, 1989.
5. Lovell WW, Winter RB: Pediatric Orthopedics. Vols. 1 and 2. Philadelphia, J.B. Lippincott Co., 1986.
6. Phillips WA: The child with a limp. Orthop Clin North Am 18(4):489–502, 1987.
7. Staheli LT: Rotational problems of the lower extremities. Orthop Clin North Am 18(4): 563–512, 1987.
8. Tachdjian MO: The Child's Foot. Philadelphia, W.B. Saunders Co, 1985.
9. Tax H: Podopediatrics. Baltimore, Williams and Wilkins Co., 1980.

11

The Geriatric Foot

Michael P. DellaCorte, DPM, Robert Caruso, MD,
and Patrick J. Grisafi, DPM

Geriatric foot problems pose a special challenge to the primary care physician. In an era when the average life expectancy is rising steadily, the need to identify and treat geriatric foot problems becomes a part of everyday practice. What may be a common foot problem or minor trauma in the middle-aged adult can be a debilitating and sometimes crippling disorder in the elderly patient. Pain-free mobility is a major factor in the general well-being of the elderly, and foot problems frequently are coupled with immobility. A normal geriatric foot is one that is asymptomatic and noncontributory to any mental, systemic, or local disorder. It has been estimated that 70% of the population over 65 years of age suffers from some kind of foot problem (Table 1).

Factors contributing to the development of foot problems in the elderly include changes in gait, past foot care and management, hereditary problems, previous foot conditions that were not treated, hygiene, emotional problems and changes in mental status, nutritional problems, systemic and local disease, hospitalization and confinement to bed, and various medications. Additional concerns and risk factors include increased susceptibility to infection, diabetes mellitus, other forms of neurovascular impairment, muscle atrophy associated with degenerative neuromuscular and musculoskeletal diseases, and worsening osteoarthritis of the lower extremity. In addition to systemic disease, obesity and increased physical activity increase the incidence of foot ailments in the elderly.

Disorders in the Elderly

Corns and Calluses

These lesions, caused by increased pressure over bone, include heloma durum, heloma molle, heloma milliare, heloma vascularis, and tyloma. Although these conditions are common in all age groups, atrophy of the plantar fat pad coupled with degenerative joint disease and decreased pain threshold predispose the elderly to an increased frequency of complaints. The pain, which is due to soft tissue inflammation, can limit the ambulation of an otherwise active senior. Commonly located dorsally on the digits (Fig. 1A) and plantarly under the metatarsal heads (Fig. 1B), these lesions often are accompanied by bursitis, capsulitis, or both. Abducted gait and shuffling are additional factors that generate increased stress and pressure on the soft tissues and lead to corns and calluses (Fig. 1C).

A heloma molle is a corn that develops between the toes. It is soft because it absorbs the moisture from the interspace. This lesion typically forms over the medial aspect of the head of the proximal phalanx of the fifth toe or the lateral aspect of the base of the proximal phalanx of the fourth toe. Without treatment, the lesion may ulcerate and become infected. Conservative treatment involves debridement of the lesion and padding to keep the toes separated. Surgical treatment of the fourth interspace soft corn is best achieved by resecting the head of the proximal phalanx of the fifth toe.

Table 1. Common Foot Ailments of the Elderly

Condition	Percentage of Elderly	Female:Male Ratio
Corns	20	4.7:1
Calluses	12	2.6:1
Keratotic lesions	32	—
Toenail problems	24	1:1
Bunions and hammer toes	8	6:1
Swelling	—	2.5:1
Burning spells	—	2.9:1
Loss of feeling	—	1.8:1
Dry skin	4	2:1
Neurovascular ulcers	6.9	—
Systemic ulcers	7	1:1

Treatments of corns and calluses range from debridement to surgery (see Chapter 20). Regarding surgery in the elderly, note that the fear of surgery often outweighs the pain caused by the corn or callus. Medical and vascular status—not age—should be the criteria for surgery. Advanced age is not, in itself, a contraindication for surgery. A healthy patient need not suffer simply because a certain age has been reached. Elderly patients should be made aware of the fact that long-standing helomas may progress to ulcerations or infections, making treatment important.

Toenail Problems

Hypertrophy (Fig. 2), or thickening and hardening of the toenails, presents problems for the elderly patient with systemic disease, impaired vision, obesity, arthritic limitations, or loss of manual dexterity. Those undergoing antithrombotic therapy (warfarin) also are at

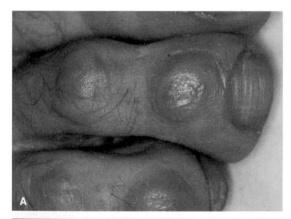

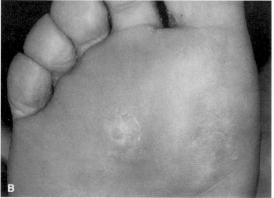

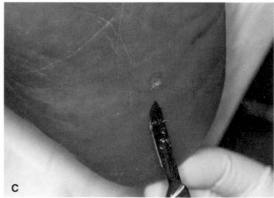

Figure 1. *A*, Digital heloma (corn). *B*, Plantar tyloma under the metatarsal heads. *C*, Plantar corn on the heel.

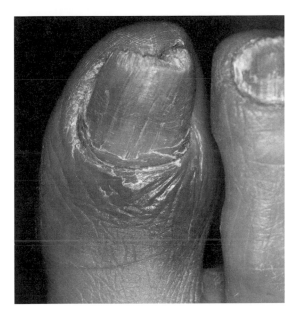

Figure 2. Thickening of the toenail.

increased risk. Due to the diminished vascular status in the elderly, preventive nail care is critical.

Onychodystrophy is caused primarily by onychomycosis, injury, or impaired circulation. If left untreated, it can result in subungual corns, ulcerations, onychia, and infections, and adjacent toes may be affected as well. Onychodystrophy may lead to excessive pressure in shoe gear with an end result of painful, unstable ambulation. Treatment of nail disorders in the elderly should be as simple as possible, consisting of debridement or grinding. Matrixectomy, given appropriate medical and vascular status, can be considered for an individual, severely symptomatic nail.

Onychocryptosis (Fig. 3), or ingrown toenail, occurs when the free edge of the nail plate penetrates the periungual soft tissue. The etiology may be trauma, a diseased nail, an ill-fitting shoe, or improper cutting of the nail. A secondary bacterial infection may occur as well as the formation of granulation tissue. Treatment is achieved by removing the offending nail spicule and granulation tissue (see Chapter 20).

Onychogryposis, or ram's horn nails, commonly are seen in the elderly who have neglected their nail care. The skin edges and the eponychium surrounding these nails are very fragile in the elderly. Care must be taken not to lacerate the surrounding soft tissue while performing debridement. In patients with circula-

tory disorders, laceration is likely to progress to infection. Appropriate wound care must be initiated with any iatrogenic injury, and documentation of the lesion and the treatment course should be ongoing until the wound resolves.

Poor nutritional status leads to toenails that are atrophic, thin and brittle, and lackluster. Marked longitudinal ridges become prominent in these cases; this condition has been termed onychorrhexis. Treatment is geared toward nutritional counseling and local nail care. Various other nail conditions along with treatments are discussed in Chapter 5.

Hallux Valgus

Bunion deformities (Fig. 4) in the elderly accompanied by peripheral vascular disease must be treated conservatively. Accommodation for the bony prominences in shoe gear is a primary concern and is accomplished with custom-molded shoes. Plaster-cast impressions for molded shoes can be taken in the office by the primary care physician, or the patient can be referred to a specialist (see Chapter 20).

Physical therapy is another method of conservative treatment for bunions in the elderly. Care must be taken with heat and cold modalities in those patients with neurologic or vascular impairments (see Chapter 20). If the patient's medical and vascular status is acceptable, surgery can be considered. Age alone should not be a criterion for foot surgery. Surgery is geared toward relief of

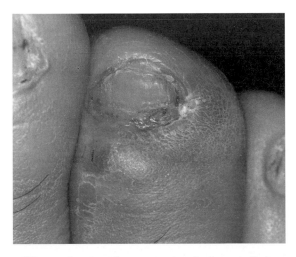

Figure 3. Onychocryptosis of a lesser digit.

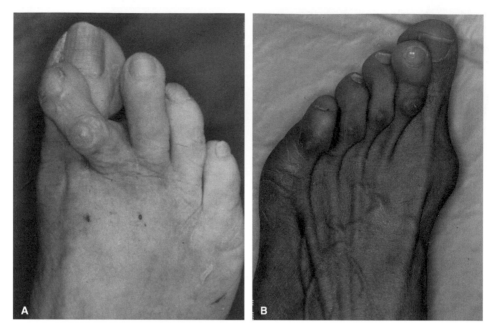

Figure 4. *A*, Mild bunion deformity with overlapping second digit. *B*, Bunion deformity with hammer toes.

symptoms—not cosmesis. Foot surgery can increase mobility and add to the quality of life. A qualified foot surgeon should be consulted in these cases.

Edema

Chronic pedal edema secondary to cardiac, renal, hepatic, and vascular etiologies may lead to discomfort in shoe gear and alteration in gait patterns and mobility in the elderly. Managing the cause medically, along with the use of support hose and elevation, should relieve symptoms. Intermittant compression devices can be helpful in venous insufficiency but not in cardiac disease.

Burning

Burning sensations in the feet can be caused by a number of ailments, such as biomechanic stress, neuroma, vascular disorders, diabetic and alcoholic neuropathies, and other systemic disorders such as hyperparathyroidism. Treatment is sometimes difficult and is geared to the underlying cause. When all else fails, physical therapy modalities such as cool whirlpool and transcutaneous electrical nerve stimulation may relieve symptoms. Oral antidepressants such as Elavil and topical prepa-

rations containing capsaicin also may reduce burning of neuropathic origin.

Xerosis

As aging progresses, skin hydration decreases and sebaceous and eccrine activity diminishes. These changes lead to dry and scaly skin (Fig. 5). Dry skin can be prevented or improved by daily hydration of the affected areas. Bathing followed by the use of a topical emollient (e.g., a lanolin preparation) retards water loss. Hydration relieves itching and prevents fissuring that can lead to infection. However, excess foot soaking or hot water dries out the skin, instead of hydrating it. There are many over-the-counter topicals such as Eucerin and prescription topicals such as Lac Hydrin and Lactinol that are helpful if used consistently.

Ulcerations

Foot ulcerations are more common in the elderly. The type should be determined prior to treatment because local ulcer care can promote injury and further functional loss, particularly with vascular and diabetic etiologies (see Chapters 16 and 18). Ulcerations may be pressure-induced, ischemic, neurotrophic, systemic, biomechanic, iatrogenic, patient-

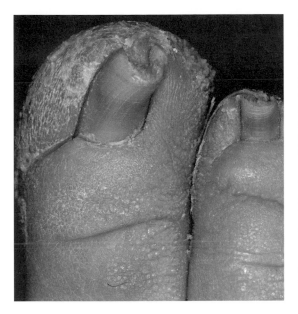

Figure 5. Dry, scaly skin—common in the elderly.

induced, or neoplastic. Note that ulcerations appear under a heloma or tyloma. Therefore, it is necessary to debride all hyperkeratotic lesions prior to making a definitive diagnosis. A noninvasive vascular exam using Doppler ultrasound should be part of the evaluation of most ulcers, with a vascular consultation as needed.

Treatment of ulcerations generally is a long process. If the primary etiology has been managed, weekly debridement and daily bandage changes (by the patient, family, or home care nurse) are necessary. If the ulcers are infected, a culture and sensitivity sample should be taken from the deepest area of the ulcer by scalpel, and not swab. Appropriate antibiotics should be administered in addition to local wound care (see Chapter 17).

Local wound care of the ulcerations consists of debridement with a scalpel or tissue nipper. Using an aseptic or sterile technique, all hyperkeratosis around the ulceration must be debrided. If the hyperkeratosis is allowed to cover over the ulceration, the epithelialization process will take much longer to complete, and the probability of infection is greater. The base of the ulceration should be debrided to a healthy bleeding level and allowed to granulate. Wet-to-dry applications of saline or dilute Betadine are applied between dressing changes; dressings should be changed twice daily. DuoDerm Hydroactive

dressings also may be used in conjunction with debridement. Areas of devitalized tissue that cannot be debrided may be eliminated by the use of enzymes such as Elase. There are a great many wound care products available, including collagen-based preparations, alginate dressings, hydrogels, and hydrocolloids. Procuren, which is made from the patient's own platelets, is coupled with debridement in wound care centers.

It should be noted that some ulcers are extremely painful, and the patient will not be able to tolerate aggressive debridement. In these cases, local anesthesia may be necessary along with oral pain medications for any post-debridement pain. The primary care physician should be cautious when trying the numerous ulcer dressings that are on the medical market because they sometimes can cause maceration and infections. They must be monitored on a daily basis.

Venous Stasis Ulcers

These commonly occur around the medial malleolus and are due to chronic venous pooling secondary to venous insufficiency. Hemosiderin deposits causing dermatitis, skin atrophy, and ultimately ulceration occur in the elderly. Treatment consists of compression therapy, possibly an Unna boot, debridement, and the above-mentioned wound care products. A biopsy of the wound occasionally is required to rule out malignancy.

Pressure Ulcers

Pressure ulcerations commonly occur in areas where bony prominences, in combination with insensitivity, lead to breakdown of overlying skin. Common sites in the foot of the geriatric patient are the skin overlying a hallux valgus or hammer digit, the skin beneath a plantarflexed metatarsal head, the plantar aspect of the fifth metatarsal base, and the area overlying a prominent navicular tuberosity. The pressure may be from the shoe or just from the repetition of normal ambulation.

If the ulcer is caused by pressure or biomechanic problems, no matter how much debridement and local wound care is performed, the ulcer will never resolve if weight is not dispersed from the affected area. Pressure ulcers have been classified into a four grade system (Table 2). The amount of damage often is in the shape of an inverted cone. Molded shoes, dispersons with felt padding, and accommodative orthotics are the best modalities to elimi-

Table 2. Classification of Pressure Ulcerations

Grade	Clinical Appearance	Prognosis	Treatment
I	Only epidermal—irregular soft tissue swelling and induration, skin reddened but unbroken	Excellent	Padding, shoe correction
II	Breach of epidermis and dermis—shallow, full-thickness ulcer	Excellent	Debridement, off-loading, padding, shoe correction
III	Deep ulcer through sub-cutaneous fat to fascia—foul smelling	Poor	Surgical debridement, zero weight bearing
IV	Deep ulcer invading fascia, bones, joints, viscera—exposed bone, drainage, necrosis	Poor	Surgical debridement all necrotic tissue and bone, possible amputation risk

Adapted from Shea DJ: Pressure sores classification and management. Clin Orthop 112:89–100, 1975.

nate or lessen the pressure to the affected area. Once the trauma or pressure has been eliminated, the ulcer is debrided as described above.

Surgical debridement is indicated for the non-healing ulcers or ulcerations with wide areas of devitalized tissue, exposed tendon, or joint capsule. If bone is exposed in an ulceration, that bone is considered to be infected. Surgical intervention is then mandatory, and the patient should be brought into the hospital operating room for surgical debridement of bone and surrounding soft tissue. A specialist should be consulted in these cases. The patient should be informed of the risks and the consequences, and possible loss of digits, foot, or limb.

Skin Atrophy

Atrophy of the submetatarsal or subcalcaneal fat pads is a common geriatric cause of a painful foot. The plantar aspect of the foot is naturally cushioned by fat. When the fat atrophies, the bony structures underlying the fat become much more prominent and are subject to increased pressure. When the resultant pain occurs under the plantar aspect of the metatarsal heads, it is called metatarsalgia. Tylomas, helomas, and bursitis are frequent complaints. The diagnosis is made on clinical exam and evaluation. X-ray evaluation may be necessary to rule out any underlying bone pathology.

Treatment consists of gentle debridement of any hyperkeratotic lesions, with padding for

immediate relief. The skin generally is very thin and tears easily; therefore, the practitioner should be cautious with the use of adhesive pads or tape. Removal may tear the skin, causing further disability. Long-term relief can be accomplished by the use of soft tissue supplements, such as Spenco or Plastazote, that can be added to the foot orthotics or inserted directly into the shoe. Many sneakers on the market today have the soft tissue supplement already in place, and their use should be encouraged as long as the bottom tread does not increase the risk of falling. A shuffling gait combined with a rough-tread shoe can cause an unexpected fall.

Osteoporosis

Osteoporosis is a condition caused by diminution of bone mass; it is very common in the elderly patient. After age 33, bone mass decreases, beginning earlier and proceeding more rapidly in women, until 20–40% has been lost by the age of 65. Decrease in bone mass in women begins prior to menopause and is accelerated in the post-menopausal state. Osteopenia and osteoporosis, in conjunction with degenerative changes, increase the likelihood of sesamoiditis. The frequency of foot fractures, therefore, is high in the elderly female population.

Note that surgical procedures involving osteotomies should be considered carefully in the elderly with osteoporosis, and medical management of any underlying systemic cause of the osteoporosis in addition to dietary counseling should be the first priorities. Evaluations every 6–8 months that include bone densitometry help monitor the condition.

Painful Heel Pad Syndrome

Heel pain is another common complaint in the elderly patient. Its primary etiology is atrophy of the subcalcaneal fat pad plus cumulative impact loading due to repetitive heel strike during walking. Once the natural cushion is gone, there is increased pressure on the inferior aspect of the calcaneus. Obesity, increased or prolonged ambulatory activity, hard floors or surfaces, and/or biomechanic abnormalities are the predisposing factors to the development of inferior calcaneal bursitis. The patient relates pain upon ambulation that is not immediately relieved by rest. Burning and throbbing also may occur. Direct palpation produces tenderness in the central aspect of the heel proximal to the medial tubercle of the calcaneus, thus distinguishing this syndrome from a heel spur syndrome.

Conservative treatment includes rest, nonsteroidal anti-inflammatory drugs (NSAIDs), and dispersion padding (U pad) or a MF heel protector. The flexible heel protector is a tight-fitting piece of plastic that cups the heel and squeezes all the fat under the calcaneus, providing more cushioning. It should be used with a rubber sole wedge-type shoe or running shoe. Over-the-counter silicone or Sorbothane-based heel cushions also are available. If this treatment is ineffective after 5 days, the calcaneal bursa should be injected (see Chapter 20). Up to four injections may be necessary to relieve symptoms, and they should be given weekly until symptoms subside. Physiotherapy modalities such as whirlpool and ultrasound also may be helpful. To prevent recurrence, shoe modifications with heel dispersion padding or foot orthotics with a calcaneal bursitis dispersion pad should be worn indefinitely.

Plantar Fasciitis

As aging progresses, the muscles and ligaments supporting the bony structures of the foot weaken, causing a decrease in the calcaneal inclination angle and the metatarsal declination angle. As the arch collapses, extra stress is placed on the plantar fascia, causing traction periostitis or strain of the fascia fibers. Coupled with obesity, increased activity, and/or biomechanical abnormalities, acute plantar fasciitis can develop. The condition is more common in men than women.

The complaint is usually pain in the morning upon first weight bearing, which gradually gets better as ambulation continues. At rest the fascia relaxes and shortens, but when full body weight is applied, the fascia overstretches, causing pain. Chronic cases of fasciitis are painful all the time. Diagnostically, dorsiflexion of the digits stretches the fascia and causes pain, as does direct palpation of the anteromedial border of the calcaneal tuberosity and medial aspect of the plantar fascia itself. Treatment, including strapping and orthotic devices, is discussed in Chapter 9.

Achilles Tendonitis

The geriatric patient may suffer from this condition as a result of a chronic overuse situation in which an already less-elastic soft tissue structure is subject to prolonged walking or standing. Equinus is a contributing factor. Direct shoe pressure at the Achilles insertion also may result in tendonitis. Not to be excluded are the more common causes, such as a direct blow, a sudden forceful contraction, or metabolic and inflammatory etiologies (gout or one of the arthritides). The condition presents with pain, erythema, and edema in the hindfoot proximal to the tendon insertion. Crepitation and nodules may be present, depending on the condition's chronicity. Management is discussed in Chapter 9.

Note: For a discussion of **Achilles bursitis,** see Chapter 9.

Posterior Tibial Tendon Dysfunction

Spontaneous strain, rupture, or degeneration of the posterior tibial tendon is acknowledged as one of the common causes of pes planus in the middle-aged and geriatric female patient. Acute valgus trauma (e.g., missing the rung of a ladder or a sudden step from a curb) results in a loss of arch height as well as a decreased ability to plantarflex and invert the foot. Pain along the tendon and some instability in gait are presenting symptoms. The pain progresses and often becomes intractable.

Physical findings verify a loss of inversion and plantarflexion of the affected foot, with pain along the course of the tendon when attempting contraction against resistance. A defect may be noted, and it may be possible to sublux the tendon anteriorly. Conservative management of a dysfunctional posterior tibial tendon includes NSAIDs, a medial arch support, and an external medial buildup at the sole and heel. In problematic cases, surgical intervention with possible tendon repair may be necessary.

For a discussion of this dysfunction relative to arthritis, see Chapter 15; to diabetes, see Chapter 16; and to the circulatory system, see Chapter 18.

Shoe Gear

Attention to shoes is an important aspect of foot care in the elderly, especially in the diabetic patient. Normal shoe gear for the geriatric patient should have an upper made of a soft material. The sole should not be too rigid and should have a good shock-absorbing heel, and the insole should be well padded for support. Laced shoes are preferred to loafers because laced shoes allow for swelling. For those patients unable to tie shoe laces, Velcro closures are available.

Extra-depth inlay shoes can accommodate arthritically contracted digits and allow insertion of an orthotic or cushioning support. Molded shoes accommodate bony prominences. For those patients who cannot afford or refuse to wear molded shoes, running shoes (sneakers) may give some relief. A good running shoe has all of the aforementioned qualities and can offer a feeling of youthfulness. Note that Medicare now reimburses for special shoes for the at-risk diabetic patient.

===

References

1. Albert SF, Jahnigen DW: Treating common foot disorders in older patients. Geriatrics 38(6): 42–55, 1983.
2. Baxter DE, Fintgors CJ: Am Acad Orthop Surg 3(3):136–145, 1995.
3. Calkins E, Davis PJ, Ford AB (eds): The Practice of Geriatrics. Philadelphia, W. B. Saunders Co., 1986.
4. Gleckman RA, Czachor JS: Managing diabetes-related infections in the elderly. Geriatrics 44(8):37–46, 1989.
5. Helfand AE (ed): Clinical Podogeriatrics. Baltimore, Williams & Wilkins, 1981.
6. Helfand AE: Nail and hyperkeratotic problems in the elderly foot. Am Fam Physician 39(2): 101–110, 1989.
7. Jahss MH (ed): Disorders of the Foot, Vol I. Philadelphia, W.B. Saunders Co, 1986.
8. Jones CD: Tendon disorders of the foot and ankle. J Am Acad Orthop Surg 1(2):87–94, 1993.
9. Mann RA (ed): DuVries' Surgery of the Foot, 4th ed. St. Louis, C.V. Mosby, 1978.
10. Yale JF: Yale's Podiatric Medicine, 3rd ed. Baltimore, Williams & Wilkins, 1987.

12

Biomechanical Abnormalities

*Patrick J. Grisafi, DPM, Michael P. DellaCorte, DPM,
and Stuart Plotkin, DPM*

Great strides have been made in the field of human biomechanics. New research coupled with computerized gait analysis has helped clarify how we walk and has revealed pathologic mechanisms of compensation (Table 1). Compensation is the biomechanical method the body employs to adjust one part to a deviation of structure, position, or function of another part.

Pronation is a subtalar joint (STJ) motion in which the calcaneus everts, the talus adducts and plantarflexes, the arch lowers, and the limb internally rotates. Excessive pronation leads to hypermobility of the foot, which causes the joints to function outside their normal range of motion. Instability of the first ray causes bunions, hammer toes, and degenerative joint disease. The flattening arch results in plantar fascia stress, plantar fasciitis, and heel spur syndrome. Excessive internal leg rotation leads to knee pain, and decreased shock absorption causes hip and low back pain. An excessively pronated foot (pes planus) is a foot with many problems.

Supination is a STJ motion in which the calcaneus inverts, the talus abducts and dorsiflexes, the arch height increases, and the limb externally rotates. An excessively supinated foot has a diminished capacity to adapt to irregular surfaces and, hence, is prone to ankle sprains. The plantar fat pad quickly atrophies from excessive pressure, causing heel pad pain, sesamoiditis, and contracted claw toes. A supinated (pes cavus) foot has its own symptomatology.

Biomechanical Disorders

Several factors can cause an abnormal angle of gait, leading to an abnormal gait cycle and associated foot problems.

Sagittal Plane Deformities

Sagittal plane motion in the foot is dorsiflexion and plantarflexion. Equinus is a sagittal plane deformity.

Equinus

If the ankle joint cannot obtain at least 10° of dorsiflexion, the patient is said to have equinus (Table 2). The etiology can be congenital, adaptive, or a combination of both. Congenital clubfoot, growth spurs in children, spasticity in cerebral palsy, trauma, and chronic wearing of high-heeled shoes all contribute to an equinus (Fig. 1).

Table 1. Symptoms of Abnormal Subtalar Joint Motion

Excess Pronation	Excess Supination
Everted heel	Inverted heel
Low arch	High arch
Bunions	Claw toes
Hammer toes	Fat pad atrophy
Hypermobility	High arch
Flatfoot	Rigidity
Spurs	Cavus foot
Chondromalacia	Callus sub 1,5*
Hip and low back pain	Heel pain
	Ankle instability
	Low back pain

*Under first and fifth metatarsal heads

Table 2. Types of Equinus

Type	Knee Joint Position	Ankle Joint Dorsiflexion
Gastroc-nemius	Knee extended	< 10°
	Knee flexed	> 10°
Gastro-soleus	Knee extended	< 10°
	Knee flexed	< 10°
Ankle*	Knee extended	< 10°
	Knee flexed	< 10°
Spastic	Observe gait	
	Calf muscle spasticity leads to early heel-off	

*A lateral foot/ankle x-ray demonstrates a tibial or talar bony block.

There are three forms of compensation for equinus: uncompensated, partially compensated, and fully compensated. In a patient with uncompensated equinus, or a "toe-walker," the heel does not touch the ground in gait. A patient with partially compensated equinus compensates first at the midfoot by unlocking

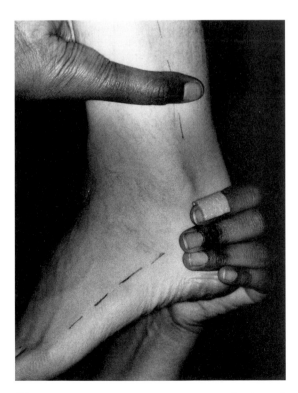

Figure 1. When equinus is present, the lateral bisection of the leg is plantarflexed in relation to the lateral bisection of the foot.

the midtarsal joint (MTJ) and then by pronating the STJ. An early heel-off is noted in gait. In a patient with fully compensated equinus, the heel remains on the ground for a normal time period, but this compensation is the cause of a great many symptoms. Compensation is possible at the midfoot, rearfoot, and forefoot. Equinus also can be compensated with a flexion of the knee or external rotation of the hip.

For treatment of acute Achilles tendonitis secondary to equinus, the patient should wear a higher-heeled shoe or a heel lift temporarily to reduce stress on the Achilles tendon. Although this practice might worsen the patient's condition on a long-term basis, it eliminates acute symptoms over shorter periods. Functional foot orthoses, an excellent conservative treatment option for all types of equinus, are fabricated with the STJ in neutral position and are designed to prevent excess pronation. A heel lift, if the equinus is not due to a bony abnormality, is added to accommodate the equinus initially. Then, in conjunction with exercises, the heel lift is gradually decreased until the equinus is resolved. Nonsteroidal anti-inflammatory drugs (NSAIDs) and ice also may be helpful.

For chronic gastrocnemius and gastrosoleus equinus, calf-stretching exercises increase ankle joint dorsiflexion (see Chapter 10, Figure 2). For bony ankle blocks, a permanent lift can be added to the shoe. For equinus deformities (e.g., spastic and ankle equinus) not responding to conservative therapy, surgery is another treatment option. Lengthening of the Achilles tendon may be necessary in cerebral palsy spasticity to allow ambulation. However, this procedure has a high recurrence rate.

Transverse Plane Deformities

Transverse plane motion in the foot is internal and external rotation. Transverse plane deformities produce an in-toe or out-toe gait. Any abnormality of the transverse plane of the lower extremity—pathology of the hip (congenital dislocation), femur (torsion), knee (ligamentous laxity), and tibia (torsion)—affects the angle of gait. Hence, a thorough examination of the lower extremity, both static and dynamic, is essential in determining the level of abnormality causing the alteration in gait. If the hip, knee, leg, and ankle are normal, a metatarsus adductus should be considered.

Frontal Plane Deformities

Frontal plane motion in the foot is inversion and eversion. There are many more deformities on the frontal plane than on the other planes.

Rearfoot Varus

A varus position is a structurally inverted position. At birth, the calcaneus is inverted relative to the talus. The posterior surface of the calcaneus undergoes an external torsion that brings it in line with the talus. If this torsion does not occur, rearfoot varus is the result (see Chapter 10). Assessment is made by placing the STJ in a neutral position and noting the heel bisector's position relative to the longitudinal bisection of the posterior leg. If the heel is inverted to the leg, then an STJ varus deformity exits.

Rearfoot varus is caused by any lower extremity deformity that allows the heel to strike the ground with greater than 2° of inversion. The patient can either compensate fully, partially, or not at all. Rearfoot varus includes tibial varus (bow leg) and subtalar varum.

Uncompensated. In uncompensated rearfoot varus, the foot strikes the ground inverted and stays inverted, leading to a chronic inversion ankle instability and rapid lateral shoe wear. The foot itself develops calluses along the lateral aspect of the heel and under the base of the fifth metatarsal. With the foot maintained in inversion, the peroneus longus muscle takes advantage of the rigid lateral column and plantarflexes the first ray, causing the patient to bear excess pressure on the tibial sesamoid. The patient also develops a hyperkeratotic lesion below the first metatarsal. Hence, the uncompensated rearfoot varus patient presents with a high arch, inverted rearfoot, and hyperkeratotic lesions of submetatarsals one and five.

In addition, this patient is prone to inversion ankle sprains due to the rearfoot being maintained in inversion. There also may be complaints of a painful heel due to poor shock absorption.

Generally, conservative treatment including palliative care of hyperkeratosis and functional orthotics to equilibrate ground reactive forces against the foot suffices. Surgical treatment to correct an intrinsic rearfoot varus (i.e., Dwyer osteotomy) usually is reserved for severe cases associated with chronic ankle sprains.

Partially Compensated. In partially compensated rearfoot varus, the rearfoot partially pronates, but not enough to get the forefoot to the ground. This causes increased motion in the forefoot, especially at the lateral aspect. Excess motion at the fifth ray leads to a tailor's bunion. With the fifth metatarsal bowing laterally, the flexor digitorum longus tendon no longer pulls the fifth toe straight, but allows it to curl inward. If the fifth ray is mobile enough, a submetatarsal four hyperkeratotic lesion may develop due to decreased weight bearing at the fifth metatarsal. Again, functional foot orthoses to equilibrate the ground forces and control pronation along with palliative care is the conservative treatment of choice. If the tailor's bunion becomes symptomatic and painful, surgery is indicated.

Fully Compensated. In fully compensated rearfoot varus, the patient is able to pronate the STJ so that the forefoot is placed totally on the ground. It is this pronation that leads to much of the foot pathology seen in a physician's office. Rearfoot pronation can cause irritation of the posterior heel, leading to a "pump bump" or Haglund's deformity. In addition, metatarsus primus elevatus can develop due to ground reactive forces pushing up on an unstable first ray after the rearfoot pronates to the perpendicular position. Because of constant pounding of the first ray during gait, a hallux limitus results, leading to a painful dorsal bunion.

Conservative treatment modalities involve functional foot orthoses to eliminate the excessive pronation. Haglund's deformity is treated according to the guidelines outlined in Chapter 9. If hallux limitus develops, then surgical intervention to remove the dorsal bunion and correct the elevated first metatarsal is indicated. If it is noted that the articular cartilage of the first metatarsophalangeal joint has undergone significant degenerative changes, then the joint must be resected (i.e., Keller bunionectomy) to eliminate the pain (see Chapter 20).

Rearfoot Valgus

With a rearfoot valgus deformity, the foot strikes the ground everted. This is caused by subtalar valgus, an intrinsic osseous abnormality in which the talus undergoes too much external rotation at birth, or by lower-extremity abnormalities such as genu valgus, a soft tissue or osseous abnormality at the knee joint causing the foot to maintain an everted relationship to the leg. In all cases, the heel strikes the ground beyond perpendicular

(Fig. 2). A flatfoot type usually is observable (Fig. 3).

Another cause of rearfoot valgus is a peroneal spastic flatfoot that usually is associated with tarsal coalition (i.e., fusion between tarsal bones) (see Chapter 10). When the patient tries to supinate the foot, pain is caused by the coalition. The peroneus brevis tries to hold the foot in an everted position to prevent pain, thus maintaining the flatfoot condition.

In forefoot supinatus associated with rearfoot valgus, with the rearfoot hitting the ground everted, the medial column of the foot is unlocked. The ground pushes up on the medial column of the foot and maintains the forefoot in a supinated position. The supinated position is held in place by soft tissue that eventually adapts and maintains the supinated attitude. These patients walk with an awkward, clumsy gait. Once subtalar pronation is eliminated, the supinatus can be reversed.

Nonsurgical treatment of rearfoot valgus includes orthotics that do not allow any motion at the STJ, so that pain is prevented during ambulation. Conservative treatment of tarsal coalition also includes orthotics fabricated to prevent motion. Surgical intervention for the painful tarsal coalition in which conservative methods have failed includes a triple arthrodesis. The rearfoot valgus foot type is a very difficult foot to manage. The practitioner must deal with the foot symptomatically and try to provide comfort. Because the patient strikes the ground in a pronated position and thus unlocks the medial column, bunions are likely to develop; yet, if corrected surgically, they are likely to recur because excessive rearfoot pronation was not addressed.

Forefoot Varus

The forefoot, at birth, should be perpendicular to the rearfoot due to intrauterine external rotation of the talar neck. When this torsion does not take place, the forefoot remains inverted to the rearfoot. A forefoot varus, a one-plane osseous deformity of the talus neck, develops (see Chapter 10). Assessment is made by placing the STJ in neutral position, maximally pronating the MTJ (loading the fifth metatarsal head via plantar pressure using the thumb), and noting the inverted relationship of the forefoot to the rearfoot.

Metatarsals one through five are inverted. Clinically, the rearfoot hits the ground and undergoes a normal amount of eversion, yet in order to get the medial column of the forefoot down, the foot must pronate beyond rearfoot perpendicular. This pronatory compensation is a severely deforming force on the foot (Table 3). Once the STJ pronates to its maximum extent, other methods of compensation may or may not come into effect.

Uncompensated. In uncompensated forefoot varus, the first ray plantarflexes as in the uncompensated rearfoot varus, but the calcaneus is perpendicular to the ground (i.e., inverted with rearfoot varus). Calluses are observed under the first and fifth metatarsal heads.

Palliative care for the calluses immediately relieves discomfort under the first and fifth

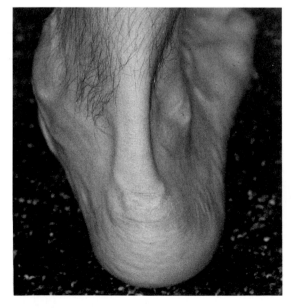

Figure 2. Valgus heel secondary to flatfoot.

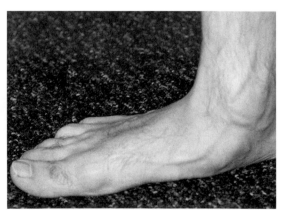

Figure 3. Severe flatfoot.

Table 3. Common Causes of Abnormal Pronation

Intrinsic to the Foot	Extrinsic to the Foot
Forefoot varus	Tibia varum
Rearfoot varus	Genu valgum
Equinus	Equinus
Tarsal coalition	Limb length inequality
Injury	Scoliosis
	Internal gait from hip or tibia
	Neuromuscular disorder

metatarsal heads. Functional foot orthoses aid in reducing and possibly eliminating the callus formation.

Partially Compensated. In partially compensated forefoot varus, the STJ and MTJ fully pronate, but do not have enough range of motion to allow full compensation. As in partially compensated rearfoot varus, a tailor's bunion, curled fifth digit, and hyperkeratosis of submetatarsal four develop because of a hypermobile fifth ray. External rotation of the leg is an extrinsic form of compensation for forefoot varus.

Functional foot orthoses fabricated with a forefoot post will, in essence, bring the ground up to the forefoot, thus eliminating the need for excessive pronation at the STJ and MTJ. Callus formation is palliatively treated through paring. If the tailor's bunion or curled fifth digit causes the patient severe pain, surgical intervention is indicated, followed by functional foot orthoses to maintain correction.

Fully Compensated. Compensated forefoot varus occurs when the STJ everts beyond perpendicular. The MTJ also compensates by pronating during midstance in an attempt to get the medial column down. The MTJ remains mobile during propulsion, causing the ground reactive forces to push the hallux into abduction, resulting in a bunion deformity. Continued hallux pressure also can cause the second digit to contract, resulting in a hammer toe or hallux overlap. Either of these situations will, in time, cause a subluxed second MPJ and development of hyperkeratosis under the second metatarsal head.

In addition, heel spur syndrome (see Chapter 9) can occur with compensated forefoot varus. When the STJ and MTJ pronate, the arch of the foot drops, leading to pulling of the plantar fascia. When the fascia is torn away from the bone, bleeding develops and more bone is deposited, leading to the formation of a spur.

The use of functional foot orthoses, fabricated in a similar manner as for partially compensated forefoot varus, is an excellent conservative treatment of choice. When the fully compensated forefoot varus deformity is discovered after a painful bunion has developed, orthotics can slow the progress of the deformity, although they cannot correct the bunion. Padding of the bunion as well as change of shoe gear (e.g., pumps to running shoes) can provide relief. Surgical correction of the bunion is reserved for intractable pain.

Forefoot Valgus

In a forefoot valgus deformity, the forefoot is everted relative to the rearfoot, and metatarsals one through five are everted relative to the calcaneus. This is a bony deformity in the talar neck. Sometimes the patient has a combination of forefoot valgus and rearfoot varus resulting in a high arched or cavovarus foot type, a static deformity. If the patient notices the arch getting higher over time, the deformity is progressive. It is prudent to look for neuromuscular problems creating a cavus foot, such as Charcot-Marie-Tooth disease or Friedreich's ataxia. A plantarflexed first ray is a localized forefoot valgus. If rigid, the gait becomes supinated, a hyperkeratotic lesion forms under the metatarsal, and lateral ankle instability occurs. Sesamoidal problems also may result.

Compensation for forefoot valgus initially occurs at the MTJ by supination, followed by elevation of the first ray, and ultimately STJ supination. In the propulsive phase, there is a rapid pronatory motion that occurs due to lateral instability.

Problems associated with this foot disorder include poor shock absorption resulting in back problems and pump bump or posterior heel irritation. Callus formation at submetatarsals one and five can appear along the plantar aspect of the foot. In time, the rearfoot may invert in an attempt to have the forefoot and rearfoot weight bearing during midstance. The chance of lateral ankle sprains increases proportionately.

Treatment options for flexible and rigid deformities include orthotics, primarily to support the deformity, palliative care for the calluses, surgical procedures to get the rearfoot out of varus, and dorsiflexory osteotomies of the metatarsals to get the forefoot out of valgus. Surgical correction of a painful bunion and heel spurs followed by application of functional foot orthoses to maintain correction are reserved for the severely painful deformity.

Forefoot Supinatus

Forefoot supinatus is a triplane, soft-tissue deformity caused by an inversion force applied to the forefoot during gait. The ground pushes up on the medial column of the foot and maintains the forefoot in a supinated position. The supinated position is held in place by soft tissue that eventually adapts and maintains the supinated attitude. These patients walk with an awkward, clumsy gait. Once pronation is eliminated, the supinatus can be reversed. Forefoot supinatus is generally caused by eversion of the rearfoot during gait.

Bunions

From a biomechanical point of view, hallux abducto valgus is caused by a hypermobile first ray. This hypermobility is due to excessive pronation which destroys the peroneus longus muscle's stabilizing ability. Shoes may exacerbate a bunion, but they are not the direct cause. As the first metatarsal loses stability it drifts medially, and the hallux drifts laterally with a valgus rotation. Degenerative changes take place in the joint and symptoms develop. See Chapter 6 for additional information on bunions.

Hammer Toes

There are two types of hammer toes: static (rigid) and dynamic. Static hammer toes are due to intrinsic osseous abnormalities, and they account for 20% of all hammer toe deformities. Dynamic hammer toes are caused by intrinsic muscle fatigue, and they account for 80% of all hammer toe deformities. There are two subtypes of dynamic hammertoes: extensor substitution and flexor stabilization.

Extensor substitution hammer toes occur when the long extensor muscles overpower the lumbricales. The lumbricales act to stabilize the digits during the swing and counteract the extensor digitorum longus pull. When weakened, as occurs with a high-arched, supinated foot, hammer toes develop.

Flexor stabilization hammer toes occur during the stance phase when the interossei muscles are overpowered by the flexor digitorum longus (FDL). When abnormal pronation occurs, the pull of the FDL is altered in the pronatory direction, causing an increased pull of the distal phalanx of toes two through five. This overcomes the stabilizing force of the interossei.

If diagnosed early, the abnormal muscle forces of dynamic hammer toes can be corrected without surgical intervention via the use of functional foot orthoses in the case of flexor stabilization. Extensor substitution hammer toes almost always require surgical intervention. Generally, the patient has a painful hyperkeratosis over the proximal interphalangeal joint, and the dynamic hammer toe becomes rigid. Conservative treatment includes routine palliation padding and extra depth shoes. See Chapter 7 for additional information on hammer toes.

Functional Foot Orthotics

A functional foot orthotic is a device that alters foot function to prevent the need for compensatory pronation. It is the treatment of choice for most biomechanical disorders. Foot orthotics generally are categorized as soft (accommodative), semi-rigid, or rigid. Soft orthotics have good shock-absorbing ability, are useful for high-arched feet, and can accommodate various plantar lesions. Semi-rigid orthotics offer more biomechanical control, are well tolerated, and are useful for sport activities. Rigid orthotics offer precise control where maximum pronatory resistance is required.

An orthotic includes a heel cup and rearfoot post, to hold the heel so the STJ functions around its neutral position; a forefoot post to prevent compensation for a forefoot varus or valgus or a plantarflexed first ray; a top cover of a shock-absorbing material; and various specialty accommodations, such as metatarsal pads, cut-outs, lifts, wedges, and designs that fit in high heels, skates, ski boots, and many other types of foot gear. An orthotic is not simply an arch support.

The casting of an orthotic is critical to its success. There are now computer scanners that digitize the foot contours and send information directly to CAD-CAM computer milling devices. Orthotics also are fabricated by hand by trained orthotists from plaster casts of the foot.

Gait Analysis

In addition to observation and history-taking (Table 4), an examination of gait is an important part of the physical exam. The head should be straight, shoulders level, and trunk erect, with arms swinging free. The knee should be on the frontal plane facing ahead, and the heel should hit the ground slightly inverted and pronating. At about 25% of the gait cycle, the STJ should start to supinate and the heel move toward inversion. Excess pronation at this point is pathologic. The heel should lift as body weight moves over the foot, and weight should transfer from rearfoot to forefoot smoothly. Finally, a propulsive force

Table 4. Signs and Symptoms Associated with Pathomechanics

Rearfoot Varus	Callus plantar to the second, fourth, or fifth metatarsal head
	Tailor's bunion
	Haglund's deformity
	Inversion ankle sprains
	Adductovarus fourth and fifth toes
Rearfoot Valgus	Callus plantar to second metatarsal head
	Fatigue of foot and leg muscles
	Plantar medial arch pain
	Hallux abductovarus
Forefoot Varus	Callus plantar to second, fourth, or fifth metatarsal head
	Fatigue of foot and leg muscles
	Tailor's bunion
	Adductovarus fourth and fifth toes
	Hallux valgus deformity
Forefoot Valgus/ Plantarflexed First Ray with Compensation by MTJ Longitudinal Axis	Callus plantar to first and fifth metatarsal heads
	Tibial sesamoiditis
	Fatigue of foot and leg muscles
	Flexion contractures of lesser toes
	Lateral knee strain
Forefoot Valgus/Plantarflexed First Ray with Compensation by Supination of the STJ and MTJ Longitudinal and Oblique Axes	Callus plantar to first metatarsal head
	Callus plantar to fourth and fifth metatarsal heads
	Tibial sesamoiditis
	Flexion contractures of lesser toes
	Lateral knee strain
	Inversion ankle sprains
	Haglund's deformity
	In-toe gait
Metatarsus Primus Elevatus	Callus plantar to second metatarsal head
	Callus plantar to hallux proximal phalanx head
	Fatigue of foot and leg muscles
	Dorsal bunion of first metatarsal head
	Hallux limitus/rigidus
Equinus in Children	Corn of fifth toe
	Abductovarus deformity of fifth toe
	Fatigue of foot and leg muscles
	Growing pains
	Osteochondritis of navicular cuneiform or calcaneus
Equinus Deformity in Adults	Callus plantar to second metatarsal head
	Adductor varus deformities of fourth and fifth digits
	Fatigue of foot and leg muscles
	Hallux abducto valgus

MTJ = midtarsal joint, STJ = subtalar joint
Adapted from Seibel MO: Foot Function—A Programmed Text. Baltimore, Williams and Wilkins, 1988.

should be generated as the hallux lifts from the floor. Any spasticity, scissoring, shuffling, weakness, or instability should be noted. Note the angle and base of gait, cadence, any hip drop, flexed knee, genu varum or valgum (bow leg or knock knee), early heel-off, or metatarsus adductus. Gait centers now have computerized and video gait analysis available.

▬▬

References

1. Jones LJ, Todd WF: Abnormal biomechanics of flatfoot deformities and related theories of bio-mechanical development. Clin Podiatr Med Surg 6(3):511–520, 1989.
2. Levitz SJ, Whiteside LS, Fitzgerald TA: Biomechanical foot therapy. Clin Podiatr Med Surg 5(3):721–736, 1988.
3. Root ML, Orien WP, Weed JH: Normal and Abnormal Function of the Foot. Los Angeles, Clinical Biomechanics Corporation, 1977.
4. Valmassy RL: Clinical Biomechanics of the Lower Extremity. St. Louis, Mosby 1996.

13

Trauma

Richard B. Birrer, MD and Michael P. DellaCorte, DPM

Injury to the foot and ankle from occupational and recreational activities is remarkably common. Sports produce higher injury rates; industry, more expensive and more serious injuries. The overall injury rate is 10–15 per 100 persons per year, most frequently involving the 17- to 44-year-old age group. Males are injured more often than females. The spectrum of injury includes abrasions and lacerations (30%), sprains and strains (23%), contusions (20%), fractures and dislocations (10%), burns (3%), and miscellaneous trauma, such as electrical or chemical injuries (14%).

While most injuries are mild to moderate in nature, severe injury to the foot may occur in association with life-threatening trauma to the patient (e.g., a motor vehicle accident). If the patient is seen during the first 20–30 minutes—the golden period—following trauma, symptoms and signs may be minimal to nonexistent. As time passes, symptoms, particularly pain, and signs such as edema and discoloration become more pronounced.

The management of the trauma patient begins with the ABCs of resuscitation (airway, breathing, and circulation) and continues with primary assessment and stabilization of life-threatening injuries (e.g., hemorrhage, sucking chest wounds, head injury). Failure to follow basic and advanced cardiac and trauma life support guidelines results in excessive morbidity and mortality. Focusing solely on pedal pathology without undressing the patient and considering nonpedal trauma may miss important associated injuries, such as entrance and exit wounds and vertebral fractures.

Once the patient is stabilized, a history of the injury should be obtained. Workers' compensation cases require an account of the injury in the patient's words. Useful questions include: What position was your foot in, relative to your body, when the injury occurred (i.e., inverted, everted, dorsiflexed, plantarflexed)? Did you hear or feel any snapping or cracking? Were you able to continue activities, or were you forced to stop because of the injury? What were you wearing on your feet at the time? (It is important to know if shoes and socks were worn and what type they were, because particles of these materials may have entered the wound during the injury if it was, for instance, a puncture wound.) Were you able to walk after the injury? Was there any treatment, and, if so, what were the results? Was the foot ever injured previously? The patient's medical and surgical history, including medications and allergies, also should be obtained and noted.

A detailed clinical examination of the foot follows. Too often lab tests and radiographs are ordered and interpreted as normal and the patient discharged without a thorough examination. The clinical evaluation should consist of inspection for problems such as erythema, ecchymosis, edema, abrasions, and breaks in the skin; palpation, checking trigger points, range of motion, and neurovascular status; and auscultation to evaluate osteophony.

Animal Bites

Lower extremity animal bites are a common cause of complaints in the physician's office (Table 1). Most animal bites come from do-

Table 1. Bite Wounds: Risk Factors for Complications

Age > 50 years
Severe crush injury and/or edema
Cat bites
Full-thickness puncture wounds
Wounds that require debridement
Hand, foot, or face wounds
Bone, tendon, joint, or ligament involvement
Wound adjacent to a prosthetic joint
Comorbid state: chronic hepatitis, embolism, presence of human immunodeficiency virus, acquired immunodeficiency disease, splenectomy, alcoholism

mestic animals and differ from human bites in that the wound contains fewer bacteria. Dogs bite less frequently than cats, but the wounds are more extensive. Cat bites become infected twice as frequently as dogs (30–40% versus 15–20%). Infection that develops in cat- and dog-bite wounds generally is due to *Pasteurella multocida.* Bite wounds developing infection after 24 hours are more likely to contain staphylococcus or streptococcus. *Capnocytophaga canimorsus* recently has been associated with dog and cat bites and sometimes leads to severe septic complications.

Treatment consists of meticulous scrubbing with a bacteriostatic agent, thorough irrigation, debridement if needed, and closure. Recent studies support primary closure of most cat- and dog-bite wounds that require repair. Puncture wounds and lacerations smaller than 1–2 cm in length should not be closed because they cannot be adequately cleaned. Bite wounds with extensive crush injuries, wounds requiring considerable amounts of debridement, and small lacerations (1–2 cm length) that are in cosmetically important locations are generally treated with delayed primary

Table 2. Tetanus Prophylaxis for Animal Bites

Over 2–3 days:
  Amoxicillin-clavulanate/Augmentin
  500/125 mg PO tid
                    or
  Penicillin VK 500 mg PO qid
                    or
  Doxycycline 100 mg PO q12 (for the penicillin-allergic patient)

closure, although no study has determined whether this results in a lower infection rate.

Tetanus prophylaxis should be given according to the guidelines in Table 2. A broad-spectrum oral antibiotic such as cephalexin, dicloxacillin, or erythromycin should be administered therapeutically—when there is contamination, associated disease such as diabetes, peripheral vascular disease, or immunosuppression, or when presentation is delayed longer than 8 hours—not prophylactically. Tetracycline covers *Pasteurella* and penicillin is good for *Capnocytophaga.* Antibiotics should not be used as a substitute for proper local wound care. Rabies vaccination is indicated in high-risk situations (e.g., bites by a raccoon, skunk, bat, fox, or an unhealthy cat or dog that is unavailable for a rabies check.

Injuries to Skin and Nails

Nail Avulsion

Partial or complete nail avulsion can be caused by indirect or direct trauma. In such cases, examine the nail bed. If it is badly lacerated, the first step is to repair it. Local anesthesia and a sterile suture tray are necessary. For the partially avulsed nail, there are two schools of thought on how to treat the injury. After x-rays have been taken to insure no bone involvement, either the nail is completely avulsed or it is put back in place and bandaged. Complete nail avulsion may cause more trauma to an already injured area. Leaving the nail on may allow it to act as a splint or guide for the new nail to follow. Some doctors feel that it may also create a deformed new nail because it blocks growth. We recommend that the amount of trauma be assessed, and if no anesthesia is necessary to avulse the nail completely, then do so; otherwise leave the nail and prescribe soaks. Re-evaluate in 2 days: if the nail is stable and asymptomatic, then leave it; if it is symptomatic, avulse it under local anesthesia.

Lacerations

The mechanism of injury is important in lacerations because it can indicate whether or not a foreign body is involved. Most glass is radiopaque, so x-rays may aid in evaluation. Treatment of a laceration associated with a foreign body consists of local anesthesia, probing and removal of any foreign bodies, and flushing of the wound. Prior to suturing the laceration, a follow-up x-ray to determine if all the foreign bodies have been removed is advised. Tetanus immunization status should be checked and tetanus toxoid 0.5 ml should be given intramuscularly (Table 3).

If the laceration does not involve any foreign bodies, after lavage, it should be sutured primarily. Simple interrupted sutures with 4-0 nylon are advised (see Chapter 20). They should remain clean and dry for 10–14 days. The wound should be examined 3, 7, and 14 days after injury for signs of infection. If the laceration is on the plantar surface of the foot, the patient should not bear any weight for 2 weeks to reduce pressure on the wound, avoiding gapping and suture disruption, and to minimize scar formation. Infected, dirty, or potentially infected lacerations should be left open to heal by secondary intention.

Note: For a discussion of **subungual hematoma,** refer to Chapter 5.

Injuries to Subcutaneous Tissue

Puncture wounds to the plantar surface of the foot often appear innocuous, but represent a diagnostic and therapeutic dilemma to the primary care physician. A total of 5.8% of lower extremity trauma involves a puncture injury,

Table 3. Guidelines for Antitetanus Treatment of Patients with Open Wounds

Tetanus Immunization History	Clean, Minor Wounds		All Other Wounds*	
	TD†	TIG	TD	TG
Unknown or 0–2 doses	Yes	No	Yes	Yes
Three or more doses	No‡	No	No§	No

TD = adult tetanus toxoid and diphtheria vaccine; TIG = tetanus immunoglobulin
* Dirty wounds include those contaminated with dirt, feces, soil, or saliva; puncture wounds; avulsions; and wounds from missiles, crushing trauma, frostbite, or burns.
† Give diphtheria-pertussis-tetanus vaccine if < 7 years old (or diphtheria-tetanus vaccine if pertussis is contraindicated).
‡ If > 10 years since last dose, give TD booster.
§ If > 5 years since last dose, give TD booster.
Adapted from Tetanus—United States, 1987 and 1988. MMWR 39:37–41, Jan 26, 1990.

with a seasonal variation favoring the warmer months. Nails are the most common wounding agent (98%), but other objects such as glass, metal, wood, sewing needles, and plastic also can be involved. Depth of penetration seems to be the most critical factor affecting outcome, although time to presentation and puncture in the metatarsophalangeal (MTP) joint area also are predictors of potential poor outcome.

Overall, puncture wounds have a low incidence of complications, but the difficulty in judging depth of penetration and the potential presence of retained foreign bodies place these wounds at a high risk. Complications include abscess cellulitis, granuloma, wound botulism, tetanus, osteomyelitis, pyarthrosis, and epidermal inclusion cyst. The infection rate appears to be 8–15%, and the incidence of osteomyelitis is less than 1%. A careful history (e.g., type of footwear and puncture object) and examination of the wound are indicated for injuries of less than 24 hours.

Puncture wounds should be managed by trimming of epidermal flaps, cleansing, and updating of the tetanus vaccination, if indicated (Table 4). Irrigation may be counterproductive, and probing for depth or a foreign body presence requires a regional nerve block and has an unknown false negative rate. Coring using a cuticle scissors, #11 scalpel blade, or 4-mm punch enhances drainage and visualization. Soft tissue radiographs, fluoroscopy, xerography, computed tomography (CT), or ultrasound should be obtained whenever there is question of a retained foreign body. Superficial foreign bodies can be soaked for a few days and then removed in the office with minimal anesthesia. The anesthesia should be placed proximal to the foreign body. If the injection is too close to the portal of entry, it may distort tissue architecture and float the foreign body. Deeper foreign bodies should be managed in the operating room, where the object can be triangulated by fluoroscopy (mini C arm) and surgically excised. Puncture wounds without lacerations should not be closed but, rather, allowed to granulate.

Antibiotics (e.g., broad-spectrum, anti-staphylococcal antibiotics such as cephalexin) for 7–10 days generally are reserved for high-risk wounds (Table 5). High-risk wounds include those untreated 24 hours after injury in patients with diabetes or peripheral vascular disease; those in patients presenting signs of local infection, draining tract, or gross contamination; or those suspected of having penetrated to bone joint space or plantar fascia.

Table 4. Management of Puncture Wounds

Type	Treatment	Comments
Superficial cutaneous	Cleansing twice daily with protective covering; non-weight bearing if painful or insensate foot	Clean wound
Subcutaneous or articular joint involvement with or without infection	Regional local anesthesia, sterile prep and drape, wound exploration and debridement. Gram stain with deep aerobic and anaerobic C&S; copious irrigation (1 L sterile H_2O); packing; twice daily cleansing with protective covering. Non-weight bearing with crutches.	Most common puncture wound (55–60%)
Established soft tissue infection including pyarthroses and retained foreign body	Repeated aspiration; surgical drainage if fluid rapidly accumulates or foreign body present. Deep cultures and sensitivities; IV antibiotics.	60% have retained foreign body. CBC and ESR may be unreliable; X-ray, bone scan helpful. Bone and joint involvement is serious complication
Foreign body penetration into bone	Surgical excision and drainage with curettage and debridement; IV antibiotics	Nail-gun injuries are common etiologies
Osteomyelitis	Surgical debridement, drainage, and biopsy. Antibiotics—IV aminoglycoside and antipseudomonal penicillin pending C&S for 6 weeks	0.6–1.8% incidence; average delayed diagnosis is 3 weeks; pseudomonas is common

C&S = culture and sensitivity, CBC = complete blood count, ESR = erythrocyte sedimentation rate

Table 5. Recommended Empiric Antibiotics for the Treatment of Soft Tissue Infection Secondary to Puncture Wounds

Antibiotic	Organism	Comment
Cefalexin	Gram (+) aerobes and anaerobes	Oral
Erythromycin	Gram (+) aerobes and anaerobes, gram (−) anaerobes	Oral
Clindamycin	Gram (+) and (−) anaerobes	Oral/IV
Dicloxacillin	Gram (+) aerobes	Oral
Amoxicillin/clavulanic acid	Gram (+) aerobes	Oral
Cefazolin	Gram (+) aerobes and anaerobes, gram (−) aerobe	IV
Ampicillin/sulbactam	Gram (+) aerobes and (−) anaerobes	IV
Ticarcillin/clavulanic acid	Gram (+) and (−) aerobes and anaerobes	IV
Vancomycin	Gram (+) and (−) aerobes	IV

The first dose should be administered intravenously, with nonweight-bearing status and 48-hour follow up arranged. If there is suspicion of joint space or plantar fascia penetration, particularly in wounds over the metatarsal heads, then the patient should be referred to a podiatric or orthopedic surgeon.

Common organisms are staphylococcus and alpha-hemolytic streptococci. Puncture wounds are clostridium-prone. Secondary infections occur in approximately 10% of all puncture wounds. Late presenters usually have an established wound infection. Oral antibiotics (e.g., antistaphylococcal penicillin) should be prescribed in conjunction with the above treatment modalities. Suspicion of a deep-space infection, failure of a cellulitis to respond to antibiotics, relapse, or a draining tract suggests a foreign body. More than 90% of osteomyelitis cases, a rare but serious complication, are caused by a Pseudomonas species derived from the inner layers of the soles of sneakers. A bone scan should be obtained rapidly because it is much more sensitive than radiographs early on.

Bursitis

A bursa is a sac or sac-like cavity that is filled with a viscous fluid and located at a frictional site in the tissues. An adventitial bursa is an abnormal bursa. Bursitis due to acute trauma or overuse often is found at the joints of the foot that are exposed to pressure from a shoe (Table 6). A highly inflamed bursa must be differentiated from infection, joint effusion, and arthritic conditions.

On examination, the area usually is elevated and circumscribed. Its surface can range from smooth and soft to firm with hyperkeratotic tissue. An acute bursa is tender to palpation and movement of the area, as well as erythematous and edematous with calor.

Treatment of acute bursitis includes elimination of the trauma and protection of the area from future irritation, aspiration, ice therapy, nonsteroidal anti-inflammatory drugs (NSAIDs), Burow's solution soaks, and injection therapy to relieve swelling and acute pain. Antibiotics are prescribed if there is a secondary infection present. In situations of chronic bursitis, surgical excision of the bursa and the underlying bone often is necessary. A consultation is warranted.

Contusion

A contusion is an injury to the soft tissue from a direct or indirect blow without disruption of the skin. Edema, erythema, ecchymosis, and warmth usually are present. Pain associated with palpation and occasionally with range of motion can occur. X-ray evaluation must be performed in order to rule out osseous pathology. The amount of visible ecchymosis or trauma does not correlate well with the possibility of fracture.

Treatment consists of rest, ice, compression, elevation, horseshoe padding, NSAIDs, analgesics, and possible non-weight bearing of the affected foot. Physical therapy should be started after the acute inflammation has subsided to reduce edema and increase painless range of motion and strength.

Dislocation

Pure dislocation is rare in the foot. The MTP joints are the ones most commonly involved in a pure dislocation. The proximal phalanx is displaced upward and backward in the vertical position, and the distal phalanx is flexed. X-ray evaluation confirms the diagnosis, with the lateral view revealing the proximal phalanx resting on the metatarsal head, and the dorsal plantar view showing the same plus a gun barrel sign of the proximal phalanx.

Immediate reduction is mandatory. Local anesthesia is administered proximal to the MTP joint on both sides of the involved metatarsal. After the area is blocked, a gauze pad is applied around the involved digit. Gripping the gauze pad and the toe firmly, the examiner pulls the toe upward and proximal; continuing the upward pull, the examiner then brings the toe distally (forward) and downward, back in place. Bone-to-bone contact, indicating that the upward distraction was not sufficient, should not be felt. Bone rubbing could also cause fractures and more trauma. A splint should be applied to the foot that will prevent recurrent hyperextension of the involved joint. Crutch walking for 2–3 weeks to prevent the

Table 6. Common Sites of Bursitis

Medial first metatarsophalangeal joint
Lateral fifth metatarsophalangeal joint
Lateral fifth metatarsal base
Dorsal interphalangeal joints of the toes
Navicular tuberosity
Plantar aspect metatarsal head
Posterior to the calcaneus (see Chapter 9)

toe-off stage of gait and further dislocation may be necessary. Physical therapy and a post-surgical shoe should be worn until symptoms resolve.

Trauma to Bone

Fractures of the foot and ankle make up 22% of all fractures, with the percentage exceeding 30% in the occupational setting.

Digital Fractures

Digital fractures generally are caused by direct trauma to the involved toe (Fig. 1). Left untreated, these fractures can result in malunion, painful bony prominences, and helomas. The most commonly fractured toe is the fifth toe. Stubbing the toe in bare or stocking feet is the usual cause. Clinically, the digit is ecchymotic, edematous, warm, and painful. Anteroposterior and lateral films demonstrate the fracture.

Treatment is determined by the degree or severity of the fracture and associated injury. A simple, nondisplaced digital fracture of the lesser digits can be treated by buddy splinting the fractured digit to the neighboring uninjured digit. Place a piece of gauze or cotton be-

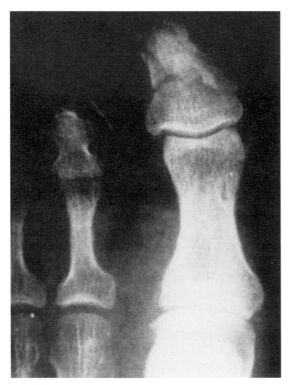

Figure 1. Nondisplaced fracture of the hallux at the distal phalanx.

tween the toes being splinted, and basket weave half-inch tape around the digits. It is important never to circumscribe the digits because the tape will act as a tourniquet around the toes and cut off circulation if there is further swelling. The basket weave, on the other hand, allows for expansion. Early ambulation in a protective shoe allows the majority of toe fractures to heal in 4–6 weeks. Amputation, however, may be necessary for fractures associated with severe crush injuries.

Careful follow-up is essential since a moderate degree of angulation or rotation of the toes produces functional disability. Posttraumatic arthritis and hammer toe deformity are perhaps the most significant disabilities and are best prevented by avoiding re-injury and carefully rehabilitating the injured foot in a progressive fashion.

Sesamoidal Fractures

The two sesamoids in the flexor hallucis brevis tendon can be fractured by direct trauma or hyperextension of the hallux. This is a common injury in athletes playing sports that require bearing weight on the toes (tennis) and in patients wearing high-heel shoes who are unaccustomed to them. The tibial sesamoid is fractured more often than the fibular (Fig. 2). Symptoms include pain, particularly when stair climbing and wearing high-heel shoes. There may be minimal to significant edema, trigger point tenderness, and tenderness and ecchymosis of the MTP joint. Contralateral x-rays are useful to rule out a congenital bipartite sesamoid. This is quite common and easily confused with a fracture (Table 7).

Treatment is determined by degree of injury. Nondisplaced fractures are treated with dispersion padding and low-heel shoes for 6 weeks. X-rays often will not demonstrate a union of the sesamoid; therefore, the degree of symptoms should determine if off-weight bearing and short-leg-cast immobilization are necessary. Displaced fractures should be casted and remain non-weight bearing for 4–6 weeks. If left untreated, sesamoid fractures may progress to painful nonunion, for which surgical excision should be considered.

Metatarsal Fractures

Metatarsal fractures (Figs. 3 and 4) may result from direct or indirect trauma. The site of the fracture (i.e., the epiphysis, metaphysis, di-

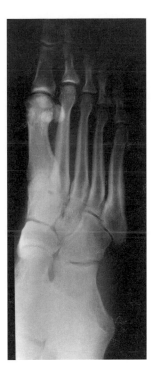

Figure 2. Fracture of the tibial sesamoid and proximal second phalanx following a crush injury.

aphysis, or joint) is important. The metaphyseal area has the best blood supply and therefore heals the quickest; the diaphysis and epiphysis have decreased vascularity, requiring longer immobilization. The diagnosis and degree of injury are determined by patient history, physical exam, and x-ray. Dorsal plantar, lateral, and oblique radiographic views are advised. The dorsal plantar x-ray shows transverse plane deviation, and the lateral demonstrates sagittal plane deviation. The five metatarsals are viewed as internal (2, 3, and 4), and external (1 and 5). The external metatarsals

Table 7. Criteria for Differentiating Multipartite Sesamoid From Sesamoid Fracture

Fracture	Multipartite
Bone callus formation	Similar findings in
Interrupted peripheral cortices	contralateral foot
	Smooth borders
Irregular, serrated, jagged separation lines	No callus formation
longitudinally or obliquely oriented division lines	

have a greater biomechanic demand (i.e., weight bearing) and generally need almost perfect alignment and rigid fixation.

Treatment should be geared to the age and physical condition of the patient. For the nondisplaced fracture without associated crush injury, a short leg cast is indicated for 4–6 weeks. The Unna boot and Ace bandage along with a shoe with a rigid shank or sole (Reece) for 4–6 weeks can be used on those patients who cannot tolerate a cast. Dorsally or plantarly displaced, angulated, or multiple metatarsal fractures, fracture dislocations, or extensive crush injuries with no bone-to-bone contact and gapping greater than 4 mm should be taken to the operating room for open reduction and internal fixation, if closed reduction fails. Fasciotomy, along with other soft tissue releases, may be required to reduce the fracture. Hospitalization and close observation are essential. If these fractures are not fixated and the patient is allowed to ambulate in a soft cast (Unna boot), the unstable distal metatarsal becomes dorsally displaced. Once healed in this position, it will bear minimal weight, subjecting the patient to possible plantar helomas under the other metatarsals now bearing more weight.

Fifth Metatarsal Fractures

There are three distinct types of fracture to the fifth metatarsal.

Type I is an acute fracture without evidence of pre-existing injury. It is subdivided into nondisplaced and displaced. Nondisplaced type I fractures are treated with a short, weight-bearing leg cast for 4–6 weeks. Displaced type I fractures should be referred for open reduction and external fixation.

Type II or the Jones fracture is a transverse, usually nondisplaced fracture of the proximal diaphyseal area, with evidence of pre-existing injury. If the individual is sedentary for the most part, a non-weight bearing cast for 6–12 weeks is appropriate. If the patient is a high-performance athlete and intramedullary stenosis is present, then referral for possible screw fixation is warranted because pseudoarthrosis occurs in 10–15% of cases. If there is no sclerosis evident, prescribe a non-weight bearing cast until the pain subsides and bony union is evident. A molded arch support in a snug shoe after casting is desirable, followed by return to play when there is clinical and radiographic evidence of union.

Type III injury involves extra-articular or

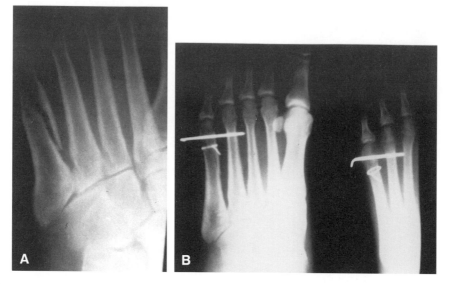

Figure 3. *A*, Fracture of fifth metatarsal. *B*, Open reduction with internal fixation.

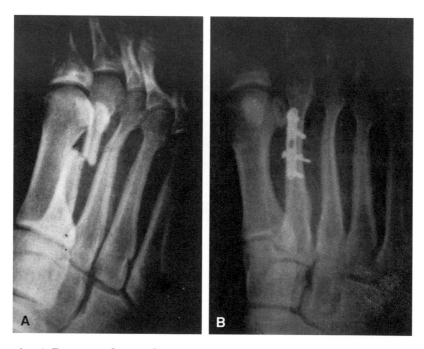

Figure 4. *A*, Fracture of second metatarsal. *B*, Open reduction with internal fixation.

intra-articular fracture of the styloid process. These are avulsion-type fractures of the metatarsal base caused by the peroneus brevis during inversion sprains. The former is managed by forefoot strapping and arch support until asymptomatic. The latter is aggressively managed in an athlete by surgical referral, or handled like a type II for a more sedentary patient.

Cuneiform Fracture

These fractures follow direct trauma and usually are associated with other injuries. The medial cuneiform is most likely to be affected. Treatment consists of compression dressing or casting, depending on the severity of the fracture. A specialist should be consulted.

Navicular Fracture

Watson-Jones classified navicular fractures into three categories: type I, fracture of the tuberosity; type II, fracture of the dorsal lip; and type III, transverse body fracture. These fractures can be caused by forceful eversion of the foot or direct trauma. It is important to distinguish tuberosity fractures from the presence of an os tibial externum, an accessory bone on the medial aspect of the navicular. Comparison x-rays are indicated, because the accessory bone is present bilaterally. Treatment consists of a non-weight bearing, short leg cast for 4–6 weeks, depending on the severity of the injury. Open reduction with internal fixation may be indicated. After immobilization, foot orthotics may be necessary.

Cuboid Fracture

This is an uncommon fracture usually resulting from compression forces or direct trauma (Fig. 5). Conservative treatment consists of cast immobilization from 4–6 weeks. A specialist should be consulted.

Talar Fracture

Although the primary care physician probably will not treat talar fractures, recognition is necessary before a specialist is consulted. The most common fractures involve the dome, neck, or body, although combination injuries

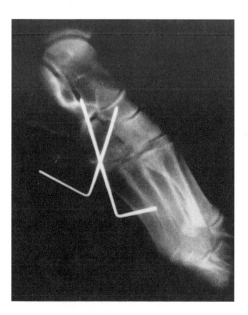

Figure 5. Cuboid fracture fixated with cross Kirschner wires.

(fractures, dislocations) are not uncommon. Talar fractures usually are associated with ankle injuries.

Talar Dome

Berndt-Harty has classified talar dome fractures into four stages: stage I, subchondral bone compression; stage II, partial detached fragment; stage III, completely detached non-displaced fragment; stage IV, completely detached displaced fragment. The mechanism of injury is inversion. The patient presents an ankle sprain that does not respond to conservative treatment. Dome fractures are difficult to visualize on standard x-ray views; a computed tomography (CT) scan or magnetic resonance image (MRI) is needed for definitive diagnosis. Treatment may involve casting, arthroscopy, and/or surgical excision of any loose fragments. A specialist should be consulted.

Talar Neck

Talar neck fractures can be caused by car accidents, falls from heights, direct trauma from falling objects, or athletic injuries. The Hawkins classification for talar neck fractures is as follows: type I, vertical fracture through the talar neck without displacement of the talar body; type II, vertical fracture through the neck with subtalar joint subluxation or dislocation; type III, vertical fracture of talar with displacement of the talar body from the subtalar and tibiotalar joint; and type IV, vertical fracture of the talar neck with talar body displacement from both subtalar and tibiotalar joint and subluxation and/or dislocation of the talar head from the talonavicular joint.

The probability of avascular necrosis of the talus increases greatly from Type I to IV. Treatment ranges from casting to open reduction depending on the degree of fracture. The average length of casting is 8–14 weeks. A specialist should be consulted.

Talar Body

Talar body fractures are not as common as talar neck fractures, and the prognosis is not as good. A small amount of incongruity caused by the injury may cause a step deformity and subsequent posttraumatic arthritis. Anatomic reduction should be attempted by a specialist, but even with good reduction, a painless joint may never be restored. Initial treatment ranges from casting to open reduction. Long-term management may require joint fusion.

Calcaneal Fracture

Calcaneal fractures (Fig. 6) are the most common of all tarsal fractures, with an incidence of approximately 60%. The thin, outer cortical shell and soft cancellous bone of the calcaneus make it easily susceptible to traumatic injuries. The majority of fractures are caused by falls from a height. Rapid egress from an upper floor window with a subsequent fall and os calcis fracture has been termed "lover's heel." Calcaneal fractures have a high incidence of associated injuries involving the spine, femur, fibula, tibia, talus, ulna, and radius.

As with most fractures, there are many classifications. On conventional radiographs, Rowe's classification of calcaneal fractures is as follows: type I, fractures of the tuberosity, the sustentaculum tali, and the anterior process; type II, beak fractures and avulsion fractures of the Achilles tendon insertion; type III, oblique fractures not involving the subtalar joint; type IV, fractures involving the subtalar joint; and type V, central depression fractures with varying degrees of comminution.

Presently almost all calcaneal fractures are evaluated with a CT scan prior to initiating treatment. The complex nature and prognosis of calcaneal fractures requires the expertise of a specialist.

Ankle Fractures

The mechanism of injury and the structures involved in ankle fractures have been classified by Lauge-Hansen. There are two terms that describe each injury. The first term describes the position of the foot at the time of injury, and the second refers to the direction

of the pathologic forces being applied to the talus (the position of the leg).

Supination adduction trauma causes a transverse avulsion fracture of the fibula at or below the ankle or a rupture of the lateral collateral ligaments (stage I). If the pathologic force continues, an oblique-to-vertical fracture of the medial malleolus occurs (stage II).

Supination eversion (supination-external rotation) injuries begin with rupture of the anterior inferior tibiofibular ligament (stage I). As the pathologic force continues, there is a spiral oblique fracture of the fibula beginning at the ankle joint (stage II) (Fig. 7), posterior inferior tibiofibular ligament rupture or posterior malleolar fracture (stage III), and finally medial malleolar fracture or deltoid ligament rupture (stage IV).

Pronation abduction trauma causes a transverse fracture of the medial malleolus or rupture of the deltoid ligament (stage I). If the pathologic force continues, a rupture of the anterior and posterior inferior tibiofibular ligaments occurs or there are avulsion fractures at the ligamentous attachment of the anterior and posterior inferior tibiofibular ligaments (stage II). Further progression to stage III causes a short oblique fracture to the fibula.

Pronation-eversion (pronation-external rotation) injury begins at the medial malleolus and as the pathologic force continues the injury progresses as follows: transverse avulsion fracture of the medial malleolus or rupture of the deltoid ligaments (stage I), rupture of the anterior inferior tibiofibular ligament and interosseous membrane (stage II), high spiral oblique fracture of the fibula (proximal extent of fracture depends on how high the interosseous ligament is ruptured) (stage III), and rupture of the posterior inferior tibiofibular ligament or avulsion fracture of the posterior malleolus (stage IV).

Stable injuries consist of one break in the mortise ring; unstable injuries consist of two or more breaks that may be any combination of fractures and ligament injuries. Symptoms include an audible pop or crack, abrupt moderate-to-severe pain and swelling, immediate disability, and delayed discoloration. Clinical signs consist of localized point tenderness, edema, positive osteophony and tuning fork tests, possible crepitus, and ecchymosis. Associated trauma (i.e., ligamentous injury) should be suspected and diligently searched for. Results of the clinical evaluation may be very similar to those associated with a sprain of the ankle. Anteroposterior, lateral, and

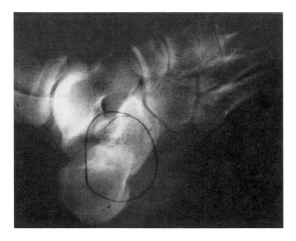

Figure 6.   Calcaneal fracture.

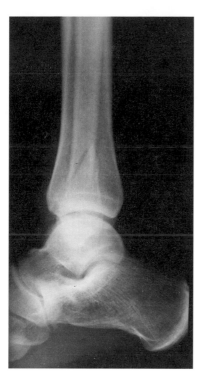

Figure 7. Spiral fracture of the distal fibula associated with a deltoid ligament tear.

mortise views are usually adequate to make the diagnosis.

Stable injuries resulting from a single fracture or ligament tear require no reduction and can be treated with a posterior splint and the RICE (rest, ice, compression, elevation) regimen, followed by a walking cast for 4–6 weeks. Unstable injuries due to a sprain, a fracture, or various combinations thereof require reduction, and a specialist should be consulted. Initially, closed manipulation, with or without local or general anesthesia, and muscle relaxants may be successful; however, open reduction often is required. Closed reduction is performed in three steps—exaggeration of the mechanism of injury, traction, and reversal of the mechanism of injury. A postreduction radiograph is essential.

The medial portion of a fibular fracture at the syndesmosis unites rapidly, though the lateral half is slower or often does not heal at all due to the interdisposition of a narrow strip of periosteum from the proximal fragment falling into the fracture line. Similarly, small avulsion fragments from the tip of the lateral malleolus, or laterally angulated comminuted fracture chips, often do not reunite and serve as a source of localized osteoarthritis. Small distal fragments of the medial malleolus tend to be less easily reduced and are a source of frequent nonunion. Fractures of the lateral tibial margin (i.e., Tillaux fractures) are a frequent source of nonunion or malunion. Posterior tibial margin fractures usually heal well, with a return of good function. One exception involves fracture of more than one third of the tibial articular surface, in which the displaced surface of the talus and tibia results in damage to the articular surface of the mortise. Despite good reduction, osteoarthritis is a frequent sequela. Compression fractures often lead to degenerative joint disease due to the profound amount of damage to the involved articular surfaces, disruption of blood supply, and infection if the fracture is open. Therefore, ongoing clinical evaluation, including radiographic examination for unstable fractures by a consultant, is essential.

Isometric exercises and a plaster cast or early range-of-motion exercises in a hinge cast minimize the harmful effects of immobilization (e.g., stiffness and muscle atrophy). Internal fixation devices generally should be removed before the athlete is allowed to return to play in contact sports. Unstable injuries tend to have a very high incidence of complication (e.g., traumatic arthritis, persistent talar instability, Sudeck's atrophy, or ossification of the interosseous membrane).

Small fragments of subchondral bone and overlying membrane cartilage can be separated from the talar dome due to compression or repetitive shearing–type loads, particularly in forced plantarflexion (e.g., a missed jump). The lesion may be located anywhere on the talar dome, but commonly involves the superomedial and lateral margins. Such injuries tend to be unilateral and often are associated with old sprains, although the cause-and-effect relationship has not been definitely established. There is a gradual onset of pain, which becomes worse over weeks and even months, intensifies with exercise, and usually causes ankle stiffness or locking. The clinical exam is, for the most part, unremarkable, except that palpation of the talar dome with the ankle in plantarflexion elicits point tenderness. Although special radiographic views may visualize the lesion, radioisotope or CT studies produce the best results. Osteonecrotic fragments tend to be unilateral, whereas osteochondritis dissecans tends to be bilateral. Arthroscopy and arthrography also are useful. Consultation should be considered because the incidence of disabling traumatic arthritis is high.

Stress Fracture

At least 30% of all stress fractures occur in the ankle and foot—up to 30% in the lateral malleolus and about 50% in the metatarsals. Repetitive microtrauma from running activities, in combination with malalignment, overweight condition, old shoes, hard surfaces, and overtraining, is a risk factor. There is a well-known correlation between this injury and eating disorders, menstrual dysfunction, and osteoporosis.

Suspect the diagnosis if there is pain on deep palpation; verify it with an x-ray study, CT scan, bone scan, or MRI. Lateral ankle pain may suggest a peroneal tendonitis or a sprain, but the onset of localized firm swelling should suggest the diagnosis. Rest with a slowly progressive training program within the limits of pain is the treatment of choice. Aquatic exercise should be considered. Underlying eating or menstrual disorders must be managed.

Tenderness and soft tissue swelling about the distal fibular epiphysis must be considered a type I Salter-Harris fracture in a youngster following trauma (see Chapter 10). Although radiographs may be normal, immobilization in a short leg cast for 4–5 weeks is appropriate. Tarsal navicular stress fracture requires immobilization for 6–8 weeks; initially, only touch-down weight bearing is allowed. Nonunion is not infrequent.

Metatarsal Stress Fracture

A stress fracture, also known as march fracture or Deutschlander's disease, is an overuse injury. Order of fracture is second, third, first, fourth, fifth metatarsal. The second and third metatarsals break midshaft and neck, whereas the first breaks proximally, the fourth breaks at the distal diaphysis, and the fifth breaks at the base, rarely the shaft. The history is notable for a change in distance, technique, training, or footwear and the absence of a traumatic event. Mild, dull pain occurs, gradually increases, and becomes incapacitating with continued activity. The foot becomes edematous and erythematous after 10–15 days. Direct palpation, dorsiflexion, or the tuning fork test causes localized pain.

X-ray evaluation in the early stages is negative; therefore it should be repeated in 10–14 days. Radiographic findings range from cortical interruptions, to thickening and callus formation around the fracture, to a complete break in the cortex. If repeat films are negative and a stress fracture is suspected, then a bone scan is indicated. The bone scan will be "hot" in the area of the fracture. The differential diagnosis includes bursitis, stone bruise, and metatarsalgia of other etiologies.

Treatment consists of NSAIDs, analgesics as needed, and a soft cast (Unna boot) wooden shoe, steel spring insert, or a Jones compression bandage for 4–6 weeks. Off-weight bearing with crutches and a short, weight-bearing leg cast thereafter may be necessary if a postoperative shoe cannot be tolerated. Gradual return to activities is then appropriate.

Combination Injuries

The potential for multiple injuries involving ligament, tendon, bone, and subcutaneous tissue is great in the trauma patient. Heightened vigilance can detect ligamentous injury with an unstable mortise or an avulsion fracture following a sprain. Such injuries should be managed in conjunction with a specialist. Tetanus immunization and antibiotics should be initiated if the clinical situation warrants.

Environmental Injuries
Burns

Collectively, the feet and ankles represent 10% of the body surface area. Because the feet are critical to all ambulatory activities, a burn can produce a disproportionate amount of disability. For one reason or another, burns of the feet often are overlooked and minimally rehabilitated. The result is a significant degree of lost wages and productivity.

Burns can occur from a variety of agents: chemicals, electricity, radiation, and thermal sources. The extent of the injury is primarily determined by the intensity and duration of contact. Less important factors, but nonetheless contributory to the overall severity of the burn, include the patient's age and health status and environmental factors such as protective gear. The details of the treatment plan depend on the type of injury agent.

Common causes of thermal burns include scalding, contact with a heat source, and fire. The individual with peripheral vascular disease due to atherosclerosis or neuropathy in association with diabetes can easily suffer contact burns from a hot water bottle due to impaired sensation. A common childhood accident is scalding by hot water. However, note that the possibility of child abuse always should be considered in any child who has suffered a symmetrical burn with a distinct line of demarcation, as from immersion. A classic child abuse scalding pattern involves the hands, feet, and buttocks. Cigarette and cigar burns have been seen on the soles of the feet, as well.

The foot frequently is involved when an electric burn occurs, serving as a site for entrance or exit of the current (e.g., from high-voltage lines, lightning strikes). The amount of injury is determined by the voltage (low versus high tension), amperage, current type (alternating current [AC] versus direct current [DC]), area of the body through which the current passes, duration, resistance of body tissue structures, and environmental factors such as water and rubber insulation. More damage occurs following contact with an AC current due to tetanic muscle contractions, which cause localized necrosis, and the fact that the victim generally is holding onto the current source.

The electric current may enter through the feet, pass through the trunk, and exit through the head, digits, or upper extremity, or vice versa. A zone of grey-white necrosis surrounding a central area of charring characterizes the entry site. A more peripheral circumferential zone is hyperemic and ischemic. Clinical signs of the exit site may be absent, but there often is extensive underlying soft-tissue and organ damage. Typically there is thrombosis of vessels, rupture of muscles, and fracture of bones. Each of the body tissues presents a different level of resistance. In diminishing order of resistance they are: skin, bone, fat, tendon, muscle, blood vessel, and nerve. The thickness of the skin enhances or detracts from resistance. With increasing amounts of resistance, greater amounts of thermal injury are induced.

Chemical injuries to the foot occur by a number of pathogenic mechanisms. Depending on the agent, there may be coagulation or liquefaction by oxidation, salt formation, corrosion, reduction, metabolic competitive inhibition, desiccation, or protoplasmic poisoning. These reactions are accompanied by a variable degree of thermal activity. The type and amount of agent, duration of contact, and local conditions determine the severity of the injury. One common cause of chemical burn is patient application of over-the-counter "corn remedies" made of salicylic acid. These can cause significant chemical burns that are especially serious in the patient with vascular impairment.

Lastly, radiation causes burns through its damage to cells by ionization. The amount of damage is related to the type of radiation (alpha, beta, or gamma particles, with the latter being the most penetrating), and the amount and duration of exposure. Acutely, death usually is due to the systemic effect of bone marrow suppression and gastrointestinal toxicity. Prolonged exposure over many years causes a number of pathologic changes, including fibrotic scarring, endarteritis obliterans, and chromosomal changes at the cellular level. The most feared development is that of neoplasia. For this reason, a full-thickness skin biopsy should be performed on suspicious lesions following radiation injury.

The management of acute burn begins with stabilization of the patient: the basic ABCs of life support. Then detailed information about the type of agent, time of occurrence, and how the burn occurred should be obtained. Rough estimates should be made of body surface area burned and depth and extent of injury. It is difficult to assess burn depth accurately. The old classification system of first, second, and third degree can be replaced by the more useful partial- and full-thickness classifications. There is no simple method to determine whether the depth is partial or full because such injuries are dynamically progressive. Careful inspection and testing for sensation by pinprick provides reasonably accurate information. A waxy appearance of skin with a denuded epidermis is highly suggestive of a full-thickness burn. An erythematous area responsive to pinprick is considered a partial-thickness injury; it can produce enough edema around the eschar to produce circulatory embarrassment.

With the exception of first-degree, partial-thickness injury, all patients with burns of the feet should be admitted to the hospital. Escharotomy often is necessary, and the dependent nature of the foot predisposes it to poor healing, infection, and circulatory compromise. The burn should be evaluated, analgesics and adequate fluids provided, tetanus prophylaxis administered according to the hospital's burn protocol, and diligent wound care begun. Cooling of the burned area with water of approximately 77° F (25° C) for 30–45 minutes is probably the safest cooling method. Systemic hypothermia, which can result from application of very cold water or ice, should be avoided because it may increase the depth and extent of necrosis.

Drying of the wound should be avoided. Vesicles should be left intact; if tense, they can be aspirated with the overlying epidermis left in place. Debridement of less necrotic tissue is acceptable, but excessive tissue removal should not occur. A protective covering of hydroactive gel, petrolatum, or antiseptic ointment (e.g., DuoDerm, Xeroform) can be used in a superficial partial-thickness injury. Deep partial-thickness or full-thickness wounds must be protected from bacteria contamination due to overlying necrosis. Such wounds should be handled in consultation with a surgeon. Grafting can be done immediately following an escharotomy, or it can be delayed. The use of antibiotic therapy depends on the severity of the burn, the overall health status of the patient, and the presence of complications (e.g., inhalation injury).

Neither topical nor systemic antibiotic therapy in burn wound management is obligatory. Usually one of the topical antibiotics—silver nitrate, mafenide acetate (Sulfamylon), silver sulfadiazine (Silvadene)—is used, although none of the three is more efficacious than the other. Up to 7% of patients are hypersensitive to mafenide acetate, which is painful on administration. Silver sulfadiazine has been known to produce neutropenia in a small number of hypersensitive individuals. Silver nitrate can cause methemoglobinemia and, of course, a profound amount of staining. It is important that serial local and systemic cultures be taken to determine the type and significance of secondary infection in the burn patient.

The total management of the burn patient consists of adequate and early rehabilitation to prevent contracture formation. Because most burns occur on the dorsum of the foot, contractures result in hyperextension and dorsiflexion of the MTP joints. Less commonly, plantar surface burns can cause deformities of the foot and toes in equinus and flexion. Such contractures follow deep partial-thickness and full-thickness burns or full-thickness burns to which autografts have been applied. Rehabilitation, when properly performed, begins during the initial care of the burn wound with the application and construction of a splint that helps prevent equinus deformity. Thereafter, a molded shoe with sufficient padding to oppose the contractile forces of the wound must be constructed to reduce scarring and fibrosis. Lastly, a carefully tailored exercise program involving passive and active range of motion is essential. Surgical reconstruction is reserved for those burns that have not responded to rehabilitation or have been subject to incomplete rehabilitation.

A brief mention should be made of the treatment for electric burns. During the acute stage, immediate escharotomy and decompressive fasciotomy are essential, particularly for high-tension injuries. These are the best methods for controlling ischemia in the electrically injured foot. When the patient's condition has stabilized, all necrotic tissue should be carefully debrided. The debridement should be performed cautiously because the full extent of the damage may be evident only after several days, particularly in the case of nerve injury.

With few exceptions (e.g., sodium metal), the application of liberal amounts of water is the best and most effective treatment for chemical injury. The use of neutralizing agents, such as a weak base for an acid or vice versa, is not to be condoned because an exothermic reaction may result, causing further damage.

Cold Injuries

As with burns, the severity and extent of tissue damage to the foot by cold temperature is proportional to the duration of exposure, the ambient temperature and humidity, the presence of environmental factors such as stockings and footwear, the overall health and activity level of the individual, and the usage of drugs such as alcohol or nicotine. Persons with Raynaud's disease or peripheral vascular disease are at increased risk.

Limited cold exposure can cause acute frostbite of the forefoot. The indigent alcoholic and the elderly, particularly in the inner city, typically are affected. The patient complains of paresthesias and a cold, numb foot with waxy skin that becomes tingling and throbbing when warmed. Treatment consists of slow, progressive thawing by passive measures such as blankets and covers of warm water 40–42° C (100–104° F). Late sequelae of frostbite include vasomotor instability in mild cases (e.g., hyperhidrosis, paresthesias) and necrosis, loss of digits, and contracture formation in severe frostbite (Fig. 8).

Related conditions include chilblains (pernio), trench foot, and immersion foot. The latter conditions were described during the world wars, although they can be seen in outdoor enthusiasts (e.g., hunters and boaters). Freezing temperatures are not required in any of these conditions. Pathophysiologically, there is chronic injury to the sympathetic nerves and the microcirculation. Trench foot usually oc-

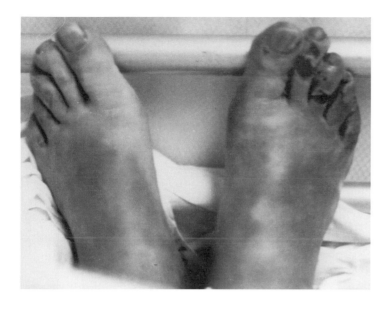

Figure 8. Necrosis and gangrene of toes following an alcoholic stupor which the patient spent in a snowdrift.

curs during limited activity in a confined space such as a foxhole in cold, damp weather. After several days there is blanching of the foot, dusky cyanosis, superficial blister formation, and pain. With longer degree of exposure, there is loss of the range of motion of the toes, diminution of sensation, and possible formation of gangrene. Immersion of the foot allows prolonged exposure to a cold, wet environment. Necrosis and maceration of the skin of the foot and leg are more significant than that seen in trench foot. Sequelae are similar though usually more severe. Treatment is supportive with conservative debridement, control of infections, rest, elevation, early rehabilitation, and prevention of further exposure.

Industrial and Occupational Foot Injuries

Numerous reports have estimated that 9–16% of occupational injuries involve the foot and ankle. The amount of compensation dollars for lost work productivity exceeds $1.2 billion each year. The majority of these injuries occur in workers doing heavy labor (49%), with the next largest single group being carpenters, who make up about 10% of the total. According to the 1977 Canadian Injury Survey of Foot and Ankle Injuries, the distribution was: ankle (32%), heel (6%), sole (6%), toes (25%), and metatarsal region (31%). The majority of such injuries occur in young, inexperienced workers, with males sustaining injuries six times more frequently than females. The type of injury is equally distributed between the genders. Twenty-five to 30% of these injuries are secondary to slips or falls, particularly while the worker is hurrying.

The recovery from a workers' compensation injury often is prolonged due to a number of psychological factors: it is difficult to resume a regular work schedule following a prolonged absence; there usually is increased pain upon return to work; the patient, through lack of understanding, often equates increased pain with increased damage and the possibility of permanent injury; and compensation payments often equal or exceed after-tax employment salary.

Regional Injuries

Toe

The majority of toe injuries occur from objects falling on the foot. The spectrum of trauma ranges from minor soft tissue contusions to severe crush injury of the phalanges. The distal phalanx of the first toe has the highest incidence of fracture injury, followed by the first metatarsal; combined, these two areas represent 50% of fractures. The fifth metatarsal is fractured 25% of the time, and the middle three metatarsal rays the remaining 25% of the time. The metatarsals also may be injured during forced plantarflexion and inversion through direct trauma—as from a blow, the most common etiology. Severe injuries, such as fracture dislocation at the tarsometatarsal joint (Lisfranc's fracture), fracture dislocation through the midtarsal joint (Chopart's fracture), and anterior crush injury, are rare. Most commonly there is soft tissue contusion, hemorrhage into the extensor digitorium brevis, and traumatic synovitis of the dorsal tendon sheaths.

Heel

Injuries to the heel are relatively uncommon in the industrial setting. The typical etiology is a fall (e.g., firemen and structural steel workers) or repetitive microtrauma (e.g., in military and marching band personnel) on a hard, nonresilient surface during ambulation. The majority of such injuries involve contusions and possibly bursitis in the heel pad, resulting in chronic fibrotic scarring that can be a continual source of pain. Such injuries must be distinguished from plantar fasciitis arising at the anterior border of the calcaneal tuberosity, which also can result from industrial injury, principally due to poorly fitting shoe wear and prolonged periods of standing and/or ambulation (see Chapter 9). Calcaneal fractures have a poor prognosis regardless of treatment methodology. An orthopedic surgeon or podiatric surgeon should be consulted.

Plantar Region

Under ideal conditions in the industrial setting, injuries to the sole of the foot are relatively uncommon due to safety boots with rigid steel shanks. Before the requirement that these boots be recommended, the incidence of puncture wounds was often as high as 30–40% of all foot injuries in construction laborers; it has now fallen to 5–8%. Unlike puncture wounds, deep plantar lacerations rarely occur and should be seen in consultation. Isolated tendon lacerations, with the exception of the flexor hallucis longus, can be repaired by the primary care physician.

Ankle

Like the dorsum of the foot, the ankle frequently is injured in the industrial setting. The etiology is a slip or trip in 50% of situations. A blow from a moving object can cause soft tissue damage, and, because of the exposed nature of the ankle above the shoe line, lacerations and burns are quite common. Fractures occur uncommonly (2–4%). "Aviator's astragalus" is fracture of the neck of the talus following a head-on crash, as originally described in British aircraft during World War I. Flexion from pressure of a rudder bar beneath the forefoot forces the talus against the anterior margin of the tibia. The respective injury can be treated according to the severity (see "Talar Fracture," page 119). Early rehabilitation of ankle injuries is essential. Note that there typically is an extended period of pain following an ankle injury.

Protection and Prevention

Of foremost concern in the podiatric management of industrial injuries is protection and prevention. The American National Standard Institute regularly publishes safety shoe guidelines. A steel toe-cap capable of sustaining a force of 75 foot-pounds is required, because 30–35% of industrial foot injuries are caused by falling objects (equipment or construction material). Currently, steel shanks are not mandatory in the United States—a number of puncture-proof devices are being constructed, but so far, no satisfactory alternate protection has been found. Other characteristics of sole design that are recommended include materials that are resistant to slippage and are nonconductive. Due to their continuous use and exposure to destructive environmental conditions, the average life expectancy for a safety shoe is about 6 months, at which time shoe wear must be replaced to be effective. The shoes in North America do not include a metatarsal shield to protect against falling objects, but such shields are recommended for steel and foundry workers and for loggers and workers in the pulp and paper industry. High boots, while decreasing the frequency of lateral ankle injuries due to direct blunt trauma, do not have a similar effect on these injuries resulting from indirect trauma.

In addition to the proper shoe wear, a number of safety measures should be undertaken. The floor and the workplace should be kept as clean and dry as possible. Rubber matting, abrasive strips, and carpeting drastically reduce slippage. Removal of nail-ridden lumber markedly reduces puncture wounds. Specific problems inherent in each department must be addressed. For instance, the proper precautions must be taken in the handling of hot fluids, chemicals, and high-voltage lines. The amount of time a worker spends on his or her feet should be addressed since prolonged standing or walking, even with a comfortable and well-fitting shoe, can produce fatigue, backache, and calluses, and also can lead to an accident.

Consideration for safety must extend to the home environment. More often than not, the use of safety equipment stops once the individual leaves the work environment. The major offender at home is the power lawn mower. The regular use of the steel-toe safety shoe prevents the majority of such injuries. Less commonly used, but equally dangerous, is the chain saw. Poor visualization, inadequate footwear, and improper technique are the usual villains in such accidents. Some workers are reluctant to use steel-toe shoes because of the possibility that a serious blow to the shoe can cause a guillotine effect—crushing or even severing the distal foot. The benefits of the protection afforded by these shoes far outweigh this risk.

══

References

1. Brackenbury PH, Muwanga C: A comparative double blind study of amoxicillin/clavulante vs. placebo in the prevention of infection after animal bites. Arch Emerg Med 6:251, 1989.
2. Brook JW: Management of pedal puncture wounds. J Foot Ankle Surg 33(5):463–466, 1994.
3. Callahan M: Controversial in antibiotic choices for bite wounds. Ann Emerg Med 12:1321–1330, 1988.
4. Chisholm CD, Schlesser JF: Plantar puncture wounds: Controversies and treatment recommendations. Am Emerg Med 18(12):1352–1356, 1989.
5. Cracehiolo A III: Office treatment of adult foot problems. Orthop Clin North Am 13:511–524, 1982.
6. Dire DJ: Management of animal bites. J Arkansas Med Soc 1(2):178–180, 1994.
7. Lavery LA, Armstrong DG, Quebedeaux TL, et al: Puncture wounds: Normal laboratory values in the face of severe infection in diabetics and non-diabetics. Am J Med 101:521–525, 1996.
8. Lewis KT, Stiles M: Management of cat and dog bites. Am Fam Physician 52(2):479–485, 489–490, 1995.
9. Paley D, Hall H: Calcaneal fracture controversies: Can we put Humpty Dumpty together again? Orthop Clin North Am 20(4):665–678, 1989.
10. Perlman MD, Leveille D, Gale B: Traumatic classification of the foot and ankle. J Foot Surg 28(6):551–585, 1989.
11. Resmick CD, Fallat LM: Puncture wounds: Therapeutic considerations and a new classification. J Foot Surg 29(2):147–153, 1990.

14

Sports Medicine

Richard Birrer, MD and Michael DellaCorte, DPM

Fifty-five to 90% of sports-related injuries occur to the lower extremity, and 15% affect the foot alone (Table 1). The physical forces and stresses to the tissues of the foot and ankle are increased two to three times during athletic activities. Foot problems are common in athletes who run, jump, and kick and in infrequent exercisers who are mostly sedentary during the work week (weekend warriors). Nine percent of injuries are associated with tennis, 11–26% with running, 4–8% with basketball, 8–14% with cycling, and 6% with volley ball. Foot injuries due to running are caused by factors that influence the distribution of the load: body weight, anatomic features, shoes, running surface, technique, and running program. Knowledge of the normal biomechanics of running (see Chapter 1) helps in preventing these injuries.

Foot injuries are not unique to sports, but they are more common in athletes. The ankle sprain is probably the single most common sports injury. Aside from structural or biomechanic abnormalities, the most common etiologies of sports-related injuries to the foot and ankle are:

1. Rapid or improper warm-up
2. Overuse or excessive training
3. Intense workouts
4. Improper footwear
5. Hardness of playing surfaces.

In addition to the routine history and physical examination, sports-related questions should be asked to elicit information about possible etiology. What is your warm-up or stretch routine? What sports do you play? How often do you play? How long do you play? What type of athletic shoes do you wear? What surfaces do you play on? Once the etiology is determined, the patient may have to be instructed to modify his/her training routine or sport to avoid further injury. The goal of treatment is to get the athlete back to the playing field as rapidly as possible and to avoid reinjury.

Sports Injuries

Black Toe (Runner's Toe)

This condition is caused by increased pressure or friction to the toenail, leading to a subungual hematoma, partial nail avulsion, or both. Symptoms include pain and burning. Clinical signs are a black or purple toenail, with or without lifting of the distal aspect of the toenail (Fig. 1). Treatment consists of drainage of the subungual hematoma (see Chapter 5), nonsteroidal anti-inflammatory drugs (NSAIDs), and soaks as needed. Also, the patient should be instructed to check his or her athletic shoes for proper size and adequate toe box to avoid further injuries.

Black Heel

Black heel, also termed calcaneal petechiae pseudochromadrosis plantaris, or jumper's or tennis heel, is characterized by variable coalescence of punctate, black dots that appear suddenly on the sides of the heels. The condition usually affects people involved in jumping activities (e.g., tennis and basketball players). The discoloration is not blood; it is melanin and a protein, located at the orifice of the ec-

Table 1. Common Foot Problems in Sports

Skin	Bone
Nail and subcutaneous tissue	Epiphysis
Contact dermatitis	Metatarsalgia
Eczema	Morton's foot
Blisters	Stress fractures
Calluses	Cavus feet
Runner's toe	Freiberg's disease
Painful heel cushion	Kohler's disease (vascular subungual exostosis necrosis of navicular bone)
Plantar fasciitis	
Hallux limitus	Sever's disease (calcaneal apophysitis)
Black heel	Symptomatic accessory navicular bone
Erythrasma	Osteochondritis dessicans
	Cuboid syndrome
Nerve	Impingement syndrome
Morton's neuroma (interdigital nerve)	
Peroneal neuropathy (superficial and deep)	Ligament
Medial plantar neuropraxia (jogger's foot)	Sprains
Motor branch to abductor digiti quinti muscle	Turf toe
Tarsal tunnel syndrome (posterior tibial or plantar nerves)	Flat feet
Sural nerve and medial calcaneal nerve entrapment	Bursa
	Metatarsal
	Plantar
Tendon	Retrocalcaneal
Ganglion	Pump bump (Haglund's heel)
Tenosynovitis	Tailor's bunion
Hammer toes	
Achilles tendonitis	
Strains	

crine glands. Treatment is conservative and consists of an adequate felt padding or similar orthotic. The differential diagnosis should include not only bleeding and coagulation but also sources of localized trauma and infection.

Blisters

Blisters are commonly caused by a repetitive shear force at the beginning of the training season, before the skin has hardened, or following a change in footwear. A horizontal tear forms in the malpighian layer of the epidermis, followed by fluid accumulation. Blisters tend to occur in regions of the foot where the skin is less mobile and somewhat adherent to the underlying fixed structure. Common sites include the posterior heel, the toes, the phalanges, and the ball of the foot beneath the metatarsal heads. Symptoms include pain and tenderness. Clinical signs are weeping and bullae filled with clear fluid.

Treatment consists of draining the bullae by needle puncture and/or aspiration, leaving the roof of the bullae intact. The optimal point of entry is at the juncture of the blister and surrounding healthy skin, so that the intact skin can serve as a biologic dressing over the sensitive underlying dermis. The blister pocket can be instilled with a small amount of antiseptic and/or anesthetic cream by injecting directly from the tube or from a syringe into the space between the two surfaces. Pretape adhesive is carefully sprayed over the blister and surrounding area, and cotton-backed adhesive tape is firmly applied. This technique allows the skin to remain in place as a natural dressing while the underlying skin heals. Treatment with padding or a donut-shaped device around the blister is not recommended, since more friction may be created, leading to further blistering.

The tape is left in place for 3 days and not removed unless necessitated by increasing pain, drainage, or signs of infection. After this period, the entire wrap is removed; the dead

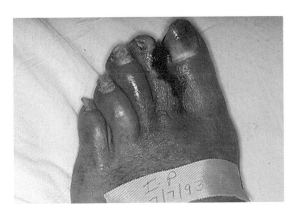

Figure 1. A severe case of black toe in an athlete who disregarded the condition and continued to exercise.

skin usually adheres to the tape and is removed with it. The underlying skin now has developed a thicker epidermal layer and should not be quite as tender as before the tape application. The edges of the blister are trimmed and beveled to prevent further blistering under the hyperkeratotic areas along the edges. Protective tape applied over the skin is left in place for another 2–3 days. If the blister area is still tender, then tape can be applied for a third time. Blood-filled blisters, which result from local trauma at the bed of the blister, are treated in the same fashion.

Infection is the most common complication in a blister due to lack of treatment or a compromised patient. Treatment of cellulitis includes warm soaks, bed rest, and appropriate antibiotics. If the blister has already ruptured, then the roof should be debrided. Cover the area with thin aseptic dressing. Instruct the athlete to wear two pairs of sanitary athletic socks—one pair of sweat socks and one pair of thin cotton socks next to the skin. Worn-out socks increase shear stress in areas where the skin and shoe come into contact and should not be used.

Graduated increases in activity level, petrolatum jelly application, and the use of toe glides (coated paper strips that fit on the bare skin and are then covered by a sock) over "hot" spots prevent most blister formation. A double-layered sock (Runique), moleskin, "second skin," tape, skin lubricant, or skin-hardening solutions (10% tannic acid or 3% salt water) also can be used for prevention.

Note: For a discussion of **athlete's foot** (tinea pedis), refer to Chapter 4.

Painful Heel Cushion

Connective tissue septae that divide the cushioning adipose tissue of the heel into small compartments can be ruptured by repeated jumping. Inflammation may occur as the fat is repeatedly microtraumatized. Symptoms include pain on hard-surface jumping, tenderness on heel palpation, and radiographically visible calcaneal cysts. The syndrome can be difficult to treat, often requiring a reduction or cessation of jumping and running activities for as long as 2–3 months. NSAIDs and a plastic heel insert with sorbothane, poron, or other shock-absorbing materials is recommended (see Chapter 9).

Ankle Sprains

Sprains are ligamentous tears caused by overstretching when a joint is forced beyond its normal range of motion or when the speed of a weight-bearing joint exceeds the musculotendinous structure's limits. There are generally three classes of sprains based on severity: grade I, mild (< 20% of fibers torn); grade II, moderate (20–70% of fibers torn); grade III, severe (> 70% of fibers torn) (Table 2). Although the grades are based on clinical findings and the results of diagnostic tests and radiographs, grading is, nonetheless, somewhat of a subjective exercise.

Eighty-five percent of all ankle sprains occur to the lateral collateral ligaments during plantar inversion. The usual scenario is an athlete who is running or skiing changes course in the direction of the ankle in question, either losing balance or being disturbed by an external force that results in marked supination (Fig. 2). In 85% of situations the anterior talofibular ligament is injured, which represents 65% of all ankle sprains. With continued force in external leg rotation, supination, and mild dorsiflexion, the calcaneal fibular ligament also is injured. Twenty percent of all ankle sprains represent combined injury to these ligaments. The posterior talofibular ligament is injured in 1% of cases due to further forced dorsiflexion. Lack of flexibility is a predisposing factor for sprains.

A careful history-taking elicits recall of a twisting motion applied to the weight-bearing joint, usually in association with internal rotation, adduction, and the foot flipping under the ankle. Relatively low-force activities such as running, walking, or stepping off curbs typically are recalled; the mechanism of injury in

Table 2. Diagnosis and Management of Ankle Sprains

	Grade I	Grade II	Grade III
Lateral Collateral Ligaments	Anterior talofibular	Anterior talofibular, calcaneal fibular	Anterior talofibular, calcaneal fibular, post-talofibular
Medial Collateral Ligaments	Deltoid ligament— superficial	Deltoid ligament— superficial	Deltoid ligament— deep
Symptoms	Minimal pain and disability	Moderate pain and disability	Severe pain, significant functional loss
Weight Bearing	Unimpaired	Difficult	Not possible
Signs	Slight edema, anterior drawer and talar tilt negative	Moderate edema, ecchymosis, anterior drawer and talar tilt positive	Severe edema, ecchymosis, anterior drawer and talar tilt positive, x-rays may show avulsion fracture
Stress	Negative	Talar tilt 5–10°, anterior drawer 4–14 mm	Talar tilt > 20°, anterior drawer > 15 mm
Initial Treatment	RICE, non-weight bearing, posterior splint or air cast, NSAIDs, and analgesics as needed.		
Long-Term Care	Weight-bearing brace or strapping for 2–3 weeks, physical therapy for 1–2 weeks	Unna boot, Jones compression bandage, weight bearing with postoperative shoe 2–4 weeks, orthotics/ strapping 1–2 weeks, physical therapy 2–4 weeks	Weight-bearing short leg cast for 3–6 weeks, then orthotics/strapping for 2–4 weeks, physical therapy 4–6 weeks. Surgery as last resort

RICE = rest, ice, compression, elevation; NSAIDs = nonsteroidal anti-inflammatory drugs

high-velocity, competitive conditions often is unknown. The athlete usually complains of a sudden, intense, localized, and transient pain. Three-quarters of patients are able to bear weight on the injured ankle, and one-third give a history of previous sprains.

Unless it is seen during the "golden period" (within about 1 hour of injury), the degree of edema generally increases with time and may involve the entire ankle. Grade II and III sprains are characterized by hemarthrosis in 60–70% of cases, and ecchymosis in 50–60% about 24 hours after injury. The edema and distortion tend to be more severe in individuals who continue to be physically active following their injury. Although the area of ligamentous injury is always tender, 30–45% of patients complain of tenderness in uninjured adjoining ligaments. Thus, palpation of the injured ankle should always begin farthest from the suspected site of injury.

Remember always to compare the clinical findings to the normal side. In addition to evaluating individual ligaments by palpation, the integrity of the fibula and tibia should be checked. Point tenderness or crepitus should raise the suspicion of an associated fracture. Active range of motion (ROM), particularly that reproducing the mechanism of injury, predictably reproduces pain. This can be confirmed by passive ROM and stress testing. Injury to the fifth metatarsal base is a common associated finding.

Inversion/Internal Rotation Injuries

Evidence of instability with lateral stress in the plantarflexion position but not in the neutral position (i.e., an abnormal talar tilt) indicates a tear of only the anterior talofibular ligament. Tears of the anterior talofibular liga-

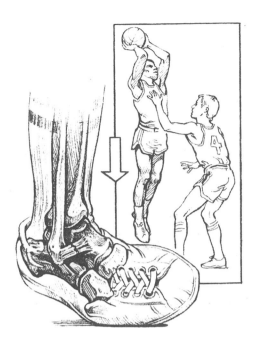

Figure 2. Spraining of the anterior talofibular ligament following forced plantarflexion and inversion.

ment *and* the calcaneal fibular ligament are suggested by instability with lateral stress in both the plantarflexion and neutral positions. The anterior drawer test demonstrates anterior displacement with tears of the anterior talofibular ligament. If there is clinical suspicion of this tear, but the drawer test is negative, inversion stress films should be taken in both a neutral and a plantarflexed position. Increased amounts of talar tilt in plantarflexion with no increase in the neutral position indicates an isolated tear of the anterior talofibular ligament. If there is increased talar tilt of greater than 5–10° in both the plantarflexion and neutral positions when compared to the normal side, tearing of both the anterior talofibular *and* calcaneal fibular ligaments is suggested.

A consultation is advised for recurrent sprains and grade III injuries. The athlete may begin training again when strength and function of the injured side are equal to that of the uninjured side. An aircast-type splint, basketweave strapping (see Chapter 20), or orthotic should be used for the first 2 weeks of training. For cases with pain present months after the injury, a talar dome fracture (see Chapter 13) must be ruled out by computed tomography (CT) scan.

Medial Ankle Sprains

Ten to 15% of ankle sprains involve the medial collateral or tibiofibular ligament complexes. A sharp cut-away from the involved ankle with severe pronation of the foot and internal leg rotation is the usual mechanism of injury. Initially the anterior portion of the superficial deltoid ligament (i.e., tibial navicular ligament), the anteriomedial capsule, and the anterior smaller portion of the deep deltoid are involved. The mortise remains stable. With progressively more stress, sequential injuries occur to the anterior inferior tibiofibular ligament, the interosseous membrane and ligament, the remaining portions of the superficial deltoid ligament, and the deep deltoid ligament (i.e., the inferior transverse ligament and the posterior inferior tibiofibular ligament), resulting in complete diastasis of the tibia and fibula. A medial sprain is generally more severe than a lateral injury.

Medial stress films assess the integrity of the deltoid ligament complex. Widening of the space between the talus and medial malleolus of greater than 2 mm indicates an unstable tear of the deep deltoid ligament. If there is separation of the distal tibia and fibula, tears of the anterior-inferior tibiofibular ligament and interosseous ligament also are present. Similarly, an anterior displacement of greater than 3 mm on draw stress radiographs indicates a complete tear of the anterior talofibular ligament.

A grade I sprain is indicated by the absence of functional or anatomic instability. Treatment is purely supportive and is aimed at the rapid restoration of normal ankle motion and strength. The RICE (rest, ice, compression, elevation) regimen should be followed for the first 24–48 hours and thereafter as needed during the rehabilitation process. Crutches or a cane should be used if there is any swelling or pain on weight bearing. The cane should be used on the contralateral uninjured side; single crutches are not recommended. Active ROM exercises within the limits of pain should be encouraged once edema has subsided, supplemented by passive ROM and progressive resistance exercises (PRE). Isometric strengthening exercises with an elastic bandage or neoprene inner tube also can be performed. Although complete anatomic healing requires

4–6 weeks, strength and ROM exercises usually permit return to play in 1–2 weeks. In the competitive situation, adhesive surgical strapping is advised to strengthen the ankle.

The RICE regimen also is adequate for grade II sprains, although it is usually continued for longer periods of time (48–72 hours). To assure immobilization, a posterior splint, Unna boot, or adhesive surgical strapping may be applied with the ankle in approximately a 90° position until the edema and pain have subsided. Thereafter, weight bearing and ROM and PRE exercises, using supplemental adhesive strapping, are initiated and supplemented by ice water or contrast soaks to promote the rehabilitation process. Supplemental adhesive strapping also should be used during training. Several weeks to months should be allowed for complete healing, and return to play should only be initiated once full range of motion and strength are restored. Some practitioners prefer cast immobilization for short periods of time. Such an approach may be useful in unstable injuries, although its routine use in stable sprains results in a considerable amount of athletic deconditioning and disuse atrophy.

Ideal treatment—nonoperative versus operative—for third degree sprains is controversial. The grade II regimen or the application of a cast for 6 weeks followed by an additional 6 weeks of ankle protection (e.g., cane, crutches, or adhesive strapping) represents the nonoperative approach. The rehabilitation process (ROM and PRE exercises) begins after cast removal and is continued until full strength and ROM are achieved, which may require 3–6 months from the time of injury. Grade III sprains often receive incorrect treatment (a conservative, grade I approach) because when there is no fracture, ligament damage is assumed to be minimal. Significant tears of the deep deltoid require surgical intervention.

The operative approach for grade III ankle sprains consists of accurate anatomic reposition of the torn ligaments and, in the case of the deep deltoid, is considered the best way to maximize joint function and restore ligament strength. Primary surgical intervention should occur within the first 7–10 post injury days. A risk of postoperative complications exists, and secondary reconstructive repairs are always possible for patients who have significant chronic symptoms. Following surgery, management is similar to that of the nonoperative approach for about 3 months. Although the incidence of chronic ankle instability in patients treated by surgery is difficult to determine, it appears to be approximately 5%.

Several words of caution are necessary concerning the management of sprains. In general it is best to err on the conservative side when it comes to diagnosis and to be liberal when it comes to treatment and rehabilitation. One of the greatest mistakes is to allow an athlete with a grade II sprain to return too early to competition and suffer reinjury or a grade III sprain. In addition to misdiagnosis, rehabilitation is commonly overlooked as a priority area. Specific ankle exercises (eversion, inversion, flexion, and dorsiflexion) should be known and taught by the practitioner. Proper warm-up and stretching exercises should be taught to the athlete. Although frequently recommended, use of high-top shoes or sneakers for routine activity as well training probably does not prevent reinjury. Remember to perform serial evaluations if the degree of injury is unclear. Finally, it is important to consider the patient's age and functional capacity when deciding the most appropriate therapy. Nonoperative approaches are usually appropriate for middle-aged individuals or occasional athletes, whereas surgery is reserved for the young, active person or older, competitive athlete. Less than adequate treatment leads to a chronically unstable ankle prone to repeated injury.

Note: For a discussion of **plantar fasciitis** and **heel spur syndrome,** refer to Chapter 9.

Turf Toe and Toe Sprain

Turf toe and toe sprain are caused by the toe, usually the hallux, jamming in the sneaker and hyperextending beyond the normal 60° of dorsiflexion, resulting in a tear of the plantar plate from its first metatarsal head origin. Risk factors include lightweight, flexible shoes on artificial turf (woven or synthetic surfaces) and sports like football, basketball, squash, and racketball. Progression of the injury can result in a tear to the joint capsule. Symptoms include pain and decreased ROM at the metatarsophalangeal (MTP) joint. Clinical signs include antalgia, edema, ecchymosis, and tenderness at the MTP joint. X-rays may reveal a small avulsion fracture from the plantar metatarsal head.

The injury can be classified as first, second, or third degree depending on severity of swelling, tenderness, reduction in motion, and extent of ecchymosis. RICE, taping, and strapping the toe in a plantarflexed position to avoid further hyperextension are recommended, along with a rigid-sole shoe with a spring steel plate or orthosis with Morton's extension to avoid dorsiflexion of the toe. Grade II injuries require rest from the activity for days to weeks. Crutches for several days are essential for grade III injuries, followed by relative rest for 3–6 weeks.

Note: For a discussion of **hallux limitus**, refer to Chapter 6.

Tendon Injuries

Tendon injuries can involve the tendon itself and its sheath or peritenon. Trauma to the tendon produces strains, whereas inflammation of the peritenon leads to tendonitis, peritendonitis, or tenosynovitis.

Extensor Tendonitis

Extensor tendonitis is an inflammation of the dorsal tendons of the foot commonly caused by overuse, short warm-ups, hill work, or long workouts. The symptoms include pain on ROM (i.e., dorsiflexion/plantarflexion), decreased ROM, and/or crepitation on ROM. The clinical signs consist of mild edema, tenderness on direct palpation, and pain on muscle and tendon function testing. RICE, NSAIDs, immobilization (e.g., strapping, Unna boot, Jones compression bandage) are the recommended treatments. Modification of training and/or athletic shoe gear is advisable.

Achilles Tendonitis

Repeated microtrauma to the Achilles tendon, caused by rigid-soled shoes, skater's and hiker's boots, faulty technique or hard landings, or the use of fluoroquinoline antibiotics, can lead to inflammation of the tendon and its sheath due to prolonged slow friction over the tendon. Acutely, there is localized pain several centimeters proximal to the insertion of the tendon into the calcaneus, pain on stair climbing, crepitus, direct tenderness, and erythema; chronically there can be marked fibrosis and calcification. The differential diagnosis should include bursitis, strain, and arthritis.

Treatment for Achilles tendonitis is conservative, consisting of NSAIDs in association with adequate periods of rest, heat application, adhesive strapping, and physical therapy for 1–3 weeks. Steroid injections are contraindicated, and consultation should be sought for truly refractive cases. Shoe modifications include cutting out the heel counter or wearing an open-back shoe. In less severe cases, a soft, cushioned heel lift accompanied by a decreased activity level suffices. In a recalcitrant or severe case, immobilization and non-weight bearing are in order.

Posterior Tibial Tendonitis

This condition is caused by repetitive microtrauma during the pronation phase of running, cutting, jumping, and so on. Symptoms include pain inferior to the medial malleolus and decreased range of motion. Clinical signs consist of edema and tenderness behind the medial malleolus or proximal to its insertion on the navicular tubercle. The pain is increased by inversion against resistance. Treatment varies according to the degree of the symptoms. Initially, RICE, NSAIDs and analgesics are recommended as needed. Long-term, a non-weight bearing, short, leg cast with the foot slightly in inversion and plantarflexion for 2–4 weeks, followed by a medial posted orthosis, can be helpful.

Peroneal Subluxation/Dislocation

The peroneal retinaculum can be torn with a direct blow to the back of the lateral malleolus while the tendons are taut in eversion and dorsiflexion. Powerful contraction of the peroneal muscles, particularly in maximal dorsiflexion, occurs most often in wrestling and downhill or cross-country skiing. Acute subluxation of the peroneal tendon is relatively uncommon and is most often confused with simple lateral ligament sprains. However, in typical lateral sprains tenderness and swelling occur over the anterolateral ankle capsule; in peroneal subluxation, tenderness and swelling are centered behind the lateral malleolus and extend proximally over the tendons.

One or both of the peroneal tendons may pop out of the groove onto the lateral malleolus. Reduction usually is spontaneous. The differential diagnosis should include an ankle sprain, contusion, and tenosynovitis. Palpation reveals direct tenderness over the tendons, which may be confused with tenosynovitis. With acute dislocation, it is not possible to displace the tendon during the examination.

Treatment is relocation, if necessary by directing pressure on the tendon posteriorly and then casting the ankle in slight pronation and flexion. The plaster should be carefully and firmly molded to the contour of the lateral malleolus or a J-shaped piece of felt used to compress the tendon in place. Surgery should be considered for failed conservative therapy or for the serious athlete for whom lost time would be critical.

Untreated acute episodes or congenital weakness results in chronic or recurrent subluxation of the peroneal tendons. There usually is a history of acute injury with appreciable soreness for many weeks followed by the recurrent feeling of something slipping out of place at the posterior portion of the ankle during foot eversion. There may be sharp pain and considerable stress noted with the condition. On physical examination, the retinaculum typically is thickened and the groove shallow. It often is possible to sublux or dislocate the tendons manually. Once again, treatment is surgical.

Peroneal Tendonitis

Persistent lateral midfoot and ankle pain, particularly after a lateral collateral ankle sprain, should suggest peroneal tendonitis. The patient complains of an occasional "giving way" sensation and lateral checking. Resisted eversion, edema, and point tenderness over the tendons are characteristic. Treatment consists of a lateral or eversion orthosis. A cast for 2–3 weeks followed by extensive rehabilitation is appropriate for severe symptoms. A corticosteroid injection should be considered for resistant symptoms.

Flexor Hallucis Longus Tendonitis

Repeated push-off maneuvers (e.g., ballet) irritate and inflame the tendon, causing pain and tenderness in the posteromedial aspect of the ankle and sometimes in the medial arch. Passive extension of the first toe is limited with the foot in neutral position and normal with the foot plantarflexed. Relief is obtained for most patients with NSAIDs, foot strapping, contrast soaks, and a longitudinal arch support. Occasionally, surgical release is necessary.

Achilles Tendon Rupture

The Achilles tendon can be ruptured at its attachment to the calcaneus, along the tendon's course, or at the musculotendinous junction (the most common site of injury). It is usually associated with a tenosynovitis. Stronger forces in a middle-aged weekend athlete, particularly a forceful drive, push-off, or

direct blow, or a landing in sudden dorsiflexion with the foot plantarflexed and extended as in basketball, racquet sports, or broad jumping, can result in spontaneous rupture of the tendon. The differential diagnosis should include strain of the calf musculature, contusion, or an ankle sprain.

Symptoms include sudden calf pain associated with an audible snap, followed by antalgia and difficulty tiptoeing and climbing. The pain may be inconsistent with the degree of injury. Clinical signs consist of a positive Thompson-Doherty squeeze test (see Chapter 2), positive heel resistance test (easy dorsiflexion of the heel and foot against plantarflexion), and positive gap sign (palpable gap in tendon which may be absent if edema is significant). Active ROM and plantarflexion are preserved due to intact peroneal, tibial, and toe flexor muscle groups.

Treatment varies with severity of injury, length of time between diagnosis and treatment, and age of patient. Nonoperative treatment consists of RICE; NSAIDs and analgesics; non-weight bearing; a long, gravity equinus leg cast for 6 weeks followed by a short, equinus leg cast for 2 weeks; and then a short walking cast for 2 weeks. For younger, active individuals, surgical repair is indicated. Nonoperative results usually are excellent and are reserved for the older athlete whose primary interests are return to work and everyday routine activities rather than athletic performance.

Strains (Shin Splints)

Because the ankle is subject to great static and dynamic forces, strains of the joint are very common in a wide variety of sports. Strains may be classified in a similar fashion as sprains. The ankle joint per se is not involved in strains. Simply switching from street shoes that have a firm medial support and a heel with a strong contour to athletic shoes that have no heel, minimal support, and a weak contour can cause a static strain of the tibial muscle. Medial strains involve the tibialis anterior (anterior shin splints). The tibialis posterior is vulnerable at its attachment to the tuberosity of the navicula or under its medial side because of its dual roles in effecting inversion and plantarflexion, as well as supporting the foot arch (posterior shin splints). Tenderness usually is palpable at the medial border of the arch, with some spread under the arch, and at the back of the medial malleolus.

The most common presentation of shin splints is a generalized pain over the anterior tibia. This comes from overuse and stress to the anterior muscle group. There often is a biomechanical component that must be addressed. There may be a muscle imbalance between the relatively strong gastrocnemius-soleus posterior muscle group and the weaker anterior group; therefore, posterior stretching and anterior strengthening exercises are necessary. Equinus is a common finding in runners.

Posterior shin splints result from overuse of the posterior tibial muscle due to excessive pronation. General RICE treatment, functional orthotics, correct running shoes, and proper training are necessary to alleviate pain. Untreated shin splints can progress to stress fractures of the tibia.

Sesamoiditis

Sesamoiditis is commonly caused by overuse of the foot in a plantarflexed position, for example in sprinting. The condition is associated with a cavus foot. The sesamoids protect the tendon of the flexor hallucis brevis, increase the mechanical advantage of the intrinsic hallux musculature, and absorb the majority of weight bearing on the medial forefoot. A cavus foot or rigid plantarflexed first ray predisposes. Symptoms include pain on ambulation in and out of shoes and sub–first metatarsal pain. Clinical signs consist of pain on dorsiflexion of the hallux, restricted motion of the first MTP joint, pain on direct palpation of the sesamoid, and mild edema.

Oblique and axial x-ray evaluations to rule out fracture of the sesamoid are advised. Remember that 30% of the general population has a bipartite sesamoid, the medial more often than the lateral. A bone scan or CT scan may be necessary to show a stress fracture. RICE, NSAIDs, felt padding, orthotic devices, and physical therapy are conservative methods of treatment. The orthoses must be worn constantly for at least 6 months, and then use should be resumed if symptoms recur. Surgical excision is rarely required.

Tibiotalar Impingement Syndrome

Repetitive microtrauma can lead to an anterior or posterior impingement syndrome. The anterior aspect of the tibia hits against the talus during deep knee bends or "drive off" from the planted foot (forced dorsiflexion) in football, rugby, and dancing. The posterior aspect of the tibia hits the posterior lateral tubercle of the talus during full weight bearing in maximum plantarflexion. Symptoms include vague anterolateral or posterolateral pain during extreme dorsiflexion (running) or plantarflexion (jumping), respectively.

The clinical signs for the anterior syndrome include point tenderness and edema over the anterior ankle and decreased dorsiflexion that produces pain. There is posterolateral tenderness particularly with forced, passive plantarflexion in posterior impingement. Radiographs visualize the spur, as well as subchondral sclerosis and pseudocysts if there are degenerative changes. Treatment is the same for both forms of the syndrome: initially, RICE, NSAIDs, and analgesics as needed. Long-term treatment includes modification of activities, appropriate stretching, injection of long-acting and short-acting corticosteroids with lidocaine, and a surgical excision for refractory cases.

Note: For a discussion of **Sever's disease,** see Chapter 10.

Cuboid Syndrome

The cuboid can sublux plantarward during dancing, marching, running, or after an inversion sprain. Eighty percent of subluxation occurs in pronated feet. There is weakness on push-off and lateral foot pain often radiating to the plantar aspect of the medial foot and anterior ankle joint. On exam, there is tenderness over the cuboid and proximal fourth metatarsal joint. The pain is worsened with plantar pressure on the cuboid. Some depression may be noted over the dorsal aspect of the cuboid, and plantarward there may be some fullness. Bone scans, x-rays and CT studies are normal.

Treatment is nonsurgical, involving manipulation. The long dorsal extensors and peronei are relaxed with deep massage. The patient is prone and the examiner's fingers are over the dorsal metatarsals and thumbs over the plantar aspect of the cuboid. The forefoot is then "whipped" plantarward while the thumbs push dorsally. After reduction, a 1/8-inch felt pad is taped under the cuboid, and the patient is taught self-mobilization.

Proper Training

Many injuries are caused by overuse and poor training. Proper running shoes should have good shock absorption, a sturdy heel counter, and pronation control. High-arched feet need more shock absorption; flat feet need more pronation control. For runners, mileage should be increased slowly. A soft running surface is important—concrete is the hardest, then asphalt, a track surface, and grass. Hill work greatly increases the risks of overuse. Low-speed jogging is a heel-toe gait, but at higher speeds only the toes contact the ground, causing increased forefoot trauma. Hamstring and gastrocnemius-soleus stretching must be done before and after exercise. Flexibility is vital to reduce injury risk. Quadriceps and anterior tibial strengthening exercises are helpful. Any biomechanical faults must be addressed with the appropriate running orthotic.

References

1. Birrer RB: Ankle injuries and the family physician. J Am Board Fam Pract 1(4):274–281, 1988.
2. Frey CC, Shereff MJ: Tendon injuries about the ankle in athletes. Clin Sports Med 7(1):103–118, 1988.
3. Garfinkel D, Rothenberger LA: Foot problems in athletes. J Fam Pract 19(2):239–250, 1984.
4. Garrick JG, Requa RK: The epidemiology of foot and ankle injuries in sports. Clin Sports Med 7(1):29–36, 1988.
5. Hawkins BJ, Haddad RJ Jr: Hallux rigidus. Clin Sports Med 7(1):37–49, 1988.
6. Lassiter THE, Malone TR, Garrett WE: Injury to the lateral ligaments of the ankle. Ortho Clin North Am 20(4):629–640, 1989.
7. McBryde AM, Anderson RB: Sesamoid foot problems in the athlete. Clin Sports Med 7(1):51–60, 1988.
8. Wojtys EM: Sports injuries in the immature athlete. Ortho Clin North Am 18(4):689–708, 1987.

15

The Arthropathies

Elizabeth G. McDonald, MD and Richard B. Birrer, MD

Eleven percent of inflammatory joint conditions affect the foot and ankle. The most common conditions include rheumatoid arthritis, osteoarthritis, gout, Reiter's syndrome, psoriatic arthritis, and ankylosing spondylitis (Table 1).

Arthritic Conditions Affecting the Foot

Gout

Arthritis of the foot can be seen in gout caused by the deposition of monosodium urate crystals (MSU) and in pseudogout caused by calcium pyrophosphate crystal deposition. Gout is a systemic metabolic disease manifested by episodic acute or chronic arthritis, hyperuricemia, MSU crystal deposits in connective tissue, urolithiasis, and, rarely, gouty nephropathy. Gouty arthritis is the most common form of inflammatory arthritis in men over 40 years of age, but it is rarely seen in premenopausal women.

Classically, the first episode of gout begins dramatically in one peripheral joint of the lower extremity. The metatarsal joint of the big toe (where gouty pain is called podagra), the ankle, the midtarsal and tarsal areas, and the knee are common areas of involvement.

Pathogenesis

Hyperuricemia is present in up to 98% of patients with gouty arthritis, and the risk of developing gout increases with the degree and duration of hyperuricemia. However, the uric acid level can be normal during the acute attack; therefore, it is not diagnostic. Gout may be a primary metabolic disease due to an inborn error in the metabolism of purine, or secondary, due to the excessive degradation of the nucleoproteins in nucleic acids.

In individuals with gout, the total miscible uric acid pool is greatly enlarged, particularly in those with tophaceous gout. As a result, the majority of dietary nitrogen is excreted as uric acid and not as urea. The increased uric acid pool is due either to decreased renal clearance of urate, presumably resulting from the defect in tubular reabsorption and/or tubular secretion, or to increased production of urate through biosynthesis of purines and/or excessive ingestion of dietary purines.

Causes of secondary gout include polycythemia rubra vera, the leukemias, and any large tumor mass that is lysed by chemotherapy or radiotherapy. Drugs such as diuretics and low-dose aspirin also induce hyperuricemia, most probably by blocking tubular reabsorption of urate. Factors that can predispose to a gouty attack include dietary excess, alcohol ingestion, hypouricemic drugs, diuretic therapy, and minor trauma.

Pathology

Urate crystals are deposited in the synovial membrane and articular cartilage as well as in the joint capsule, subarticular bone, and surrounding tissue (Fig. 1). The inflammatory process begins with the ingestion of urate crystals by polymorphonuclear leukocytes, which have been attracted by activation of the complement cascade and kinin system. The result is lysis of the white cell membrane and release

Table 1. Comparison of Inflammatory Joint Conditions

	Rheumatoid Arthritis	Osteo-arthritis	Gout	Reiter's Syndrome	Psoriatic Arthritis	Ankylosing Spondylitis
Erosions	Marginal	N/A	Central and marginal Martel's sign	N/A	N/A	N/A
Sex Ratio	Female 2 or 3:1	No predilection	Male 20:1	Male 5:1 to 50:1	N/A	Male 9:1
Joint Space	Symmetric narrowing, loss of cartilage	Asymmetric narrowing	Narrowing in chronic gout	N/A	N/A	N/A
Joint Subluxation	Common	Common	Rare	N/A	N/A	N/A
Joint Involvement	Polyarticular small joints of hands, feet, and cervical spine	Knee, hips, spine, distal IPJ	Mono or oligo-trophic	Ankle, STJ, IPJ, hallux, oligo-arthritis	Feet, knees, sacroiliac	Hips, shoulders, sacroiliac, insertion of Achilles tendon
Enthesopathy	Yes	N/A	N/A	Yes (classic)	Yes (classic)	Yes
Sausage Toe	N/A	N/A	N/A	Yes	Yes	Yes
Capsular Osteophytosis	N/A	Soft tissue atrophy	Osteo-porosis	Yes	Yes	Yes
Spondylo-arthro-pathies	Yes	N/A	N/A	Yes	Yes	Yes
Special Characteristics	Bony ankylosis of tarsus, synovitis—1st stage synovial cysts	N/A	N/A	N/A	N/A	N/A

IPJ = interphalangeal joints, STJ = subtalar joints

of lysosomal enzymes that initiate inflammatory reactions characteristic of gout. Intense pain, swelling, erythema, and warmth occur due to cell necrosis. The articular surface and subchondral bone can be destroyed, and urate crystals deposited in connective tissues form tophi, particularly in the bursae, ligaments, tendons, and subcutaneous tissues of the skin.

Clinical Manifestations

Gouty arthritis attacks are intermittent and asymmetric in presentation. The attack usually begins suddenly and resolves within 72–96 hours, but the ensuing asymptomatic or intercritical period may last for several days to

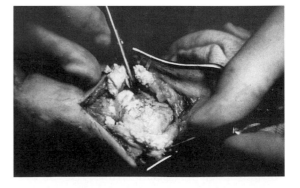

Figure 1. Urate crystals form tophi in gout at the first metatarsophalangeal joint.

years. Pain during an acute attack increases in intensity over the first 24 hours and is associated with edema, warmth, and erythema of the involved joint. The pain tends to be gnawing and throbbing in nature and may be so severe as to prevent walking and necessitate the removal of footwear from the affected area. The patient may be febrile during the attack. A monoarticular arthritis of the first metatarsophalangeal (MTP) joint is involved in 75–80% of cases (Fig. 2). Ten to 20% of patients present with multiple inflamed joints during their first attack.

Although the diagnosis of gout often can be made on clinical grounds, the identification of MSU crystals in the synovial fluid is pathognomonic. A tuberculin or insulin syringe with a 22–23 gauge needle can be used to enter the joint aseptically and aspirate a small amount of synovial fluid. Preloading the syringe with sterile saline is not recommended since water containing solutions can dissolve crystals. The fluid aspirate should then be examined under a light microscope or polarizing lens to determine if crystals are present. The type of crystal can be evaluated further with the use of a compensating lens. Urate crystals are characteristically needle-shaped and produce strongly negative birefringence.

Chronic tophaceous gout can affect the foot and usually appears after years of gout that has not been treated or treated ineffectively. Tophaceous deposits of urate also have been noted, without any evidence of inflammation, in elderly women with renal insufficiency who are on chronic diuretic therapy. Tophaceous gout tends to present as symmetric nodules that may involve any area of the body, but most frequently involve the extensor surface

of the hand and elbow, the first MTP joint, the heel (particularly the Achilles tendon), and the ear. Since tophi can be confused with rheumatoid nodules, needle aspiration of the tophus should be performed to search for crystals.

Acute episodes of pseudogout, or calcium pyrophosphate deposition disease (CPPD), characteristically involve the knee, wrist, and, less commonly, the first MTP joint. As in the case of gout, trauma, surgery, and medical illness can precipitate an acute arthritic attack. Examination of the synovial fluid reveals an inflammatory fluid with weakly positive birefringent, rhomboid-shaped crystals. The presence of crystals does not exclude the possibility of infection, as CPPD crystals and septic arthritis can coexist. If there is clinical evidence for septic arthritis, the fluid should be sent for the appropriate cultures.

Treatment

The therapeutic management of gout is twofold: (1) the treatment of an acute attack, and (2) the long-term prevention of acute gouty attacks and tophaceous gout. Nonsteroidal anti-inflammatory drugs (NSAIDs) are effective for treatment of the acute gouty attack (Table 2). Anti-inflammatory doses of a drug such as indomethacin 50 mg three times a day with food, or the equivalent dose of another NSAID, can be given over 3–5 days. NSAIDs have largely replaced oral colchicine for the management of acute gout. When using NSAID therapy, the potential side effects of gastrointestinal (GI) bleeding, azotemia, and drug-drug interactions must be considered—particularly in the elderly patient. Pseudogout also responds well to NSAID therapy. Corticotropin (ACTH), 40 units given by intramus-

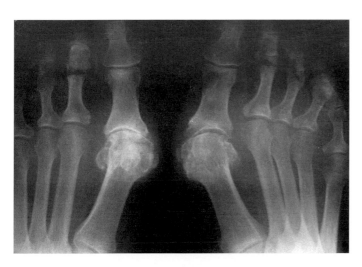

Figure 2. X-ray shows arthritic changes secondary to gout at first metatarsophalangeal joint.

Table 2. Nonsteroidal Anti-Inflammatory Drugs

Class*	Availability	Doses Per Day	Maximum Dosage (mg)
Proprionic Acids			
Fenoprofen	200, 300, 600	3 or 4	3200
Flurbiprofen	50, 100	2–4	300
Ibuprofen	200, 300, 400, 600, 800	3 or 4	3200
Ketoprofen	25, 50, 75	3 or 4	300
Naproxen	250, 375, 500, 125/5 ml	2 or 3	1500
Oxaprozin	600	1	1200
Indoles			
Indomethacin	25, 50, 75, 25/5 ml	2–4	200
Sulindac	150, 200	2	400
Tolmetin	200, 400	3 or 4	2000
Fenamates			
Meclofenamate	50, 100	4	400
Mefenamic acid	250	4	1000
Napthylalkanone			
Nabumetone	500, 750	1 or 2	2000
Oxicams			
Piroxicam	10, 20	1	20
Pyranocarboxylic Acid			
Etodolac	200, 300, 400	2–3	1200
Phenylacetic Acids			
Diclofenac sodium	25, 50, 75	4	200
Salicylates			
Diflunisal	250, 500	2 or 3	1500

*If clinical response is not seen after 3–4 weeks of treatment, another drug from a different class should be considered.

Warnings

Hypersensitivity reactions: anaphylactoid reaction among patients allergic to aspirin.

Gastrointestinal effects: serious toxicity such as bleeding, ulceration, and perforation can occur at any time, with or without warnings or symptoms, in patients treated with NSAIDs long term. Contraindicated in patients with peptic ulcer.

Central nervous system effects: indomethacin may aggravate depression, other psychiatric disturbances, epilepsy, and parkinsonism, and therefore must be used with caution. Headaches are common.

Renal effects: many forms of renal dysfunction occur due to prostaglandin inhibition. Contraindicated in renally impaired patients. May decrease the effects of diuretics and therefore must be used with caution in hypertensive and cardiac patients.

Miscellaneous: safety of drugs not established in pregnancy; they are excreted in breast milk. Must be used with caution among elderly patients more prone to adverse effects. Tolmetin, naproxen, and ibuprofen have been approved for use in children with juvenile arthritis.

cular injection, has rapid onset of action equivalent to that of indomethacin.

An effective dose of oral colchicine for acute gout also causes GI symptoms. Oral colchicine is administered 1 mg initially, followed by 0.5 mg every 2 hours to a maximum of 8 mg, until GI symptoms develop or the pain subsides. This dosage regimen may prove to be toxic in patients with hepatic or renal impairment. Colchicine also can be given intravenously if the patient is unable to take oral medications. A dose of 1 mg diluted in 20 ml of normal saline can be administered slowly (over not less than 10 minutes) as a single dose to a maximum of 2 mg. It is imperative that the drug be given with utmost care as extravasation can cause local tissue necrosis. It is recommended that after intravenous administration of colchicine, no more be given by any route for 7 days. Contraindications to intravenous colchicine include renal or hepatic insufficiency, extra hepatic biliary obstruction, and depressed bone marrow function.

NSAIDs and colchicine can be given in maintenance doses to prevent future attacks of gout, but they have little effect on urate load. The treatment of tophaceous gout and/or chronic gouty arthritis often consists of a combined pharmacologic and surgical approach. Elevated levels of serum uric acid can be reduced by increasing uric acid excretion through inhibition of tubular reabsorption. Uricosuric agents such as probenecid 0.5 gm twice a day or sulfinpyrazone 100 mg three times a day have this effect. These agents are helpful in preventing the occurrence of chronic gouty arthritis as well as in avoiding the formation of tophaceous deposits or decreasing their size. Uricosuric agents are ineffective in patients with a low glomerular filtration rate (less than 20–30 ml/min).

Allopurinol is a potent inhibitor of xanthine oxidase and inhibits the formation of uric acid, effectively decreasing both serum and urine uric acid levels. Indications for allopurinol therapy include tophaceous gout, chronic gouty arthritis, and uric acid urolithiasis. When allopurinol is given in a dose of 100 mg two to three times a day, it can prevent the formation of tophaceous deposits and renal stones. Allopurinol should never be started during an acute attack of gout, because the rapid lowering of uric acid levels can precipitate an episode of polyarthritic gout.

Occasionally, surgical management is required to remove tophaceous deposits that have not responded to medical therapy. A number of authors have recommended surgery for gout involving the foot when any of the following conditions are present:

- Large tophi that compress nerves, vessels, and tendons
- Tophi in weight-bearing areas or tophi that interfere with footwear
- A tophus with a draining sinus
- Painful destruction or deformity of the toe joints.

With the exception of tophi involving the superficial soft tissues, such surgery is not within the purview of the practicing primary care physician, and the patient should be referred to a consultant. Superficial tophi usually are encapsulated by fibrous tissue and should be shelled out by careful dissection and curettage. Prophylactic colchicine should be initiated prior to a planned operation because surgery can precipitate a gouty attack.

Osteoarthritis

The loss of articular cartilage is the primary pathology in osteoarthritis. These changes are manifested radiographically by joint space narrowing due to loss of cartilage and reactive bone formation or osteophytic spur development at the articular margins. Hallux rigidus is the term used for the involvement of the first MTP joint of the foot. Clinically, patients with osteoarthritis present with insidious onset of joint pain that increases with activity. Women are more commonly affected than men. Examination typically reveals loss of extension and bony enlargement of the joint. The bony enlargement may in turn lead to impingement against footwear and cause secondary skin and tendon inflammation. Joint aspiration is rarely helpful as this is a noninflammatory process. When the diagnosis of osteoarthritis is suspected clinically, it can be confirmed by characteristic radiographic changes (Fig. 3).

Treatment should be directed at any mechanical dysfunction that exacerbates the stress placed on involved joints. Well-fitted footwear with a stiff sole or longitudinal arch support may offer relief. Analgesics such as acetaminophen and low-dose NSAIDs may be prescribed for symptomatic relief. Surgical intervention such as silicone implant arthroplasty, osteotomy, or arthrodesis should be considered if symptoms fail to improve.

Rheumatoid Arthritis

Rheumatoid arthritis (RA) is a systemic disease with inflammatory changes throughout the connective tissue of the body. The foot is the initial site of RA in 12–20% of patients, and throughout the course of the disease the incidence of foot involvement may reach 90%. At the joint level there is chronic proliferative inflammation (pannus) of the synovial membrane that causes an irreversible change in the joint capsule and articular cartilage. X-ray findings consist of joint space narrowing, periarticular osteopenia, marginal erosions, and subluxed deformed joints (Fig. 4).

The diagnosis of RA is made clinically in the setting of inflammatory symmetric polyarthritis, usually involving the hands, wrist, and feet. The proximal interphalangeal (PIP) joint and MTP joints are most commonly affected. MTP joint involvement can result in hallux valgus,

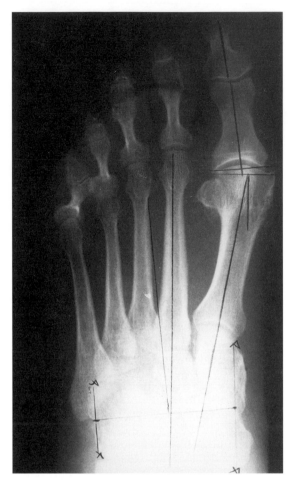

Figure 3. Osteoarthritis of first metatarsophalangeal joint with uneven joint narrowing, spur formation, and subchondral sclerosis.

hammer toe deformities, and spreading of the forefoot. RA causes the soft tissue pad normally beneath the metatarsal head to displace, resulting in pain on the plantar surface of the foot when walking. Calluses and skin ulceration can develop on the plantar surface of the metatarsal heads and the dorsum of the PIP joints. The deformities—subluxation and fibular deviation—generally are in the small joints of the feet. When RA affects the midtarsal joint (65%) and the subtalar joint (35%), it can lead to a flatfoot deformity and a valgus hindfoot. Rheumatoid nodules may form over bony prominences such as the heels.

Rheumatoid arthritis is more prevalent in females than males (3:1). The diagnosis is made clinically, based on the history and physical examination. The erythrocyte sedimentation rate may be moderately to markedly increased. Confirmatory blood tests of rheumatoid factor positivity (present in 85% of patients) and characteristic x-ray changes also are important. An inflammatory picture is characteristically found on synovial fluid analysis. The patient must meet at least four of the following criteria to be diagnosed with RA:

- Morning stiffness for at least 1 hour
- Soft-tissue swelling (arthritis) of three or more joints observed by a physician
- Swelling of the PIP, metacarpophalangeal, or wrist joints
- Symmetric arthritis
- Subcutaneous nodules
- Positive rheumatoid factor
- Radiographic erosions or periarticular osteopenia in hand and wrist joints.

This list is the American Rheumatism Association's revised criteria (1987) for the classification of RA.

Treatment

The objective of therapy in treating patients with RA is to decrease inflammation, minimize pain, and improve functional status. Patients may benefit from a combination of medical, surgical, and rehabilitative services. Various medications are used depending on the stage of the disease. NSAIDs are used early on in combination with intra-articular steroids to reduce pain and inflammation (see Table 2). For more persistent disease, drugs prescribed may include antimalarials, oral steroids, gold salts, and methotrexate. Rheumatologic consultation is warranted prior to initiating therapy with these drugs, because complications can develop from their use, and there is a need to monitor for drug toxicity.

Debridement and padding of any hyperkeratotic lesions may afford relief of underlying bursitis. Plastazote inserts, accommodative orthotics, running shoes, and molded shoes also can be helpful. Once the arthritic changes have completely destroyed the cartilage and there is dislocation of the joints in the forefoot, surgical management should be considered. Evaluation for vascular integrity and infected skin ulcerations should be performed preoperatively. Indications for surgery include painful calluses and corns, ulcerations at pressure points, severe pain when weight bearing, and painful hallux valgus. Classic procedures for the RA patient with a bunion and subluxed hammer toes at the MTP joint range from first MTP joint arthroplasty to arthrodesis and panmetatarsal head resection. These proce-

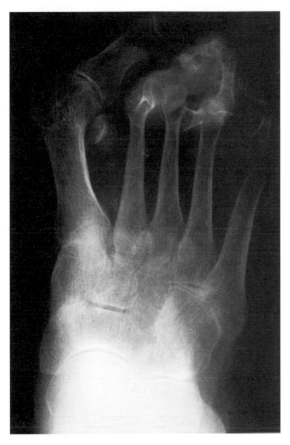

Figure 4. X-ray findings in rheumatoid arthritis.

dures are not cosmetic; they are purely accommodative.

The recovery period may be prolonged, particularly if the patient is on corticosteroid therapy. The use of casts and crutches for 4–5 weeks in these patients is often complicated by arthritic involvement of the hands. Rest and physiotherapy following surgery is mandatory. The prognosis for pain-free ambulation in normal foot gear is excellent. Due to bone removal, some modification of shoe gear may be necessary.

Reiter's Syndrome

Seronegative arthropathies are disorders characterized by inflammatory arthritis, male predominance, and the absence of rheumatoid factor. This group of disorders includes Reiter's syndrome, psoriatic arthritis, and ankylosing spondylitis.

Reiter's syndrome is a reactive arthritis distinguished by inflammation that follows an infectious process. Genetically susceptible individuals who are human leukocyte antigen

(HLA)-B27 positive may acquire this syndrome after exposure to certain genitourinary (Chlamydia) or enteric pathogens. The clinical triad of symptoms includes conjunctivitis, urethritis, and arthritis, and the syndrome most commonly affects young adult males. The synovial fluid is inflammatory in nature and nondiagnostic; however, examination and culture of the synovial fluid may be necessary to exclude a septic process or crystalline arthroplasty. Management of the disease involves a combination of NSAIDs, exercise, and physical therapy. Injectable corticosteroids may relieve articular, bursal, or tendon inflammation locally.

Psoriatic Arthritis

Psoriatic arthritis, also seronegative, affects up to 7% of patients with psoriasis of the skin. The majority of patients are diagnosed with psoriasis prior to developing arthritis. The most common presentation is asymmetric and involves peripheral joints—namely, the distal and proximal interphalangeal joints of the hands, feet, knees, hips, and ankles. There are other rheumatoid-like presentations with arthritic involvement of the wrists and hands. The absence of rheumatoid factor and x-ray evidence of erosive arthritis with bony ankylosis of peripheral joints is typical of psoriatic arthritis.

Resorption of the distal phalangeal tufts—so-called "penciling" of the digit—is a classic sign of psoriatic arthritis. Symptomatic control of the arthritis usually can be achieved with NSAID therapy. Methotrexate is used in more severe disease because it is efficacious for both skin and joint involvement. Surgical intervention should be initiated with caution due to the Koebner phenomenon (i.e., the appearance of psoriatic lesions in areas of trauma or surgical incisions).

Ankylosing Spondylitis

Ankylosing spondylitis, which is closely linked to HLA-B27, is characterized by enthesopathy, anterior uveitis, and inflammation of the spine, sacroiliac joints, and axial joints. The disorder is common in adolescent males, and onset is accompanied by symptoms of low back pain and stiffness. Enthesopathy, inflammation at the site of tendon or ligament insertion, also is common early in the course of the disease. Heel pain due to plantar fasciitis or Achilles tendonitis may be the presenting problem. Radiographic evidence of bilateral sacroiliitis and calcaneal spurs is characteristic. Treatment includes physiotherapy, proper footwear, and NSAIDs, with indomethacin being the most widely used agent.

Septic Arthritis

Joint infection may follow surgery, trauma, or hematogenous spread from a remote infection. It occurs most frequently in children, the elderly, immunocompromised patients, and patients with previously damaged joints (i.e., those with chronic RA). Abrupt onset of pain and swelling of one joint is most common, and the arthritis may be accompanied by systemic complaints of fever and chills. Blood cultures, complete blood count and chemistry, and arthrocentesis with analysis and culture of the synovial fluid are necessary. Plain x-rays should be obtained to exclude the presence of osteomyelitis or a foreign body, but the x-rays rarely show abnormalities acutely. If an infection is suspected, the patient should be admitted to the hospital, blood cultures and synovial fluid cultures should be sent, and parenteral antibiotic therapy should be instituted. Immediate diagnosis and treatment are essential to avoid joint damage.

References

1. Axelrod D, Preston S: Comparison of parenteral ACTH and oral indomethacin in the treatment of acute gout. Arthritis Rheum 31:803–805, 1988.
2. Becker MA: Clinical aspects of monosodium urate crystal deposition disease. Rheum Dis Clin North Am 14(2):377–394, 1988.
3. Coughlin MJ: The rheumatoid foot. Post Grad Med 75(5):207–216, 1984
4. Egan R, Sartoris DJ, Resnick D: Radiographic features of gout in the foot. J Foot Surg 26(5):434–439, 1987.
5. German DC, et al: Hyperuricemia and gout. Med Clin North Am 70(2):419–436, 1986.
6. Kitaoka HB: Rheumatoid burdfoot. Ortho Clin North Am 20(4):593–604, 1989.
7. Mann RA: The painful foot. Post Grad Med 86(3):121–132, 1989.
8. Schumacher HR (ed): Primer On The Rheumatic Diseases, 10th ed. Atlanta, Arthritis Foundation, 1993.
9. Terkeltaub RA: Pathogenesis and treatment of crystal induced inflammation. *In* McCarty DJ (ed): Arthritis and Allied Conditions, 12th ed. Philadelphia, Lea & Febiger, 1993.
10. Wallace SL, et al: Therapy in gout. Rheum Dis Clin North Am 14(2):441–457, 1988.

16

Foot Lesions in Diabetic Patients

Richard B. Birrer, MD

In the United States, 5–6% of the population suffers from diabetes mellitus. Because of the remarkable consequences of their disease, diabetics are vulnerable to foot complications. Rampant and often widespread arteriosclerosis of the lower extremity combined with peripheral neuropathy make these patients susceptible to foot ulcerations, infection, and gangrene. Not uncommonly, a foot ulcer, recurrent fungal infection, or paronychial abscess is the first clue to chemical or clinical diabetes.

The following facts illustrate the severity of diabetic complications in the lower extremities:

• Gangrene of the lower extremities occurs 53 times as frequently in diabetic men and 71 times as frequently in diabetic women as in their nondiabetic counterparts.

• The risk of lower extremity amputation in diabetic patients is 15 to 30 times greater than in nondiabetic patients.

• 50–70% of all nontraumatic amputations are performed in diabetics.

• 50% of patients who have a unilateral amputation develop a limb-threatening complication in the opposite extremity within 2 years of the amputation.

• 25% of all diabetic hospital admissions are due to foot complications.

• The 3 year survival rate for diabetics who have undergone amputation is only 50%.

• Two billion dollars were spent in 1988 for hospital care related to diabetic amputations.

• 85% of diabetic amputations can be prevented with early detection and treatment in a multidisciplinary approach.

• More in-hospital days are spent treating foot infections than any other complication of diabetes.

The need for an aggressive and multidisciplinary approach to prevent limb loss is of paramount importance and may reduce these figures by 50%.

Pathophysiology

Complex and interrelated, the pathogenic effects of diabetes in the foot are threefold: angiopathy, neuropathy, and immunopathy (Fig. 1). Combined with environmental factors (e.g., poor hygiene), comorbid states (e.g., dehydration, malnutrition), trauma (e.g., poor shoe gear), and pathomechanical deformities (e.g., Charcot joints and mal perforans), ulcers lead to superinfection, gangrene, and limb loss through a viscous reinjury cycle of repeated ulcer formation.

Angiopathy

In diabetic patients, the gross and microscopic pathology of advanced arteriosclerosis is quite similar to that seen in nondiabetics. However, the disease is much more prevalent in diabetics as a group, and is more widespread and rapidly progressive in the individual with diabetes. Diabetics are found to have microangiopathy that begins with increased platelet adhesiveness and aggregation; this, in combination with endothelial injury, may be the most significant factor contributing to the increased prevalence of atherosclerosis. Lipoprotein oxidation and glycation have been clearly demonstrated in vitro to destroy endothelial, smooth muscle, and fibroblast

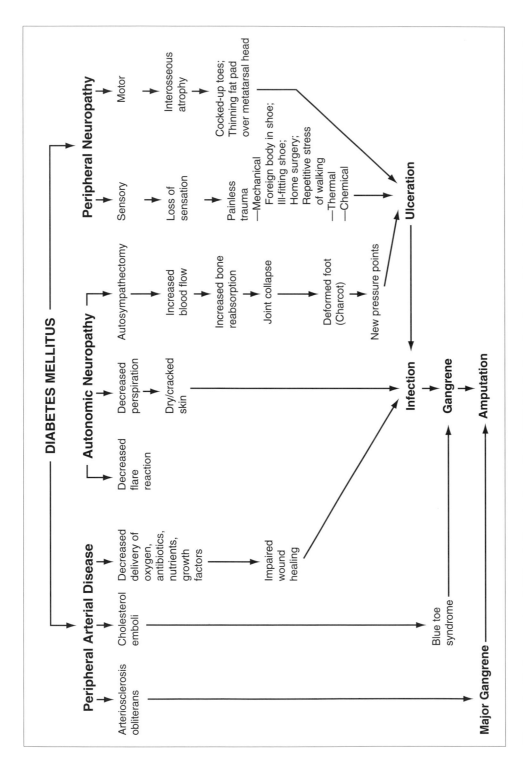

Figure 1. Pathogenesis of diabetic foot lesions. (Levin ME: Medical evaluation and treatment. *In* Levin ME, O'Neal LW, Bowker JH (eds): The Diabetic Foot. 5th ed. St. Louis, CV Mosby, 1993, with permission.)

cells as well as transform macrophages into foam cells. Once the platelets adhere to the area of intimal disruption, they stimulate the proliferation and migration of smooth muscle cells from the medial area of the vessels into the lumen. Plaque formation begins with the subsequent accumulation of lipids including cholesterol, fatty acid, and foam cells, and these plus calcium make up the atheromatous plaque. Denervation of the vasa vasorum supplying the tunica media of the artery may lead to diffuse linear calcification—a common finding in diabetics that is directly related to how long the disease has been present. Platelet aggregation continues to increase, leading to inadequate blood flow, arteriovenous shunting (capillary bypass), leakage of albumin and other proteins, and arterial wall stiffening. Resultant complications of decreased nutrition, oxygen tension, delayed immune response, and infection ensue. Risk factors such as smoking, hypertension, and hyperlipidemia exponentially worsen the atherosclerotic process. "Small vessel disease" and microvascular occlusion probably are not causes of ischemia.

As a general rule the severity of the angiopathy is directly related to the degree of the chemical diabetes and to the level of control of the serum glucose as well as the duration of disease. The prognosis for pedal infections is directly related to vascular disease, which also exacerbates the attendant neuropathy. Arteriosclerosis most often is the underlying cause of gangrene (ischemic necrosis)—one of the most feared complications of diabetes. The incidence of vascular disease is 8% at the onset of diabetes, rising to 15% after 10 years and 45% after 20 years of disease. Diabetics appear to have more pronounced disease in the distal vasculature involving the metatarsal vessels. Occlusion tends to be multisegmental, with a higher predilection for the infra geniculate vessels.

Neuropathy

Virtually all diabetic patients develop histopathologic changes of neuropathy in time. Direct metabolic damage to the Schwann cells results in segmental loss of the myelin sheath. Neuropathy is believed to be secondary to axonal degeneration that involves both small and large myelinated and unmyelinated fibers due to microangiopathic changes in the vasonervorum. Acute infections lead to

rapid onset of asymmetric mononeuropathy or mononeuritis multiplex. Biochemical abnormalities including depletion of axonal *myo*-inositol, accumulation of intraneural sorbitol and fructose, and impairment of intra-axonal vesicle transport are likely responsible for distal symmetric polyneuropathy.

Diabetic neuropathy encompasses a wide spectrum of neurologic conditions affecting sensory, motor, and autonomic functions. Mononeuropathies frequently are asymmetric and acute. Symmetric polyneuropathies are more common (50%), usually are bilateral and gradual in onset, and are classically described with a sock-glove distribution. Sensory impairment with loss of proprioception and touch, vibration, pain, and temperature perception usually precedes motor dysfunction. The latter affects intrinsic muscles of the foot, leading to alteration in shape and a change in gait pattern. Autonomic nervous system abnormalities yield a picture analogous to sympathectomy: the foot is warm, dry, and very susceptible to cracks and fissures, which often develop in a vague and nonspecific manner.

Osteopenia and stress fractures secondary to arteriovenous shunting eventually lead to the "rocker-bottom sole" or "bag of bones" of end-stage diabetic neuropathy, called Charcot's neuropathic osteoarthropathy. The biomechanical alterations and decreased sensation that result from neuropathy are the most common underlying causes of ulceration and infection. Neuropathy is present in over 80% of diabetic foot wounds. Bacteria localize in areas of increased compression and sensory loss, allowing the infection to progress without alerting the patient (Table 1).

Immunopathy

Recent research indicates that abnormalities in the diabetic immune system may be synergistic with vascular and neural pathophysiology. Autoimmunity in the form of low-density lipoprotein–containing immune complexes may underlie the development of macrovascular complications in diabetes. The complexes bind to the endothelium, perhaps promoted by an infectious etiology, and initiate the atherosclerotic process. Granulocyte function, as measured by phagocytosis and complement fixations, is impaired, leading to increased risk and severity of infection. Fibroblast replication and collagen production also are decreased, promoting poor wound healing

Table 1. Diabetic Neuropathy in the Foot

Types of Infection	Prevalence (%)
Intact skin	4
Ulcer	
Superficial	20
Deep	9
Gangrene	
Forefoot	27
Whole foot	7
Osteomyelitis/abscess	33

Sites of Osteomyelitis	Prevalence (%)
Ankle	3
Hindfoot	7
Metatarsals	38
Phalanges	51

and skin breakdown. Recently, glutamate de-carboxylase and ganglioside antibodies have been associated with neural injury in diabetes.

Clinical Evaluation

The most important aspect in evaluating the diabetic foot is the clinical examination. A careful dermatologic, neurologic, orthopedic, and vascular examination must be performed to assess patients at risk for foot problems.

Dermatologic Examination

The lower extremity is by far the most commonly affected skin area in diabetes. Infections of the toe nails, nail beds, and adjacent structures compose an important and frequently encountered group of problems.

Onychomycosis is among the most common dermatologic manifestations in the diabetic foot. The fungal infection is recognized by its yellowish-white, opaque appearance. It is, for the most part, asymptomatic; however, the nails become very thick, and subungual ulcerations can sometimes result from increased shoe pressure on the thickened nail. Often, the patient with mycotic nails has an associated chronic dermatophytosis (tinea pedis). The organisms that cause both the skin and nail infections are *Trichophyton mentagrophytes, Trichophyton rubrum,* and *Epidermophyton floccosum. Candida albicans* is less commonly found.

Onychocryptosis or ingrowing nail is a common and usually painful condition that is aggravated by tight shoes and improper nail care. The inflamed nail fold must be addressed by excising the offending nail. Without immediate and proper attention, this can quickly develop into a paronychia, followed by cellulitis and sepsis.

The interstitial web spaces of the diabetic, particularly the fourth space, may become macerated and white. The differential diagnosis must include tinea pedis, moniliasis, white psoriasis, soft corns, and bacterial infections from single or mixed organisms such as Proteus, Corynebacterium, Bacillus, Staphylococcus, Bacteroides, Clostridium, and Pseudomonas. Cultures for fungi, candida, and aerobic and anaerobic bacteria are essential for diagnosis of nail and skin infections. Proper and immediate attention is necessary to prevent more serious sequelae.

Hyperkeratotic lesions are no more frequent in the diabetic than the nondiabetic. However, such lesions in the ischemic or neuropathic foot can, if left untreated, lead to subkeratotic ulcerations, hematomas, and sinus tracts. As the pressure increases, the microcirculation becomes impeded and frank ulceration occurs (mal perforans). Fifteen to 20% of diabetic patients develop a foot ulcer during their lifetime; of these, 60–70% are neuropathic, 15–20% are vascular, and 15–20% are mixed in origin.

There are many other cutaneous lesions associated with diabetes that present in the lower extremity. Granuloma annulare, idiopathic hemmorhagic bullae, xanthochromia, xanthoma, and necrobiosis lipoidica diabeticorum should raise the clinician's suspicion of underlying diabetes. Pruritis is a common finding due to dryness of skin resulting from autonomic dysfunction.

Neurologic Examination

A simple exam can detect neuropathy in 30–40% of patients. Neuropathy develops slowly, and initially consists of paresthesias and night cramps, progresses to loss of vibration sense and perception of pain and light touch, and finally leads to loss of deep tendon reflexes. A simple monofilament wire (e.g., Semmes-Weinstein 5.07 gm) applied to several sites on the foot can be used to diagnose the hypoesthesia characteristic of peripheral sensory neuropathy. These clinical findings are a reflection of the fact that the more distal portion of the nerve exhibits greater demyelinization than the proximal portion. Evidence of peripheral autonomic dysfunction is exhibited by a brittle keratoses, atrophy of the fat pads, and loss of sebaceous gland function.

Since motor nerves also are involved, diabetics often develop a weakness in the intrinsic muscles of the feet leading to a disruption of the normal fine balance between the toe flexors and extensors. The result is claw and hammer-toe deformities with extensor subluxation of the toes, concomitant plantar prominence of the metatarsal heads, and proximal migration of the metatarsal fat pads. Weight bearing shifts to the unprotected metatarsal heads, and the now more prominent dorsally contracted toes are impacted into the shoe. In response to the trauma, the body reacts by producing excessive amounts of hyperkeratotic tissue or corns (heloma dura) and calluses (tylomata).

In addition to these structural changes, severe longstanding neuropathy can lead to a neuropathic arthropathy or Charcot joint. Due to the loss of proprioceptive sense, excessive and abnormal ranges of motion can develop in a joint. The result is a tearing of supportive ligaments and soft tissue, destruction of the joint cartilage, and microfractures of bone. The foot may appear grossly deformed, with typical rocker-bottom subluxation of the midtarsal region or subluxation of the metatarsophalangeal (MTP) joints. In an acute Charcot joint, the foot is erythematous, quite warm to the touch, and shows signs of anhidrosis. Almost always the pulses are bounding, and the patient relates a history of relatively mild to absent pain.

Orthopedic Examination

The importance of recognizing areas of potential breakdown due to altered weight-bearing patterns and bony prominences cannot be overemphasized. After observing gait pattern, structural deformities must be assessed. Hallux valgus deformity can lead to ulceration of the medial eminence; hallux rigidus or degenerative joint disease of the first MTP joint produces excessive motion and ulceration at the distal interphalangeal joint of the hallux. Hammer toe and cavus foot claw deformities can lead to ulcerations at the proximal interphalangeal joint, the distal interphalangeal joint, or both. Prominent metatarsal heads lead to hyperkeratotic tissue and, in combination with atrophied or anteriorly displaced fat pads, predispose to plantar ulcerations. A rocker-bottom or Charcot foot, characteristically appearing as a dorsiflexed and abducted forefoot, tends to cause midfoot plantar ulcerations. Patients with prior amputations will also have altered weight bearing and areas of increased pressure predisposing to breakdown.

Collectively, the neuropathic, angiopathic, and structural changes; defects in the skin barrier; wound healing chemotaxis; and phagocytosis predispose the diabetic foot to easy and often serious infection.

Vascular Examination

Assessing the role that ischemia plays in the diabetic foot requires a clinical examination and the use of noninvasive testing (Table 2). Inspection of an ischemic limb reveals skin pallor that is more pronounced on elevation, hair loss, and subcutaneous and dermal atro-

---

Table 2. Risk Factors for Lower Extremity Amputation in Diabetic Foot

Absent protective sensation
Vascular insufficiency
Foot deformity causing foci of high pressure
Autonomic neuropathy causing integument and osseous hyperemia
Limited joint mobility
Poor glucose control causing advanced glycosylation and impaired wound healing
Poor footwear causing or inadequately protecting from tissue breakdown
History of lower extremity amputation
History of foot ulceration
Obesity
Impaired vision

phy. These features plus nocturnal claudication are the most common symptoms of macroangiopathy. Paresthesia also is frequent. Claudication is 4 to 5 fold greater in incidence than in nondiabetics, and there is increased thickness of the nails. Dependent rubor is present in advanced stages of ischemia. Upon palpation the foot may be cool to cold, and the absence of pedal pulses (popliteal often strong and palpable) confirms the presence of arteriosclerotic occlusive disease. Paralysis represents irreversible tissue ischemia.

The measurement of flow velocity with Doppler apparatus allows for a more accurate assessment of peripheral perfusion. Because of incompressibility of the tibial vessels in diabetics, ankle pressure can be falsely elevated. A more accurate assessment is made by recording toe pressure. A normal toe/brachial index is 0.75; 0.25 represents severe occlusive disease. By calculating the toe/brachial index and measuring segmental pressure (absolute toe systolic pressure < 45 mmHg or ankle < 70 mmHg), the practitioner can evaluate the level of obstruction on the arterial tree between the femoral vessels and the digital arteries. Transcutaneous oxygen pressure of < 40 mmHg indicates significant disease; < 20 mmHg is associated with only a 20% chance of ulcer healing; and < 5 mmHg is an indication for amputation.

Radiographic Findings

Differentiation must be made between the noninfectious osseous alterations in the diabetic foot and osteomyelitis. It is crucial to note that using the radiograph as an isolated entity without an in-depth clinical evaluation can easily lead to misdiagnosis.

Osteolysis is a common noninfectious finding in the diabetic. Resorption of bone usually begins as a sharply defined lesion in the metatarsal or phalangeal region or both. The metatarsal shaft takes the appearance of a "pencil" or "candlestick" deformity. The remaining bone appears sclerotic, giving the lytic process a burned-out appearance. Acute osteomyelitis rarely shows areas of sclerosis. In addition, osteolysis does not exhibit the extensive periosteal elevation that is seen in osteomyelitis. There is minimal or no soft tissue inflammation, and the patient may be asymptomatic.

Osteoporosis, which is diffuse loss of bone mineral content, is another finding in the diabetic foot. Clinically this is important because it predisposes the patient to fracture.

Neuropathic joint (Charcot joint) produces the classic picture of bone lysis with marked fragmentation and eburnation. The joint space is decreased, the articulating bone margins are irregular, and osteophytes and bone resorption may be seen. There may be a tendency toward disarticulation and dissolution of the joints as well as calcification in and around the involved joints. The foot becomes shorter and wider.

Osteomyelitis has a radiographic appearance that is similar in the diabetic and nondiabetic patient. Characteristic changes include soft tissue swelling, osteolysis, periosteal reaction, and sequestrum formation (see Chapter 17).

Often the radiographic changes lag behind the clinical evidence; therefore, in addition to conventional radiographs, technetium 99m, gallium 67, and indium 111 scans used separately or together may assist in making an earlier diagnosis. Note that the health outcome may not justify the expense. Technetium scans are preferred since they can be positive as early as 48 hours after the onset of infection, and they detect reactive bone formation. Invasive diagnostic modalities such as arteriography, performed either conventionally or using digital computerized (subtraction) technology, are indicated for patients deemed candidates for vascular reconstruction. As a general rule, arteriography is indicated when there is a foot ulceration, with or without neuropathy, and when foot pulses are absent. Patency of the distal vessels must be arteriographically demonstrated before proceeding with bypass; careful selection with special follow-up is necessary because of the risks associated with the contrast media. Magnetic resonance angiography has the distinct advantage of avoiding any injection of contrast material. Osseous changes may be accompanied by the presence of gas in soft tissue—the end result of the metabolism of organisms such as *Escherichia coli, Acinobacter aerogenes,* Pseudomonas, and Klebsiella.

At the completion of the evaluation, the physician should be able to classify the diabetic patient with foot pathology into one of the following categories: neuropathic foot, ischemic foot, or combined ischemic and neuropathic foot with or without superinfection.

Management

Although this discussion concentrates on diabetic foot problems, such considerations are only part of an overall management plan for the diabetic. Clearly, other physiologic systems must be evaluated, particularly the serum glucose. The clinical objective is to convert the patient to the lowest possible category of pathology (Table 3). Prophylactic surgery generally is performed if the foot cannot be safely accommodated in prescription shoe wear. The keynote to the treatment of the diabetic foot is prevention.

The pain associated with polyneuropathy can be managed initially with simple analgesics (Table 4). It is essential to recognize that pain associated with diabetic neuropathy is either an exclusive diagnosis after ischemia has been ruled out or a chronic condition that spontaneously resolves when hypoesthesia becomes the dominant feature in the clinical picture.

Ischemic ulcers in diabetics should be recognized by clinical examination, evaluated by preoperative angiography, and revascularized if anatomically and technically feasible. If no reconstructible distal vessel is detectable on angiography, a below-knee amputation may be unavoidable.

Neuropathic ulcers can be subdivided into mild, moderate, or severe, depending on the depth of the ulcer, the presence or absence of bone involvement, and the presence of associated cellulitis or abscess (Table 5). Essential guidelines that should be adhered to in the treatment of neuropathic ulcers are:

1. Non-weight bearing is mandatory.

2. Soaking the wound macerates the tissue but does not debride the necrotic tissue and should be avoided.

3. Enzymatic chemical debridement and whirlpool soaks are not useful.

4. Although dextran polymer (Debrisan) may help in cleaning the wound, a wet or moist dressing of dilute povidone-iodine, Dakin's solution, or normal saline solution changed twice daily combined with thorough wound debridement is the safest and most effective method of wound care.

5. A fine-mesh, dry, sterile, nonadherent gauze dressing is preferred to either plain gauze or occlusive or semi-occlusive dressings.

6. Topical antibiotic solutions or ointments effective against methicillin-resistant strains of staphylococci sp. are nontoxic to most cells.

7. The use of vasodilators should be abandoned.

8. Hemorrheologic agents (pentoxifylline) have a limited role to play in patients with claudication due to diabetes associated with chronic occlusive arterial disease. These agents have no scientifically proven role to play in the treatment of diabetic foot ulcers.

9. Mature lyophilized (freeze dried) type 1 bovine collagen is a cost-effective primary dressing for all types of ulcers (infected and noninfected) that accelerates epithelialization, has minimum recurrence rates, and is superior to other dressings (hydrogels, hydrocolloids, calcium, and dextranomer products).

Surgical treatment is indicated for severe claudication, intractable rest pain, necrosis, or nonresponding ulcerations. Surgical options include arterial reconstruction (angioplasty or in-situ or reversed vein bypass), thromboembolectomy when applicable, and, rarely, sympathectomy. Three-year patency rates are 85–90%, with comparable limb salvage rates. Excellent results in the treatment of arterial insufficiency follow dedicated, aggressive medical treatment and improved surgical techniques, such as angioscopy, balloon or laser angioplasty, and atherectomy catheterization.

Amputation (1% incidence per year among diabetics) is the treatment of last resort in end-stage vascular disease (Table 6). Initial mortality after amputation is 20%; 60% of patients survive 3 years and 45% are alive at 5 years. Within 3 years, 49% of surviving patients have a second amputation; within 5 years, 55–60%.

10. Topical application of growth factors (twice a day for 8 weeks) derived from the patient's peripheral blood improves granulation and epithelization.

11. Total contact casting every week for 3–9 weeks is beneficial because it allows equal distribution of weight over the entire foot surface due to snug fitting (see Chapter 20).

12. Prepare yourself and the patient for a prolonged treatment plan, since healing is often slow.

Diabetic ulcers are a limb-threatening complication of the disease, and they require a very aggressive approach to avoid the potential risk of limb loss. All ulcers should be probed with a sterile instrument to determine involvement of underlying structures. Because osteomyelitis is strongly associated once the

Table 3. Diabetic Foot Classification and Management

Category	Treatment
0—Minimal pathology present • Patient diagnosed with diabetes mellitus • Protective sensation intact (Semmes-Weinstein 10 gm wire detectable) • Ankle brachial index (ABI) > 0.80 and toe systolic pressure > 45 mmHg • No history of ulceration	Tri-annual visits to assess neurovascular status and foci of stress Possible shoe accommodations Patient education Medical management
1—The neuropathic foot • Category 0 characteristics PLUS • No history of diabetic neuropathic osteoarthropathy (Charcot's joint) • Protective sensation absent (Semmes-Weinstein 10 gm wire not detectable) • No foot deformity	Same as category 0 PLUS Possible shoe gear accommodation insole (pedorthic/orthotist consultation) Follow-up visits every 6 months
2—Neuropathy with foot deformity • Category 1 characteristics PLUS • Foot deformity present (focus of stress)	Same as Category 1 PLUS Pedorthic/orthotist consultation for possible custom-molded/extra-depth shoes Possible prophylactic surgery to alleviate focus of stress Follow-up visits every 3–4 months.
3—Demonstrated pathology Category 2 characteristics PLUS • History of neuropathic ulceration • History of Charcot's joint • Foot deformity present (focus of stress)	Same as Category 2 BUT Follow-up visits every 1–2 months
4A—Neuropathic ulceration • Noninfected neuropathic ulceration	Same as Category 3 PLUS Pressure reduction program Dressing change program Debridement program Weekly to bi-weekly follow-up visits as needed
4B—Acute Charcot's joint • Category 4A characteristics PLUS • Acute diabetic neuropathic osteoarthropathy (Charcot's joint)	Same as Category 3 PLUS Pressure reduction program; possible total contact cast Weekly to bi-weekly follow-up visits (as per contact casting regimen)
5—The infected diabetic foot • Protective sensation may or may not be present • Infected wound • Charcot's joint may be present	Same as Category 4 (A and B) PLUS Debridement of infected, necrotic tissue and/or bone, as indicated Possible hospitalization, antibiotic treatment regimen

Table continues on next page.

Table 3. Diabetic Foot Classification and Management (*continued*)

Category	Treatment
6—The ischemic limb • Protective sensation may or may not be present • Ankle brachial index (ABI) < 0.80 or toe systolic pressure < 45 mmHg or pedal transcutaneous oxygen tension < 40 mmHg. • Ulceration may be present	Vascular consultation, possible revascularization If infection present, treatment same as for Category 5 Contact casting generally contraindicated

wound probes to bone, it should be included in the initial assessment of all patients with infected pedal ulcers. Special roentgenographic and radionuclide tests are unnecessary if bone is palpated on probing. Early referral to podiatry and vascular surgery specialists is necessary to limit the progression of the pathology.

Prevention

Although pathogenic complications of diabetes mellitus such as angiopathy and neuropathy cannot be prevented, the resultant ulcerations and infection can. The patient must take an active role in the management and constant monitoring of his or her feet to decrease the risk of serious foot problems. Patient education is crucial, and a list should be provided as a constant reminder of do's and don'ts (see Appendix II at end of book).

The feet must be inspected daily for signs of erythema, cuts, scratches, abrasions, blisters, or the buildup of callus. A family member may need to assist if the patient's vision is inadequate. If any of the above are noticed or any other abnormality is seen, the patient should contact a doctor. The patient should not cut his or her own nails, corns, or calluses. The feet should be washed daily with a mild soap and dried carefully, especially between the toes.

Table 4. Common Analgesics for Diabetic Neuropathy

Tricyclic antidepressants	Inhibits ascending serotonin pathway Lower dosage range usually sufficient Dosage range 25–75 mg (max 100–200 mg/day) Adjunctive therapy with phenothiazine often helpful in refractory cases (fluphenazine 1–6 mg/day)
NSAIDs	First-line agent May inhibit aldose reductase inhibitors
Local anesthetics	IV lidocaine hydrochloride good for up to 3 weeks; cost effective; be wary of cardiac side effects Mexiletine < 10 mg/kg/day
Anticonvulsants	Clonidine 100–500 mg Carbamazepine is effective but serious side effects (100 mg tid starting at 1–1.5 g/day) Clonazepam appears to be effective; valproic acid (250–1500 mg/day) Phenytoin not useful
Hemorrhagic agents	Pentoxifylline may be helpful (400 mg tid)
Capsaicin cream	Locally depletes substance P; transient effects; expensive and significant dermatologic side effects; apply tid or qid
Aldose reductase inhibitors	May be useful in selected cases Metoclopramide 10 mg tid

NSAIDS = nonsteroidal anti-inflammatory drugs, tid = three times a day, qid = four times a day

Table 5. Classification and Management of Neuropathic Ulcers in Diabetes

Category	Clinical Appearance	Treatment
Mild	Superficial No cellulitis No osteomyelitis	Rest Culture and sensitivity Antibiotics (oral) Orthotics appliances Careful follow-up
Grade 0 (Wagner Brodsky)	No ischemia No open lesions Bony deformities and/or hyper- keratoses present	Observation

Moderate
  Grades 1–3 (Wagner)
  Grades 2 (Brodsky)
	Deep ulcer extending into tendon
	  and/or joint capsule with possible
	  bone involvement
		Admission to hospital
		Culture specific
		Antibiotics (IV)
		Surgical debridement
		Local dressings?
		Amputation?
		Bypass
		Orthotic appliances
		Careful follow-up

Severe
  Grades 4 and 5 (Wagner)
  Grade 3 (Brodsky)
	Deep ulcer
	Osteomyelitis
	Cellulitis > 2 cm
	Gangrene
		Admission to surgery
		Culture specific
		Antibiotics (IV)
		Surgical debridement
		Local wound care?
		Amputation?
		Bypass
		Orthotic appliances
		Careful follow-up

Daily lubrication with a nonperfumed, lanolin-based lotion helps to avoid dryness and fissuring. Sometimes an antifungal preparation may be needed if dryness and peeling are due to dermatophytosis, but this should be prescribed by the patient's physician. Thick socks without seams should be worn, preferably wool. Shoes must be inspected daily for foreign objects.

Reduction of abnormal forces by means of orthoses and proper shoe gear is mandatory in the foot at risk of developing ulcerations. One type of orthosis is an insole used mostly to redistribute the plantar weight forces acting on the metatarsal heads, distal tips of the digits, and other plantar bony prominences which have a tendency to build excessive hyperkeratotic tissue and eventually ulcerate. The orthotic also can be designed to add support to the longitudinal arch of the foot and to the greater and lesser tarsus, especially for those diabetics with Charcot changes. Another type of orthosis is the prescription foot orthotic.

The advantage of a custom-fabricated orthotic is that it allows for more biomechanical control of the entire foot. Once the appropriate insert or orthotic is fabricated, certain precautions must be taken to avoid causing lesions on other areas of the foot. A break-in period and constant observation for irritation or other problems, especially in the neuropathic foot, are essential.

In addition to foot orthoses, the prevention of soft tissue damage from continuous or intermittent pressures can be achieved by the selection of proper shoe gear (Table 7). An inappropriately fitting shoe (e.g., too tight) can cause increased pressure and resultant soft tissue breakdown at the site of irritation. A shoe that is too loose can increase friction as the foot slips, resulting in ulcerations at bony prominences. The diabetic patient should be made aware that new shoes should not be worn for more than 2 hours at a time, and after each usage the foot must be examined for areas of irritation. The bunion last shoe, with

Table 6. Indications for Amputation

Excessive tissue destruction obstructing weight bearing and ambulation
Dissemination of infection
Failure to heal with prolonged (3- to 4-week) therapy (antibiotics and local wound care)
Recurrent ischemic ulceration in a patient with surgically untreatable ischemic disease
Osteomyelitis associated with severe ischemia; gangrene in diffuse presentation

an increased medial width, prevents friction and ulceration over the medial eminence. Molded shoes also have been used to prevent or treat neuropathic ulcerations. These shoes are made from a cast of the patient's foot to assure proper fit and to redistribute the forces of weight bearing more evenly. However, specialized footwear is expensive, often not covered by insurance, and may not be easily available.

Alternatively, specific materials can be used to directly alleviate pressure areas and disperse the weight-bearing pattern of the foot. These materials must be used cautiously because certain adhesives may be deleterious to the skin of a diabetic; moreover, any device placed around the toes or foot must be placed loosely, if at all, to avoid strangulation of tissue and further serious complications. Proper shoes, insoles, and orthotic devices along with appropriate foot care and hygiene serve as adjuncts to good diabetic control in preventing pedal ulcerations.

The Septic Foot

Life threatening infections such as sepsis, gangrene, and myonecrosis occur in 1-5% of diabetic patients. Often these patients present to the emergency department in ketoacidosis with signs of systemic sepsis. A complete examination of the patient reveals a swollen foot draining pus from an ulceration on the plantar surface. The dorsal location of the swelling is often misleading since most of the pathology is originating from the sole of the foot. An unexplained loss of glucose control in any diabetic patient should prompt a thorough examination of the feet. The complete blood count and erythrocyte sedimentation rate may be normal except in the presence of a glaring infection. For additional information on infections, see Chapter 17.

Microbiologic studies are mandatory to guide the antimicrobial therapy accurately (Table 8). The average number of isolates is 3.2 bacterial species per patient. The best technique for routine culture is the swab method, after debridement and sterile saline wipe, with careful attention to anaerobic cultures. Sixty five to 70% of pathogenic bacteria are identified. Cultures obtained by curettage of ulcers or needle aspiration more nearly match culture results obtained surgically

Anaerobes are more prevalent in chronic wounds. Gram-negative or anaerobic infections are suggested by the presence of foul smelling pus or gas in deeper tissue. Complicated infections are more frequently caused by Pseudomonas and Enterobacteriaceae species. The presence of multiple organisms or gram-positive, gram-negative, aerobic, or anaerobic strains underlines the importance of broad-spectrum antibiotic coverage upon admission. Combinations are usually preferred over single drug regimens. Bactericidal agents are preferred over bacteriostatic ones due to granulocyte dysfunction.

The diabetic patient with a septic foot rep-

Table 7. Footwear Guidelines for Diabetic Patients

1. Good fit (excess width or length causes friction leading to blistering and probable infection)
2. High toe box and a round toe (to accommodate hammer toes, orthoses, and interdigital heloma)
3. Rigid counter to support heel
4. Rigid shank to support arch
5. Soft insert to act as soft-tissue supplement and to accommodate any plantar lesions
6. No cracks or breaks in the inserts or seams
7. Soft leather upper

Table 8. Organisms Typically Found in Foot Ulcers of Diabetic Patients

Organism	Percentage Found in Ulcer
Gram-negative, aerobic	
Proteus species	55
Escherichia coli	30
Klebsiella species	20
Pseudomonas aeruginosa	15
Gram-positive, aerobic	
Streptococcus fecalis	45
Staphylococcus aureus	35
Streptococci (non-group A or D)	35
Staphylococcus epidermidis	25–30
Gram-negative, anaerobic	
Bacteroides fragilis	45
Bacteroides melaninogenicus	35
Gram-positive, anaerobic	
Peptostreptococcus species	20–25
Clostridium species	35
Propionibacterium species	25

resents an absolute surgical emergency requiring hospital admission. Initial management must focus on the correction of the systemic aspects of sepsis:

1. Correction of hypovolemia
2. Control of hyperglycemia
3. Correction of metabolic acidosis
4. Administration of broad-spectrum antibiotics
5. Control of cardiovascular instability.

Within 8–12 hours, the patient should undergo surgical drainage of the purulent collection. If the foot is well perfused with present pedal pulses, wide debridement of all infected tissue is necessary, along with toe amputation if osteomyelitis is present. Secondary wound coverage is performed when all sepsis has been controlled and good granulation tissue appears in the wound.

Charcot's Joint

Charcot's joint in the acute stage is managed by rest and total non-weight bearing on the affected foot, typically for a minimum of 8 weeks. Serial radiographs and physical exam aid in determining how long the patient requires non-weight bearing. Gradual weight bearing with a diabetic orthotic (accommodative) or cast brace can be initiated if there is radiographic evidence of coalescence, no crepitus on range-of-motion exercises, and no markers of acute inflammation. Weight bearing is progressive if symptoms are not exacerbated. Weight bearing is discontinued if symptoms recur. Full ambulation is achieved in 4–5 months on average for midfoot disease, and, more importantly, progressive deformities are avoided.

Chronic Charcot's joint and Charcot's disease of the heel and ankle are frustrating and difficult to manage. Depending upon the degree of deformity or dislocation, treatment ranges from molded orthotics or shoes to bone simulators to promote healing, cast immobilization, and surgical intervention. Surgery is indicated for removal of plantar exostosis resulting in chronic ulcerations or for incision and drainage of infected ulcers. Joint fusions are not universally recommended.

Conclusion

The pathobiology of the diabetic foot lesion is complex. Aggressive diagnosis and treatment are essential to maximize chances for limb salvage. The primary care physician must understand these important aspects and coordinate a multidisciplinary effort to optimize the diabetic's foot life and avoid long-term disability.

References

1. American Diabetics Association: Diabetic Foot Care. McLean, Virginia, ADA, 1990. (1970 Chain Bridge Rd, McLean, VA, 22109-0592. Telephone 1-800-ADA-DISC, extension 363)
2. Bulat T, Kosinski M: Diabetic foot: Strategies to prevent and treat common problems. Geriatrics 50(2):46–55, 1995.
3. Eckman MH, Greenfields S, Mackey WC, et al: Foot infections in diabetic patients. JAMA 273(9):712–720, 1995.
4. Giurini JM, Chrzan JS, Gibbons GW, et al: Charcot's disease in diabetic patients. Postgrad Med 89(4):163–169, 1991.
5. Grayson ML, Gibbons GW, Balogh K, et al: Probing to bone in infected pedal ulcers. JAMA 273(9):721–723, 1995.
6. Gruinfield C: Diabetic foot ulcers: Etiology, treatment, and prevention. Adv Intern Med 37:103–32, 1992.
7. Kaschak TJ, et al: Radiology of the diabetic foot. Clin Podiatr Med Surg 857, 1988.
8. Keyser JE: Foot wounds in diabetic patients. Postgrad Med 91(4):98–109, 1992.
9. Pecoraro RE, Reiber GE, Burgess EM: Causal pathways to amputation: Basis for prevention. Diabetes Care 13:513–521, 1990.
10. Pliskin MA, Todd WF, Edelson GW: Presentations of the diabetic foot. Arch Fam Med 3:273–279, 1994.
11. Siller TA, Calhoren JH, Mader JT: Diabetic foot infections. J Musculoskeletal Med 13(11): 43–55, 1996.
12. U.S. Dept. Of Health and Human Services: Lower extremity amputation prevention (LEAP) program. Carvel, Louisiana, Bureau of Primary Health Care, USDHHS, National Clearinghouse for Primary Care Information, 1995. (Telephone 703-821-8955, extension 248 [$15.00 for LEAP])

17

Infections of the Foot

Harrison Donnelly, MD and Michael P. DellaCorte, DPM

The foot is predisposed to a variety of infections that reflect both functional and environmental factors. Stress to both the skin and subcutaneous structures causes blisters, hematomas, inflammation, and fissures that often progress to superficial and sometimes deep tissue infections. Exposure to the elements can cause breakdown of the skin, giving access to causative agents. Shoes and socks or stockings, functioning primarily for protection, produce a closed environment that deprives the foot of light and fresh air and generates moisture from increased heat production and perspiration. The cause of the infection may not always be obvious, and the classic signs of infection may be misleading. The differential diagnosis should include gout, stress fracture, infection (both bacterial and fungal), dermatitis, and arthritis.

Under ideal circumstances (hospital, clinic, office), a complete blood count with differential, culture and sensitivity testing of the wound base, and a chemistry panel should be obtained. The antibiotic prescribed should be narrow spectrum and specific for the causative bacteria (as noted on the culture report). Practically speaking, such lab work may not be readily available to office-based practitioners, and the culture and sensitivity require 24–48 hours. Therefore, an educated guess (empiric) for the choice of antibiotic is necessary (Table 1).

Traditionally, penicillin (e.g., Pen-Vee K) has been the drug of choice; it is inexpensive and effective. However, penicillinase-producing bacteria (i.e., *Staphylococcus aureus*) require the use of synthetic penicillins, such as di-cloxacillin or cloxacillin. Such agents are not very broad spectrum, and they are expensive. A broad-spectrum antibiotic, such as a cephalosporin (e.g., cephalexin, cefadroxil) is a reasonable alternative. Cephalexin, 500 mg given orally every 6 hours for 7–10 days, has a spectrum of coverage consisting of *S. aureus,* Streptococcus group A, Klebsiella, *Escherichia coli,* and Proteus. Cefadroxil has a similar spectrum, but dosage is 500 mg given twice daily or 1 gram daily. Once culture results are available, the antibiotic therapy is adjusted based on sensitivities. If the wound is improving clinically, the initial antibiotic generally is continued for 10 days. Intravenous antibiotics, along with hospitalization, are warranted if no clinical improvement is noted, if systemic symptoms and signs are noted, or if there is history of poorly controlled diabetes or peripheral vascular disease.

Skin Infections

Cellulitis

Cellulitis is an acute, severe, rapidly spreading skin infection. The two most common agents causing cellulitis are group A *Streptococcus pyogenes* and *S. aureus*. The severity of the disease is variable but warrants rapid diagnosis and treatment. Clinical presentation is characterized by hyperemia, edema, pain, increased local temperature, and decreased function. The causative microorganism and its by-products can travel proximally along anatomic pathways such as subcutaneous tissue spaces, tendon sheaths, fascial spaces,

Table 1. Antimicrobial Drugs of Choice

Infecting Organism	Drug of Choice	Usual Adult Dose	Alternative
Gram-positive cocci			
Staphylococcus aureus or *epidermidis* (non-pencillinase)	Penicillin G, V	V: 1-2 g/day PO Q6h G: 2-20 million units IV Q4-6h	Cephalosporin, vancomycin, clindamycin
S. aureus or *epidermidis* (penicillinase) Methicillin resistant	Penicillinase-resistant penicillin (cloxacillin, dicloxacillin) Vancomycin with or without rifampin and/or gentamicin	2-4 g/day PO Q6h 2-12 g/day IV Q4-6h 1-2 g/day IV Q6-12h	Cephalosporin, vancomycin, clindamycin, trimethoprim/sulfamethoxazole, ciprofloxacin, imipenem
Streptococcus—groups A, B, C, G; *bovis; milleri; pneumoniae;* or *viridans*	Penicillin G, V	As above	Cephalosporin, vancomycin, clindamycin, erythromycin
Streptococcus group D, enterococcus	Ampicillin + gentamicin	2-8 g/day IV Q4-6h 1-2 g/day PO Q6h 0.75-2 g/day PO Q6-8h	Vancomycin, imipenem, penicillin, aminoglycoside
Gram-positive bacilli			
Bacillus anthracis Cornybacterium species *Listeria monocytogenes*	Penicillin G, V Erythromycin Ampicillin Gentamicin Ciprofloxacin Doxycycline	As above 1-4 g/day IV Q6h 1-2 g/day PO Q6h 3-5 mg/kg/day 500 mg PO Q12h 100 mg PO Q12h	Erythromycin, penicillin G, trimethoprim/sulfamethoxazole
Gram-negative cocci			
Neisseria meningitides *Neisseria gonorrhoeae*	Penicillin G Ceftriaxone, cefaxime	As above As above	Ceftriaxone, ofloxacin, ciprofloxacin
Gram-negative bacilli			
Escherichia coli	Beta lactamase inhibitor Cephalosporin	3-5 mg/kg/day IV or IM Q8h 250-500 mg PO QID	Cephalosporin, trimethoprim/sulfamethoxazole, imipenem, aztreonam, ciprofloxacin, norfloxacin
Klebsiella	Cephalosporin with or without aminoglycoside	As above	Aminoglycoside, trimethoprim/sulfamethoxazole, piperacillin, mezlocillin, imipenem, ticarcillin, clavulanate, aztreonam, ciprofloxacin, norfloxacin, amoxicillin-clavulanate

Table continues on next page.

Table 1. Antimicrobial Drugs of Choice (*continued*)

Infecting Organism	Drug of Choice	Usual Adult Dose	Alternative

Morganella morganii	Imipenam
	Aminoglycoside
	Ciprofloxacin/
	  norfloxacin
		3–5 mg/kg/day IV or
		  IM Q8h
		750 mg PO BID
			Amikacin,
			  aztreonam,
			  antipseudomonal
			  penicillin,
			  ticarcillin,
			  amoxicillin,
			  clavulanate

Enterobacter aerogenes or *cloacae*	Aminoglycoside
	Cephalosporin—
	  third generation
		As above	Aztreonam,
			  imipenem,
			  trimethoprim,
			  sulfamethoxazole,
			  antipseudomonal
			  penicillin,
			  ciprofloxacin

Citrobacter freundii	Imipenem, trime-
	  thoprim/sulfame-
	  thoxazole, amino-
	  glycoside, ciproflo-
	  xacin, norfloxacin
	Aminoglycoside
	  (gentamicin)
		1–4 g/day IV Q6h
		
		3–5 mg/kg/day
			Tetracycline,
			  cephalosporin—
			  third
			  generation

Pseudomonas aeruginosa	Antipseudomonal
	  penicillin (carben-
	  icillin)
		3–5 mg/kg/day IV or
		  IM Q8h
		8–40 g/day IV Q4–6h
			Aminoglycoside,
			  cefoperazone,
			  imipenem,
			  ceftazidime,
			  aztreonam,
			  ciprofloxacin

Pseudomonas cepacia	Trimethoprim/
	  sulfamethoxazole
		2–20 mg/kg/day PO
		  or IV Q6–8h
			Chloramphenicol,
			  ceftazidime

Pseudomonas mallei	Streptomycin +
	  tetracycline
		1–2 g/day IM	Chloramphenicol,
			  streptomycin

Pseudomonas maltophilia	Trimethoprim/
	  sulfamethoxazole
		2–20 mg/kg/day PO
		  or IV Q6–8h
			Ticarcillin-
			  clavulanate

Proteus mirabilis	Ampicillin	2–8 g/day IV Q4–6h
		1–2 g/day PO Q6h
			Aminoglycoside,
			  trimethoprim/-
			  sulfamethoxazole,
			  aztreonam,
			  imipenem,
			  ciprofloxacin,
			  antipseudomonal
			  penicillin,
			  cephalosporin—
			  third generation

Proteus vulgaris	Cephalosporin—
	  third generation
	  (cefoperazone)
	Aminoglycoside
		2–8 g/day IM or
		  IV Q8–12h
			Trimethoprim/
			  sulfamethoxazole,
			  aztreonam,
			  oxacillin,
			  imipenem,
			  amoxicillin,
			  ticarcillin,
			  clavulanate,
			  ciprofloxacin

Table continues on next page.

Table 1. Antimicrobial Drugs of Choice (*continued*)

Infecting Organism	Drug of Choice	Usual Adult Dose	Alternative
Pasteurella multocida	Penicillin G	2–20 million units IV Q4–6h	Tetracycline, erythromycin, cephalosporin, ampicillin
Haemophilus influenzae	Amoxicillin/ clavulanate Cephalosporin— third generation (cefoperazone) Trimethoprim/ sulfamethoxazole	2–8 g/day IM or IV Q8–12h	Chloramphenicol
Anaerobes			
Bacteroides fragilis group	Metronidazole Clindamycin, cefoxitin, imipenem, ticarcillin Clavulanate	0.75–2 g/day PO Q 12h	Cefotan, chloramphenicol, oxacillin, ampicillin, sulbactam
Clostridium species	Penicillin G, clindamycin	As above	Chloramphenicol, metronidazole, erythromycin, clindamycin, oxacillin, penicillin
Clostridium difficile	Vancomycin (oral) Metronidazole (oral)	1.0 g/day PO Q6h 100 mg/day PO Q6h	Bacitracin (oral), cholestyramine
Peptostreptococcus	Penicillin G	2–20 million units IV Q4–6h	Clindamycin, metronidazole, cephalosporin, chloramphenicol, erythromycin, vancomycin, imipenem
Actinomyces israelii	Ampicillin or penicillin G	2–20 million units IV Q4–6h	Clindamycin, tetracycline, erythromycin

BID = two times daily, h = hours; IM = intramuscularly; IV = intravenously; PO = orally; Q = every; QID = four times daily

muscles, lymphatics, and bone. The result may be bacteremia or septicemia. Both erythema and interdigital fungi with maceration can mimic a cellulitis. The diagnosis is sometimes difficult in these cases.

Acute cellulitis also can be caused by coliform bacteria, e.g., *E. coli,* Klebsiella, or Enterobacter. Treatment varies depending on the severity of the infection and the susceptibility testing, when available. Mild to moderate staph/strep infection is treated with cephalexin 250–500 mg PO qid, dicloxacillin 250–500 mg PO qid, clindamycin 300 mg PO qid, erythromycin 250–500 mg PO qid or amoxicillin-clavulanate 250–500 mg PO tid until the third day after the acute inflammation disappears.

Severe staph/strep infection requires nafcillin 1–2 g IV q4h for 7–10 days. Cefuroxime axetil 250–500 mg PO q12h, cefuroxime sodium 750 mg–1.5 g IV q8h, and clarithromycin 500 mg PO q12h are reserved for gram-negative cellulitis.

Note: For a discussion of **unguis incarnatus** (paronychia), refer to chapter 5.

Infected Blister

Blisters result from the stress of constant friction in one area of the foot. The pain that accompanies the blister formation usually forces the patient to change gait pattern or to rest the foot. Without relief, further stress can open the blister and expose the underlying tissue to bacteria; the end result is a localized painful infection. Treatment consists of debridement, dispersion padding, and warm soaks or compresses; antibiotic therapy can include cephalexin 250–500 mg PO qid.

Infected Fissures

Fissures are cracks in the skin that can be caused by fungus, dry skin conditions (e.g., xerosis), biomechanical abnormalities, or long-standing tylomata. Left untreated, the fissure progresses through the skin and into the subcutaneous tissue, causing pain and infection. Once infected, progression to cellulitis is rapid; therefore, aggressive treatment is necessary. In addition to management of the infection, treatment consists of debridement of the fissure with a scalpel or tissue nipper to remove any hyperkeratotic or necrotic tissue. Dispersion padding and modifications in shoe gear may be necessary to relieve pressure. Modifications include cutting the shoe to relieve pressure and/or padding inside the shoe. Weekly debridements may be necessary until the condition resolves completely. When the etiology is biomechanical, foot orthotics may be indicated to prevent future infections.

Infection Laceration

The clinician should obtain a history of how and when the laceration occurred, along with any pertinent medical history (i.e., medications, diabetes, peripheral vascular disease). The patient should be questioned about constitutional symptoms, such as fever, general malaise, chills, and tetanus immunization sta-

tus. Vital signs are recorded, and the wound is carefully inspected, measured, and palpated. A drawing of the wound should be noted in the chart.

Treatment consists of rest, elevation, heat, debridement, lavage, and a broad-spectrum antibiotic. A dosage of 0.5 ml of tetanus toxoid should be administered intramuscularly according to the guidelines in Chapter 13. Warm water soaks in Burow's solution or epsom salt may be effective in draining open wounds. Dry, sterile dressings should be applied to the wound after the soaks. Elevation above heart level has been the standard of care for allowing an edematous area to drain. In cases in which the pedal circulation is marginal, leaving the foot level relative to the heart increases tissue perfusion and antibiotic blood levels. The wound should not be sutured; secondary closure or delayed primary closure is the usual treatment.

Osteomyelitis

Osteomyelitis (OM), or infection of the bone, historically has been classified or described as:
- Hematogenous—spread of micro-organisms via the bloodstream
- Contiguous—spread of infection from adjacent soft tissue
- Direct inoculation secondary to trauma or surgery
- Vascular insufficiency—generally caused by poor tissue perfusion.

A four-stage system noting the clinical presentation is outlined below:
1. Simple infections, consisting of cellulitis in soft tissue, medullary OM in bone, and acute septic arthritis in joints
2. Superficial infections, consisting of ulcers in soft tissue, superficial OM in bone (no medullary involvement), and septic arthritis with chondrolysis in joints
3. Localized infections, consisting of abscesses in soft tissue, localized OM in bone, and septic arthritis with localized OM in joints
4. Diffuse infections, consisting of gangrene in soft tissue, diffuse OM in bone, and joint infections producing instability.

The system is based on the status of the host: good immune system and good local tissue perfusion; immunocompromised and compromised tissue perfusion; or not a surgical candidate.

Although a definitive diagnosis of osteomyelitis can be made only by bone culture, the clinical and radiographic evaluations can aid the clinician in ruling out this complicated bone infection. Grayson, et al. have reported a bedside technique for the diagnosis of osteomyelitis. A hand-held, sterile probe is introduced into the ulcer site and directed at the underlying bone: the test is positive if bone is encountered underlying the ulcer base without the apparent presence of intervening soft tissue; it is negative in the absence of this finding. Exposed bone in this instance is considered clinical osteomyelitis, and it behooves the clinician to treat the patient aggressively until the definitive diagnosis can be made.

Radiology Findings

Three radiologic methods are available to assess OM: conventional x-ray, radionuclide studies, and magnetic resonance imaging (MRI). Plain films of the noninfected foot and/or previous films of the involved foot are helpful for a comparison analysis.

Radiographic appearance of OM is evident on conventional x-ray when there is 50–60% loss of bone mass, on radionuclide studies using Tc 99 (three-phase bone scan) or gallium 97 when there is 20% loss of bone mass, and on MRI when there is 10% loss of bone mass. The first sign of OM on conventional x-ray is deep soft-tissue swelling; the first sign of bone involvement is periosteal lifting (Codman's triangle or areas of radiolucency) which can occur in 1–2 weeks. The chronic phase of OM is noted by the formation of sequestra, which are highly opaque, smooth islands of bone that usually are surrounded by areas of decreased bone density. The three-phase bone scan may be positive in all three phases—flow, blood pool, and delayed—but even this does not allow a definitive diagnosis. The usefulness of the gallium-97 scan can be compromised because of masking of bone involvement due to concurrent uptake of the nuclide by inflamed soft tissues. Thus, in equivocal OM cases, the Tc-99 scan (with a half-life of about 24 hours) can be followed, in a day, by a gallium-97 scan (with a half life of 48–72 hours) to aid in differentiation between bone and soft-tissue-only involvement (see Chapter 3).

Treatment of Osteomyelitis

Hospital admission often is mandatory. A complete blood count with differential, erythrocyte sedimentation rate (ESR), HbA_{1c}, and cultures of both soft tissue and bone are essential. Two sets of blood cultures should be obtained immediately and can be repeated based on clinical conditions. Superficial wound cultures are discouraged because both colonizing and infecting organisms are recovered; hence, either deep wound or debrided tissue cultures should be obtained. Vascular evaluation is essential prior to surgical intervention. Debridement with resection of infected bone usually is indicated. Preservation of digits/rays is a goal, but amputation often is necessary.

In the operating room, deep tissue for culture and sensitivity (C&S) along with bone from the remaining proximal bone margin for both pathology (histology and gram stain) and C&S must be obtained. This is to insure that all the infected bone has been removed.

Empiric therapy with ticarcillin-clavulanic acid 3.1 g IV q4h for calculated creatinine clearance of 60 ml/min or greater (q6 or q8 for impaired renal function) is appropriate for uncomplicated OM. In cases of limb- or life-threatening conditions, imipenem 500 mg IV q 6 may be used plus an aminoglycoside (gentamicin 1.5 mg/kg q8 or 4.5 mg/kg single daily dose or amikacin 5 mg/kg q 8 or 15 mg/kg single daily dose; tobramycin is expensive). If an aminoglycoside is used, 3 days of close attention to renal function is mandatory. Once-daily dosing of aminoglycosides does not require peak and trough measurements. The initial, empiric treatment regimen can be modified as necessary based on the culture results.

The optimal duration of antimicrobial therapy after surgical debridement of infected bone has not been established. There has been considered opinion that antimicrobial therapy does not cure OM in the diabetic foot. The traditional regimen for acute OM has been 7 weeks parenteral therapy; for chronic OM, several months. One regimen for the chronic case has been parenteral therapy until the ESR is one-half the initial value, then oral therapy for 4–6 months. Home parenteral therapy should be considered as an alternative to long-term hospitalization.

If, after amputation, the proximal remaining-bone margin is found to be free of OM (hence, the value of this invasive diagnostic approach), then the local tissue infection can be treated for 3–5 days parenterally. OM remaining at the proximal site may be an indication for further debridement; clinical assessment and patient wishes are to be considered. The culture results of the bone biopsy sent for C&S should be evaluated in light of the pathology/history of the concurrent sample; frequently, the bone C&S provokes positive culture results that reflect carry-along infected soft tissue rather than infected bone. In the face of further necrotic/devitalized tissue, subsequent tissue debridement may be necessary.

══

References

1. Cierny G, III: Classification and treatment of adult osteomyelitis. *In* Evarts CM (ed): Surgery of the Musculoskeletal System, 2nd ed. New York, Churchill Livingston, 1990.
2. Gorbach SL, Bartlett JG, Blacklow NR: Infectious Diseases. Philadelphia, WB Saunders Co, 1992.
3. Grayson ML, et al: Probing to bone in infected pedal ulcers. JAMA 273(9):721–723, 1995.
4. Sanford JP, Gilbert DN, Moellering Jr RC, Sande MA: Guide to Antimicrobial Therapy, 27th ed. Vienna, Virginia, Antimicrobial Therapy, Inc., 1997.

18

Peripheral Vascular Disease

Neil Mandava, MD and Richard B. Birrer, MD

Due to the growth of the elderly population in the United States, peripheral vascular disease has become common and a major source of morbidity. Over 100,000 lower extremity vascular reconstructions are performed each year in this country. Over the last decade there have been significant advances in our understanding of the pathogenesis of peripheral arterial disease (PAD) as well as in the areas of noninvasive diagnosis and treatment. Advances in noninvasive evaluation of the lower extremity include duplex ultrasonography, color-coded flow studies, magnetic resonance angiography, and spiral computed tomographic angiography. Advances in treatment include endoscopic-in-situ bypass, angioplasty, intravascular stents, and thrombolytic therapy.

This chapter discusses the primary care approach in evaluating and managing patients with lower extremity ischemia. While most patients with limb ischemia can be managed nonoperatively, knowing when to refer is important.

Pathophysiology

In order to select optimal therapy for PAD, we must first understand the pathophysiology of the disease. The major underlying disease process is atherosclerosis of the arterial tree. The relatively insidious process of narrowing of the artery becomes clinically significant only when the diameter of the vessel has been reduced by 75% or more. Despite the slow progression of the disease, 15–30% of patients with intermittent claudication show progression within 5–10 years. Stages of atherogene-

sis are: (1) activation of endothelial cells by circulating vasoactive substances, (2) alterations in permeability of smooth muscle, (3) lipid accumulation in extracellular and intracellular space in the form of foam cells, (4) widening of the tunica intima and underlying tunica media, (5) tissue reaction with platelet buildup and sclerosis, (6) outward bulging of plaque with luminal narrowing, and (7) complications such as plaque disruption, hemorrhage, ulceration, fissuring, and thrombus deposition.

Atherosclerotic occlusive disease is defined as being located above or below the inguinal ligament. Above the inguinal ligament, the distal abdominal aorta and iliac bifurcation are the most common sites of pathology, and atherogenesis here is referred to as "aortoiliac occlusive disease." Because it impedes flow to the lower extremity below the groin, it also is referred to as "inflow disease." Below the inguinal ligament, the most common site of arterial occlusive disease is in the superficial femoral artery at the Hunter's canal. The distal arteries also can be affected, namely the popliteal artery or its distal branches and the anterior tibial, posterior tibial, and peroneal arteries. These vessels commonly are affected in diabetes, but the digital arteries of the toes generally are spared. Arterial occlusive disease below the knee is referred to as "outflow disease."

Clinical Evaluation

History

The history taking should include interrogation for risk factors such as smoking, hypertension, diabetes mellitus, hypercholesterolemia, and heart disease.

Pain is the cardinal symptom in arterial insufficiency. Anaerobic metabolism sets in due to arterial ischemia, resulting in accumulation of metabolic end products such as lactates and pyruvates, which are the mediators of pain. Occlusion of an artery can be gradual or sudden. Sudden onset of ischemia is due to total occlusion of an artery resulting from an embolism, trauma, or progression of thrombus. In 80% of cases, the heart is the source of the embolus. More insidious onset of ischemia almost always is due to atherosclerotic narrowing of large- or medium-sized vessels. When there is a history of pain, information about its distinctive character, location, duration, and precipitating and relieving factors is sought to assist in making the diagnosis.

Intermittent claudication is a characteristic calf, thigh, or buttock pain associated with exercise or walking and relieved with rest. It is the only complaint in the majority of patients with PAD. Location of the pain is related to the level of critical stenosis. Atherosclerosis in the aortoiliac region results in buttock, hip, or thigh pain, whereas femoropopliteal atherosclerosis results in calf pain. "Claudication distance" is the term used for how far the individual can walk before having to rest to get relief from pain. This distance may be significantly less if the individual walks rapidly or on an incline. Progression to pain during rest or gangrene occurs in 7.5% of patients with claudication in the first year and 2.2% annually thereafter.

Ischemic rest pain always is experienced in the forefoot and also may involve the toes or the heel. Rest pain is worse at night because blood pressure and cardiac output decline, so there is less force to drive blood through stenotic vessels. Often the pain is relieved by dangling the extremity over the bedside. Hyperemic skin, a condition known as "dependent rubor," is a characteristic of ischemic rest pain. Any cuts, burns, or infections in an extremity with rest pain can precipitate events that can lead to limb loss. Patients with rest pain are candidates for urgent work-up and revascularization, since 95% of patients require amputation within 5 years if the condition is left untreated.

Physical Examination

The physical examination includes inspection of legs and feet for signs of ischemia, palpation of peripheral pulses and abdomen for aneurysm, and auscultation of neck and abdomen for bruit and heart for murmur. The signs and symptoms of arterial insufficiency are referred to as "the six P's" (Table 1). Fingers should be examined for clubbing, which is indicative of underlying pulmonary disease or neoplasm. Examination of vessels for pulse quality and symmetry should include the carotid, brachial, radial, femoral, popliteal, posterior tibial, and dorsalis pedis arteries. Pulses should be palpated for thickening, hardening, and tortuosity which occurs due to arteriosclerosis.

The femoral pulse lies below the inguinal ligament, two finger-breadths lateral to the pubic tubercle. The popliteal pulse is palpated with the patient in a supine position and the knee partially flexed. The posterior tibial pulse is palpated behind the medial malleolus, and the dorsalis pedis pulse is palpated on the dorsum of the foot between the first and second metatarsals. Congenital absence of a dorsalis pedal pulse is seen in 10–15% of the population. In addition to the loss of palpable pulses, some signs of chronic arterial insufficiency are brittle nails, shiny skin, hair loss, and cold feet.

Auscultation over carotid, renal, and aortoiliac arteries should be done for bruit, which results from turbulence of blood flowing through narrowed arteries. In general, the louder, longer, and higher pitched the bruit, the worse the stenosis. Bruit extending into diastole also signifies tighter stenosis. Bruit-like turbulence in a river is conducted downstream; similarly, the site at which the abnormal sound is *first* heard when the stethoscope is moved along the artery indicates the site of stenosis.

Ulcers are another sign of chronic arterial insufficiency (Table 2). Ischemic leg ulcers are small and shallow with irregular edges, tender to touch, and located distally on the feet or the anterior aspect of the leg. Absence of granulation tissue is a characteristic finding with ulcers due to arterial disease. Conversely, ve-

---

Table 1.   Six P's of Arterial Insufficiency

Pain
Pallor—waxy appearance
Paresthesias—numbness
Pulselessness—no pulses below blockage
Paralysis—weakness
Polar—cold to touch

Table 2. Signs and Symptoms of
Chronic Arterial Insufficiency

Absent pulses on palpation
Blanching of skin on elevation of feet
Cold feet
Dependent rubor
Pain relieved by dependency
Delayed capillary refill
Hair loss on feet and toes
Thickened and brittle toe nails, often with
    fungus
Shiny appearance of skin from atrophy of
    subcutaneous fat
Skin breakdown, ulceration or gangrene
Intermittent claudication
Nocturnal and rest pain
Impotence

nous stasis ulcers occur on the anteromedial
aspect of the leg just above the medial malleolus, are large in size, usually painless, indolent
in nature, and associated with stasis dermatitis and varicose veins.

A thorough neurologic evaluation for any
motor and sensory deficits completes the
physical examination of the vascular patient.

Differential Diagnosis

Neurogenic Claudication

This is claudication pain resulting from
nerve entrapment due to degenerative bone
and joint disease around the spinal foramina
or spinal stenosis. It often is difficult to differentiate neurogenic claudication from pain due
to vascular insufficiency. However, in claudication of neurogenic origin, pain is distributed
along a dermatome and often lasts 30–60 minutes, unlike intermittent claudication of vascular origin which usually lasts only a minute
or two.

Arthritis

Pain due to osteoarthritis of the hip can
present in a manner similar to intermittent
claudication of the buttock. Pain from degenerative arthritis can present at night while resting or as morning stiffness that improves with
movement. Joint pain leads to difficulty in going up and down the stairs, whereas intermittent claudication occurs while climbing stairs
and never when going down.

Varicose Veins

Patients with venous valvular incompetence
can have pain after exercising. This occurs due
to increased blood flow in a limb with poor venous tone, leading to increased venous pressure and distention of the varicosities. The
pain is rarely as severe as with arterial insufficiency, and inspection reveals obviously dis-
tended veins.

Causalgia

Causalgia is a pain syndrome of the peripheral nerves that usually follows partial nerve
injury of a major proximal nerve. Usually the
nerve injury is incomplete, with partial sensory
loss in the involved painful extremity. Symptoms may be temporarily relieved by blocking
the sympathetic ganglion of the involved limb.
Patients often complain that emotional problems aggravate the pain.

Imaging Studies

Ultrasonography

Continuous wave Doppler ultrasonography
consists of sound waves, produced by electrical stimulation of a piezoelectric crystal, that
reflect off flowing blood and are transformed
to an audible signal. The pencil-size probe is
inexpensive and portable. In claudicants, the
ankle-brachial index (ABI), which is the ratio of
the ankle to arm systolic pressure (normally
greater than 1), is 0.5–0.8. Patients with rest
pain or impending tissue loss have ABI's of 0.3
or less (Table 4). The ABI usually has an inverse
relationship with the severity of the vascular
disease. Patients with end-stage renal disease
and diabetes mellitus, however, have rigid, calcified vessels; hence, falsely high ABI ratios can
be misinterpreted even in the face of severe ischemia.

Table 3. Differential Diagnosis of
Peripheral Vascular Disease

Radiculopathy
Compensatory gait changes
Myxedema
Myalgia
Anemia
Trauma
Arthritis
Achilles tendonitis
Varicose veins
Causalgia

Duplex ultrasonography is a combination of real-time brightness mode image and pulsed Doppler ultrasound. The two modalities combined provide better and simultaneous evaluation of the vessel wall and blood flow. Color coding of blood flow aids in diagnosing blood flow disturbances and offers better definition of the arterial wall. Atherosclerotic plaques and intraluminal thrombi causing luminal narrowing can be differentiated easily.

Angiography and Other Diagnostic Modalities

Angiography requires an arterial or intravenous puncture and injection of radiocontrast material to visualize the vascular tree. It can be performed via the femoral, axillary, or translumbar routes. Digital subtraction techniques can enhance the quality of the images via computer image reconstruction. Allergic reactions to the contrast medium and renal failure can be reduced significantly by using noniodinated contrast material. Magnetic resonance angiography, using gadolinium for contrast, visualizes distal run-off better than conventional angiography; however, it cannot be used in individuals with pacemakers and metal clips. Spiral CT angiography, performed while the patient is moved through a continuously rotating gantry and the contrast material is infused intravenously, can visualize an entire vascular region in 30–40 seconds.

Management

Risk Factor Modification

Nearly 75% of PAD patients can be managed conservatively if they stop smoking and receive adequate therapy for associated medical problems (see Table 4). PAD is particularly virulent among smokers, and 70–90% of patients with PAD are smokers. Patients who continue to smoke have an amputation rate approximately 10 times greater than those who quit. Conservative medical management for PAD is successful in 85% of patients who have quit smoking versus 20% of patients who continue to smoke. Behavior modification, hypnosis, and acupuncture can help patients discontinue smoking. Use of nicotine patches or gum and counseling produces long-term abstinence in 30% of patients. More intensive programs with use of nicotine substitutes, biofeedback, group therapy sessions, and frequent follow-up calls by nurse practitioners may improve this number to 60%.

In the Framingham study, Sagie et al. reported in 1993 that one third of claudicants were hypertensive. Hypertension is known to accelerate atherosclerosis in various animal models. Treatment of hypertension may not directly reduce the progression of PAD, but it helps reduce other systemic illnesses typical in claudicants, such as coronary artery disease (CAD) and renal failure. CAD accounts for 30–70% of deaths in PAD patients, with the risk of mortality ranging from two to 15 times greater than in the healthy population.

The incidence of PAD is 8% at the onset of diabetes, 15% by year 10, and 45% by year 20. Patients with diabetes are at an increased risk of limb loss. Risk of amputation (6/1000 patients per year) is increased five-fold and risk of gangrene is increased 17-fold in diabetics. Strict control of blood sugar promotes wound healing, controls infection, and helps normalize triglyceride levels (Table 5).

Table 4. Evaluation and Management of Peripheral Vascular Disease

ABI	Capillary Refill	Signs and Symptoms	Plan
> 1	10–15 sec	Normal	Regular preventive care, diet, smoking cessation, and exercise
0.8–1.0	15–20 sec	Minimal or no symptoms	Regular preventive care, diet, smoking cessation, and exercise
0.5–0.8	20–30 sec	Claudication	Regular preventive care, diet, smoking cessation, and exercise
0.3–0.5	30–40 sec	Rest pain	Regular preventive care, diet, smoking cessation, and exercise; selected surgery
< 0.3	40+ sec	Impending tissue loss	Surgery

ABI = ankle-brachial index; sec = seconds

Table 5. Comparison of Diabetic and Nondiabetic Peripheral Arterial Disease

	Diabetic PAD	Nondiabetic PAD
Clinical	More common	Less common
	Younger patient	Older patient
Male:female	2:1	3:1
Occlusion	Multisegmental	Single segment
Vessels adjacent to occlusion	Involved	Not involved
Collaterals	Involved	Usually normal
Lower extremities	Both	Unilateral
Vessels involved	Tibials, peroneals, small vessels, arterioles	Aortic, iliac, femoral
Gangrene	Patchy areas of foot and toes	Extensive

Approximately half of PAD patients have hypertriglyceridemia. Reduction of serum cholesterol can induce regression of atherosclerosis. The low-density lipoproteins should be reduced to 100 mg/dl or less and the high-density lipoproteins increased to 45 mg/dl or more. Fasting serum triglyceride should be kept below 200 mg/dl. Dietary counseling, an exercise program, weight reduction, and use of lipid-lowering agents are all integral in management of this risk factor.

Conservative Strategies

This is the only option in individuals in whom revascularization is not possible due to either poor vessels or the patient's general condition. Treatment includes local debridement of nonviable tissue to allow re-epithelialization, wet-to-dry soaks, pain control, rest, treatment of infection with antibiotics, keeping the extremity warm, systemic anticoagulation, and pentoxifylline.

Most patients can double their claudication distance in 3 months by following a carefully prescribed exercise program. This may be due to better joint mobility and neuromuscular function and improvement in cardiac status and local blood flow. The usual prescription for a walking program is a 30–60 minute walk, 4 to 5 days a week at a pace of two miles per hour, with patients taking a break for moderate pain.

Vasodilator agents have been essentially useless in treatment of PAD because the ischemic limb is already maximally vasodilated from local hypoxia. However, it is possible that by preferentially vasodilating collateral vessels, some new agents such as potassium channel agonists may have efficacy.

Aspirin inhibits production of thromboxane A_2, which is a powerful vasoconstrictor and

platelet activator. One 81 mg baby aspirin a day is probably sufficient to obtain the benefits with minimum side effects.

Antioxidants such as Vitamin E, C, and β-carotene prevent free radical injury to the endothelial cells, thereby retarding the cascade of events that lead to atherosclerosis.

Surgical Treatment

Percutaneous transluminal angioplasty (PTA) is the localized dilation of an atherosclerotic plaque with balloon catheters. Fracture of the plaque and dissection of the underlying media increases the intraluminal diameter. Adjunctive therapy with heparin, nitroglycerine, papaverine, nifedipine, and/or aspirin helps to retard vascular thrombosis and platelet aggregation which may reproduce the blockage. Patency of iliac and femoropopliteal vessels with PTA at 2 years is 81% and 67%, respectively. PTA is sparingly used for infrapopliteal disease because long-term results are not available.

Certain types of lesions in the vascular tree are associated with high elastic recoil. PTA is unsuccessful in maintaining long term patency for these lesions. Stents placed within the diseased segment provide a rigid framework and maintain patency by mechanical means. Wall-stents and Gianturco stents are housed within a sheath, and they self-expand into a stenotic arterial segment when the sheath is retracted. Palmaz and Strecker stents are balloon-mounted stents that are released into position when the balloon is inflated. The cost of intravascular stenting is about one third that of open vascular reconstruction. Short segments of stenosis are ideally suited for correction by this modality.

Predictors of perioperative cardiac morbidity include advanced age, symptoms of angina, history of previous myocardial infarction, valvular heart disease, arrhythmias, cigarette smoking, and diabetes mellitus. The most commonly used tests to identify high-risk patients are electrocardiogram, stress test, Holter monitoring, echocardiography, dipyridamole thallium scintigraphy, and cardiac catheterization. Patients who have threatened limbs or are severely symptomatic cannot afford the time involved in obtaining these additional tests. However, these special studies can reduce the risk of a perioperative myocardial infarction by identifying those who need to undergo cardiac revascularization prior to peripheral vascular surgery. They also may identify individuals who require further optimization with fluids or ionotropic agents and/or perioperative hemodynamic monitoring with pulmonary artery catheters and arterial lines.

Surgical Procedures

Embolectomy is an emergency procedure for acute arterial occlusion secondary to an embolus from a proximal source that may include an aneurysm (popliteal, femoral, or aortic), dislodged arteriosclerotic plaque, or a piece of thrombus from the left atrium in a patient with atrial fibrillation. A 5000 unit heparin bolus is given preoperatively as soon as the diagnosis is established. Some patients may need continued anticoagulation after embolectomy. This procedure usually is done under local anesthesia and often requires a completion angiogram.

Vascular reconstruction techniques provide long-term definitive control of the complications associated with PAD. Endarterectomy is a procedure done to excise atherosclerotic plaques and lesions of intimal hyperplasia that are causing significant occlusion. Long segments of narrowing are better suited for bypass rather than endarterectomy. Extra-anatomical bypass (axillofemoral or femorofemoral) might be indicated in high-risk patients and often can be performed under local anesthesia. Diseased femoropopliteal segments are reconstructed by either a femoropopliteal or femorotibial bypass procedure. An autogenous saphenous vein, either in-situ or reversed, is the preferred conduit for vascular reconstruction. Synthetic grafts made of polytetrafluoroethylene are used for above-the-knee bypasses or when a suitable vein graft is not available. The 5-year patency rate

for a bypass using a vein graft is 68%, compared to 38% for a synthetic graft.

Endoscopic in-situ bypass is a femoropopliteal procedure using an in-situ saphenous vein with valves rendered incompetent by an angioscope. At operation, the proximal femoral artery and saphenous vein are mobilized for enough length to perform an anastomosis. An angioscope is passed down the saphenous vein, and venous side branches are marked on the skin. Valvulotomy is performed under angioscopic guidance so that the blood can flow forward in the arterialized vein. Coils are placed in venous tributaries of the saphenous vein and confirmed to be occluded by Doppler analysis. Vascular anastomosis is performed proximally and distally. The hospital length of stay for endovascular in-situ bypass is 4.2 days versus 11.6 days for the classic in-situ bypass. Other benefits include fewer wound-related complications and a shorter disability period.

Lumbar sympathectomy has lost its popularity over the years. Now it primarily is performed for patients with causalgia and other vasospastic disorders. It occasionally is used in patients with small ischemic foot ulcers if they are not candidates for reconstruction due to poor vessels.

Lower-extremity amputation is often the end result of progressive vascular disease. It is performed to control sepsis and to relieve pain. Diabetic foot infections often lead to minor amputations, such as single digit amputations and transmetatarsal amputations, that are associated with excellent functional results. Below-knee and above-knee amputations are much more debilitating and carry a 10% perioperative mortality, which is probably due to concomitant illnesses. Nonambulating patients and patients with contractures are not candidates for vascular reconstruction. Elderly patients with a contracted knee should undergo an above-knee amputation rather than a below-knee amputation. Survival in major amputation is only 50% in the 3 years following surgery.

Thrombolytic Therapy

Tissue plasminogen activator, urokinase, and streptokinase comprise a group of proteins that can dissolve fibrin clots. Lysis of the clot requires contact of the thrombolytic agent with the fibrin within the thrombus. Intra-arterial catheter placement into the peripheral arterial thrombi with direct administration of the lytic agent is necessary for the treatment of large, lower-extremity, occlusive clots. A multihole catheter must be pushed distally as the clot dissolution occurs.

Contraindications to the use of lytic therapy include patients with bleeding tendency, recent gastrointestinal hemorrhage, active peptic ulcer disease, major surgery within 2 weeks, and cerebrovascular accident within 6 months. During treatment, patients must be monitored in an intensive care setting. The majority of patients who undergo successful thrombolysis are treated with an adjunct operative procedure to correct the underlying stenotic lesion. Lysis of distal, small-vessel clots improves perfusion and run-off, thereby increasing the success rate of any subsequent bypass procedure.

Conclusion

PAD is a slowly progressive disease. Annual evaluation including a careful history, physical examination, and ABI assessment by the primary care physician can determine whether these patients should have surgery or more conservative treatment. While the majority of PAD patients respond to an exercise program, smoking cessation, and dietary therapy, surgical intervention is appropriate for patients with rest pain or tissue loss. Vigilance for an acutely threatened limb is paramount.

━━

References

1. Criqui MH, Langer RD, Fronek A, et al: Mortality over a period of 10 years in patients with peripheral arterial disease. N Engl J Med 326:381–386, 1992.
2. DeWeese JA, Leather R, Porter J: Practical guidelines: Lower extremity revascularization. J Vasc Surg 18:280–294, 1993.
3. Radach K, Wyderski RJ: Conservative management of intermittent claudication. Ann Intern Med 113:135–146, 1991.
4. Rutherford RB: Vascular Surgery, 4th ed. Philadelphia, W.B. Saunders Co., 1995.
5. Sabiston DC: Textbook of Surgery, 15th ed. Philadelphia, W.B. Saunders Co., 1997.
6. Schwartz SI: Principles of Surgery, 6th ed. New York, McGraw Hill Inc., 1994.
7. Vogt MT, Wolfsen SK, Kuller LH: Lower extremity arterial disease and the aging process: A review. J Clin Epidemiol 45:529–537, 1992.

Miscellaneous Conditions

Richard B. Birrer, MD, Patrick J. Grisafi, DPM,
and Michael P. DellaCorte, DPM

Tumors of the Foot

Malignant tumors of the foot are rare, and benign tumors and tumor-like lesions are uncommon (Table 1). On the other hand, deformities, swelling, and protuberances of a nontumorous etiology are quite common. Confusion of nontumorous lesions with tumorous ones often leads to a delayed diagnosis and inappropriately conservative therapy.

Symptoms usually include swelling, pain, deformity, and dysfunction. The physical exam confirms the presentation, but more detailed laboratory and imaging studies usually are required. Lab tests may involve a complete blood count and an automated chemistry panel including calcium, immunoglobulin, and serum enzyme levels (phosphatases). Imaging studies may include tomography, angiography, radioisotopic scanning (technetium phosphate), computed tomography, and magnetic resonance imaging. Definitive diagnosis is made by a biopsy. The technique can be incisional, excisional, or by curettage, and can be performed with a needle or by an open excisional approach. Whenever possible, the latter approach is preferred, because adequate tissue is obtained and the risk of local and systemic contamination is minimized. Normal tissue must always be included in the sample. A qualified pathologist should review all biopsy specimens by permanent section in order to make a definitive diagnosis. Consultation with a surgeon and oncologist is advised for all malignant and complex benign tumors.

Neurologic Disorders Affecting the Foot

Diagnosis of neurologic disorders affecting the foot is difficult due to the complexity of the nervous system and the variable, often subtle manifestations of neurologic disease (Table 2). These neurologic problems encompass a vast collection of complaints, symptoms, and etiologies for which a proper referral to a neurologic specialist is essential in early podiatric management of such patients.

Clinical manifestations of neurologic disorders affecting the foot generally arise from the peripheral nervous system. Central nervous system disease often is secondary to spinal cord compression, convulsions, stroke, and coma and is infrequently seen in the foot. Disorders of peripheral nerves may affect the foot in several ways, including paresis, paralysis, sensory defects, pain, and contractures. When these changes occur quickly, the patient usually notices and reports a change in function. However, when deficits develop slowly, the patient may ignore the reduced sensation or motor power. Pain resulting from peripheral neuropathy may be the most devastating symptom.

Treatment often requires pharmacologic, physiotherapeutic, psychologic, and surgical intervention, especially in posttraumatic cases. Associated manifestations of peripheral neuropathies include calf weakness (from paralysis of the posterior tibial nerve) and foot drop or an equinus deformity (from peroneal nerve paralysis). The sympathetic nervous sys-

Table 1. Types of Foot Tumors

	Benign	Malignant
Tumors and lesions of skin	Nevi Viral lesions Keratosis Keratoacanthoma Eccrine poroma Epidermal inclusion cyst Keloids	Melanoma Verrucous carcinoma Squamous cell carcinoma Basal cell carcinoma Malignant sweat gland tumors
Tumors of fibrous tissue and fat	Fibroma Nodular fasciitis Plantar fibromatosis Juvenile aponeurotic fibroma Lipoma	Fibrosarcoma Dermatofibroma protuberans Liposarcoma
Tumors of muscle, tendons, and joints	Leiomyoma Rhabdomyoma Giant cell tumor of tendon sheath Ganglion cyst Digital mucous cyst	Leiomyosarcoma Rhabdomyosarcoma Malignant giant cell tumor Synovial sarcoma Clear cell sarcoma
Tumors and lesions of nerves	Neuroma Neurofibroma Neurilemmoma Myoblastoma	Malignant neurofibroma Malignant neurilemmoma Malignant schwannoma
Tumors and lesions of blood vessels	Capillary hemangioma Cavernous hemangioma Venous hemangioma Hemangiopericytoma Glomus	Angiosarcoma Malignant hemangiopericy-toma Kaposi's sarcoma
Tumors and lesions of cartilage	Chondroblastoma Chondromyxoid fibroma Enchondroma (most common tumor in digits) Juxtacortical chondroma Osteochondroma	Chondrosarcoma Myxosarcoma
Tumors and lesions of bone marrow		Myeloma (most common malignant bone tumor) Ewing's sarcoma Reticular cell sarcoma Malignant lymphoma
Tumors and lesions of bone	Osteoma Osteoblastoma Osteoid osteoma	Osteosarcoma (most common malignant foot tumor) Acrometastases Giant cell tumor
Tumor-like lesions of bone	Solitary bone cyst Aneurysmal bone cyst Giant cell tumor Myositis ossificans Fibrosis dysplasia, nonossifying Fibroma body abscess Eosinophilic granuloma	

tem also should be evaluated in patients with pain, with special reference to absence of sweating and poor response to hot and cold, indicating sympathetic degeneration.

The examination of the patient with suspected neurologic disease should be thorough and include sensation, strength, reflexes, coordination, and gait (see Chapter 2).

Entrapment Neuropathies

Tarsal tunnel syndrome is caused by entrapment of the posterior tibial nerve as it passes behind the medial malleolus. The entrapment can be caused by inflammatory collagen vascular diseases, trauma, tumors, varicosities, ganglion cysts, chronic flexor tenosynovitis, or chronic severe pronation. The most common cause is fibrosis related to trauma.

Symptoms consist of a burning sharp pain, or paresthesia, that begins under the medial malleolus and radiates into the sole of the foot toward the toes. The symptoms are intermittent, but increase with prolonged activity. Clinically, there is a positive Tinel's sign (i.e., percussion of the posterior tibial nerve at the level of the medial malleolus, causing paresthesias distal to the toes). The definitive diagnosis is made by nerve conduction velocities and electromyographic studies.

Once the diagnosis is confirmed, treatment is geared toward the severity of symptoms and the etiology. Rest, strapping, and nonsteroidal anti-inflammatory drugs (NSAIDs) are indicated initially. Injection therapy and orthotic control of abnormal foot function are recommended thereafter. No more than six injections should be given.

If conservative therapy fails, then surgical intervention to decompress the nerve is indicated. Surgical decompression involves complete exploration of the tarsal tunnel with release of the flexor retinaculum and its fibroses bands and resection and ligation of any thrombosed or enlarged veins in the area.

Lateral Plantar (Calcaneal) Nerve Entrapment

Approximately 10–15% of athletes with chronic unresolved heel pain have entrapment of the lateral plantar nerve between the deep fascia of the abductor hallucis muscle and the medial caudal margin of the quadratus plantar muscle. Although running and jogging are the major causes, soccer, tennis, dance, and track and field events also are provocative. There

usually is chronic heel pain for 1–2 years that is dull, aching, or sharp in character. The pain may radiate into the ankle and is intensified by walking or running. There is point tenderness over the first branch of the lateral plantar nerve deep to the abductor hallucis muscle. The lateral plantar nerve to abductor digiti quinti muscle may cause a vague burning pain in the heel pad.

Nerve conduction studies usually are not helpful. The Tinel's sign is infrequently positive, and a hypermobile foot may be noted. While stretching, NSAIDs, injection therapy, and orthotics should be tried, their variable success rates often lead to surgical neurolysis.

Peroneal Nerve Entrapment

The deep peroneal can be entrapped in several locations, most commonly under the inferior extensor retinaculum (anterior tarsal tunnel syndrome). The superficial peroneal nerve can be entrapped at its exit point from the deep fascia. While acute trauma in the form of recurrent ankle sprains is the major culprit underlying these neuropathies, repetitive microtrauma from running, soccer, tennis, dancing, skiing, and hockey subjects the nerve to recurrent stretching.

Deep peroneal involvement is suggested by dorsomedial foot pain that is dull, aching, sharp, or spasmodic in nature and may radiate to the first toe web. There is decreased sensation in the first toe web and reproduction of the pain with either dorsiflexion or plantarflexion. Superficial neuropathy is suggested by pain, paresthesias, or numbness over the outer border of the distal calf, dorsum of the foot, and ankle, but sparing the first web space. There may be point tenderness and a fascial defect where the nerve emerges from the deep fascia. Activity worsens both conditions, and there is usually a history of recurrent sprains or trauma. Nerve conduction studies are helpful.

Treatment includes conservative modalities such as NSAIDs, physical therapy, orthotics, and injection therapy. Neurolysis is reserved for cases of intractable pain and atrophy (deep peroneal neuropathy).

Sural Nerve Entrapment

Running activities can lead to entrapment of the sural nerve anywhere along its course. There is usually a history of an acute twisting

Table 2. Clinical Manifestations of Neurologic Disorders Affecting the Foot

Disorder	Area of Primary Pathology	Etiology	Pedal Manifestations
Hereditary peripheral neuropathies Charcot-Marie-Tooth	Peroneal muscle atrophy and intrinsic muscle atrophy	Inherited, dominant or recessive	Pes cavus Clawing of digits "Stork leg" Muscle wasting Paresis Steppage gait Drop foot deformity Decreased/absent ankle jerk and vibratory sensation
Dejerine-Sottas disease (hypertrophic interstitial polyneuropathy)	Enlargement of peripheral nerves (peroneal nerve) Distal macular weakness	Inherited, autosomal recessive	Pes cavus Foot drop Loss of tendon reflexes Distal sensory disturbances
Roussy-Levy syndrome	Peripheral nerves	Inherited, dominant	Essential tremor Acquired cavus deformity Clumsy gait Absent tendon reflexes Foot atrophy
Refsum's disease (heredopathia atactic polyneuritiformis)	Nerves	Inherited, autosomal recessive	Progressive paralysis Drop foot Pes cavus Ankle reflexes are decreased
Friedreich's ataxia	Cerebellum Cord Peripheral nerve	Posterior and caudal spinal cord degeneration Usually recessively inherited but also reported by dominant and partially sex-linked transmission	Pes cavus Ataxia Drop foot Peroneal nerve paresis Lurching Trendelenburg gait Babinski response
Cerebral vascular accident (stroke)	Cerebrum Ischemia to brain, with infarction	Hemorrhage Thrombosis Embolism to brain	Spastic contractures Equinovarus Claw-toe deformity Spastic equinus deformity Drop foot Babinski response

Condition	Structure Affected	Cause	Signs/Deformities
Muscular dystrophy (Duchenne's)	Muscle fibers (dystrophism)	X-linked inherited	Ankle equinus; Equinovarus; Paresis; Loss of reflexes; Secondary contractures; Unusual enlargement of muscles from fatty deposition
Spinal cord abnormalities	Lumbar and sacral areas	Failure of neural arch to close during development	Depends on level and extent of involvement
Spina bifida with meningocele (meninges and sac protrude through defect), myelomeningocele (additional element of spinal cord and nerve root protrusion), or myelocele (most severe: skin failed to close over neural elements); spina bifida occulta (all neural elements remain in spinal canal)			Pes cavus; Equinus; Equinovarus; Valgus deformities; Mild neurologic deficits (spina bifida occulta)
Poliomyelitis	Viral infection of anterior horn cells of spinal cord; Paralysis of innervated muscle	Viral infection; Destruction of anterior Horn cells (enterovirus)	Paralysis of tibialis anterior (tender and painful muscles); Permanent lower motor neuron paralysis with paralytic-type polio; Muscle contracture; Muscle wasting; Limb length discrepancy
Cerebral palsy		Brain lesion; Congenital neuromuscular disease	Ankle equinus; Spastic equinus
Spastic (most common)	Frontal lobe	Congenital maldevelopment of brain	Flexion, adduction, internal rotation of hip, knee, genu valgum
Athetoid	Basal ganglia	Cerebral anoxia during perinatal period	Scissors gait or knock-knee gait
Ataxic	Cerebellar and 8th cranial nerve	Trauma during birth	Secondary talipes equino-valgus; Talipes calcaneus; Pes cavus; Hallux valgus; Hammer toe deformities
Rigid	Basal ganglia		
Tremor	Basal ganglia and cerebellar		
Dystonic	Combination of the above		

Table continues on next page.

Table 2. Clinical Manifestations of Neurologic Disorders Affecting the Foot (continued)

Disorder	Area of Primary Pathology	Etiology	Pedal Manifestations
Diabetic neuropathy	Peripheral nerves (at vasonervosum and posterior column) Autonomic nerves	Hyperglycemia Metabolic changes Segmental demyelination Loss of Schwann cells	Stocking/glove distribution Decreased sensation of pain, temperature, and touch Impaired proprioception Sluggish or absent deep tendon reflexes Denervation of intrinsic muscles (atrophy) Hammer toes Charcot joints Malperforans ulcers
Sciatica	Distribution of sciatic nerve	Sacralization of 5th lumbar vertebrae Arthritis of the interarticular joints Spondylitis Tumor, especially cauda equina Infection Hernia	Steppage gait Dorsiflexion of foot Increased pain (Bragardis sign) Flexion of great toe Increased pain (Sicardi's sign) Achilles reflex lost or decreased Pain on straight-leg raise (Lasegue's sign)
Peripheral neuritis	Peripheral nerves	Alcohol Beriberi Arsenic	Painful hyperesthesias of the soles of feet Short, painful steps Gait has limping, halting character with feet rotated to avoid walking on painful portions
Cerebral arteriosclerosis	Circle of Willis	Senility	Short-stepped, shuffling gait
Parkinson's disease (paralysis agitans)	Basal ganglia	Arteriosclerosis Encephalopathy Senility	Loss of automatic swing of arms Difficulty in starting and stopping gait Gait slow and shuffling
Dystonia musculorum	Basal ganglia	Idiopathic Infection Vascular disease of brain Toxic conditions Tumors	Gait characterized by severe contortions; ludicrous, bizarre appearance

injury and recurrent ankle sprains. Shooting pain and paresthesias typically extend to the lateral foot border and are confirmed by local tenderness, a positive Tinel's sign, and, occasionally, an area of hyperesthesias. A trial of NSAIDs, orthotics, physical therapy, and injection therapy should be tried, although surgical release usually is definitive.

Note: For a discussion of **Morton's interdigital neuroma,** see Chapter 8.

Medial Calcaneal Nerve Entrapment

This condition is most commonly known as jogger's or runner's foot. Entrapment of the medial calcaneal branch of the posterior tibial nerve causes acute irritation and inflammation and chronic fibrosis and neuroma formation. The patient, usually a runner, jogger, or avid walker, complains of aching pain along the medial border of the heel that is more severe on weight bearing but does not radiate further forward into the foot. A planovalgus deformity or foot hyperpronation tends to aggravate the condition further. Anti-inflammatory agents with a custom-molded orthotic are good conservative therapies. If the patient does not respond to these modalities after several months, operative neurolysis should be considered.

▬

References

1. Campbell CJ: Tumors of the foot. *In* Jahss MH (ed): Disorders of the Foot. Vol. 1. Philadelphia, W.B. Saunders Co., 1982, pp 979–1013.
2. Schon LC, Baxter DE: Neuropathies of the foot and ankle in athletes. Clin Sports Med 9(2): 489–510, 1990.
3. Schubiner JM, Simon MA: Primary bone tumors in children. Orthop Clin North Am 18(4): 577–596, 1987.

General Treatment Guidelines

Michael P. DellaCorte, DPM, Patrick J. Grisafi, DPM, and Richard B. Birrer, MD

The goals of any treatment plan are to relieve symptoms and, if possible, cure the illness. Unfortunately, many illnesses cannot be cured, so treatment plans must be structured to maximize function. The purpose of this section is to discuss the indications, contraindications, methodologies, and outcomes of common podiatric procedures and devices.

Common Procedures

Paring

Indications

Paring is done for temporary relief of pain associated with tyloma and heloma. The patient should be made aware of the underlying cause of the corn and be informed that paring is not a permanent treatment.

Contraindication: severe peripheral vascular disease.

Procedure

Paring is a conservative, noninvasive technique done with a scalpel. The novice may wish to start with a No. 15 or No. 10 blade that fits a No. 3 handle, while the more experienced practitioner may use a No. 20 blade with a No. 4 handle. The scalpel blade should always be sterile. The patient's feet should be elevated to a comfortable level, and the practitioner should be seated. The nondominant hand supports the foot, while the other debrides the corn or callus (Fig. 1). The scalpel blade is held firmly between the thumb and index finger, positioned almost parallel to the lesion (Fig. 2). With a slicing, semicircular motion, superficial

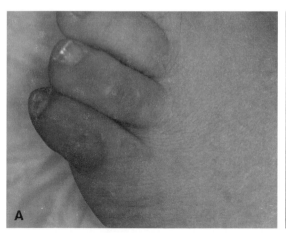
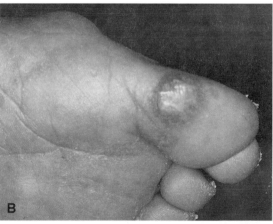

Figure 1. A, Heloma (corn)—discrete area of hyperkeratosis with a central core. B, Tyloma (callus)—diffuse area of hyperkeratosis.

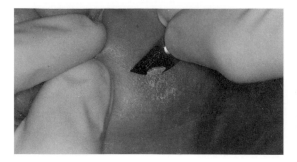

Figure 2. Paring of tyloma.

amounts of corn or callus are debrided repeatedly until healthy, pink tissue is noted. For safety, the cutting edge of the scalpel is always moving away from the practitioner; digital corns require a backhand stroke to accomplish this (Fig. 3).

After the superficial debridement of the corn is complete, the central core must be removed to relieve symptoms. This deeper core is removed with the tip of the scalpel blade in a circular manner. Care must be taken to avoid cutting into the underlying healthy tissue. The practitioner should realize that the procedure is time consuming, and rushing through it may cause unnecessary iatrogenic lesions. Bursitis underlying a corn may warrant a local injection of lidocaine prior to debridement. Debridement of a callus may uncover hidden corns, foreign bodies, or ulcerations. The treatment plan may have to be altered depending on the findings.

Outcome/Prognosis

This procedure offers 6–8 weeks of relief from the pain associated with heloma and tyloma. After this period, the process is repeated.

Padding

Indications

Padding offers temporary and immediate relief of pain associated with bursitis, fasciitis, and tendonitis, as well as dispersion of pressure around bony prominences.

Contraindications: allergies to tape or adhesives, diabetes, or peripheral vascular disease.

Procedures

The general rules for applying tape or adhesives to the skin also apply to the feet. The skin should be healthy, well hydrated, and noninfected. Hair overlying the area should *not* be shaven, so as to avoid irritation and folliculitis; use of a prewrap prior to taping elimi-

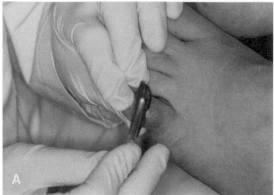

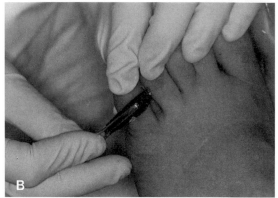

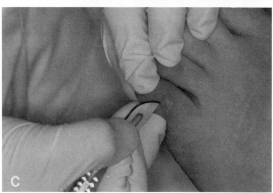

Figure 3. *A* and *B,* Debridement of heloma with backhand stroke. *C,* Removal of central core of heloma.

nates the need for shaving and pretape sprays. The materials generally used for padding are: adhesive felt or foam of 1/4-inch or 1/8-inch thickness, moleskin, roll foam, and tape. Most pads come prefabricated from the suppliers and have adhesive backing.

Bunions. Bunion pads are fashioned with thicker felt materials. A "U" or donut pad is placed over the dorsomedial bump, and the pad is covered with two or three strips of tape to hold it in place for 2–4 days. Alternatively, roll foam, fashioned to cover the hallux and the dorsomedial eminence, can be used (Fig. 4).

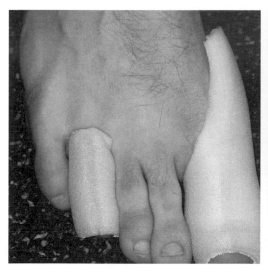

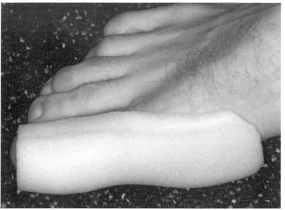

Figure 4. Roll foam bunion pad.

Bunion splints are over-the-counter or prescription devices that relieve mild to moderate bunion pain. Static splints are worn without shoe gear to hold the hallux straight and stretch the lateral muscular and capsular structures of the first metatarsophalangeal (MTP) joint. They are effective but limit the patient's ability to ambulate freely. Interdigital spacers hold the hallux straight and allow the patient the freedom of ambulation in and out of shoes. Dynamic splints are distributed as single, removable devices or mitten-like socks (e.g., Dynamic Splint Bunion Socks, available from Doctor's Choice; see Appendix IV). They allow full range of motion in all planes while holding the hallux straight and are easily worn in shoes. Pediatric bunion deformities are a prime indication for bunion splints.

Lesser digits. This is another common area for padding. A smaller U-shaped or donut-shaped pad is placed over the corn and secured in place by tape or small digital covers (Fig. 5). The digit should never be circumscribed with tape or digital covers due to risk of constriction and circulatory impairment. Roll foam also can be used on digits for dis-

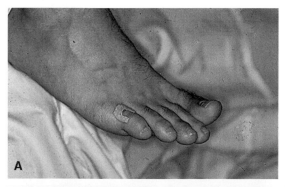

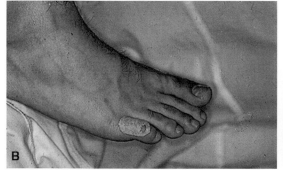

Figure 5. *A* and *B,* Digital corn pads. *C,* Cover to secure padding.

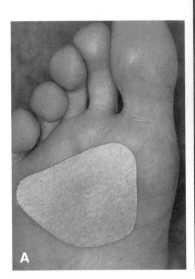
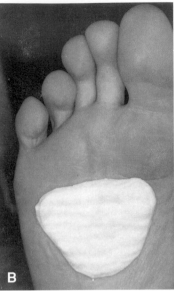

Figure 6. *A,* Submetatarsal padding with 1/4-inch felt placed proximal to the metatarsal heads. *B,* Submetatarsal padding with moleskin placed directly over the metatarsal heads.

persion. Lamb's wool, also called angel hair, can be wrapped around the affected digit for temporary relief. The advantage here is that the patient can repeat the procedure daily, and there are no adhesives.

Temporary relief of submetatarsal pain also can be afforded with padding, which is placed to disperse pressure from any or all of the metatarsal heads (Fig. 6). The padding usually is covered with strips of two-inch tape. Moleskin padding is applied directly over the metatarsal heads to relieve friction burning and diffuse callus.

Heel spurs. The pain of heel spurs can be relieved temporarily by padding or strapping. The heel spur pad (Fig. 7) is made of thicker felt padding and fashioned in the shape of a U. It is applied directly to the affected heel and is covered with two or three strips of two-inch tape. This pad is designed to disperse weight from the central and more painful part of the heel.

Plantar fasciitis. For relief of plantar fasciitis, a pad made of 1/4-inch felt is fashioned to fit the longitudinal arch (Fig. 8). It is then covered with two-inch adhesive tape, which relieves symptoms by taking tension off the plantar fascia. Combinations of these pads also can be used.

Outcome/Prognosis

The patient is instructed to leave the pads on for 1–3 days. If the pads become wet, they should be removed to avoid skin maceration.

Padding generally is used as an adjunct to other treatment modalities, such as paring, injections, and nonsteroidal anti-inflammatory

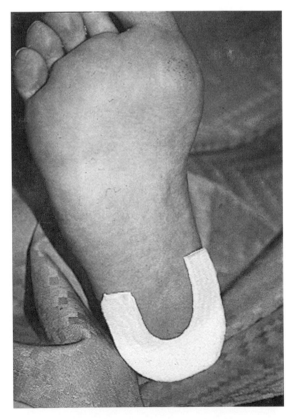

Figure 7. Heel spur padding.

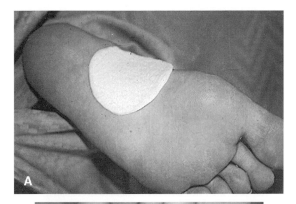

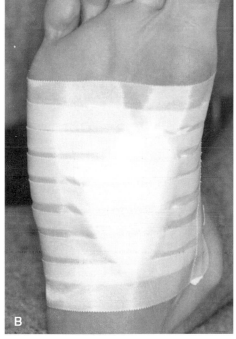

Figure 8. A, Long arch pad of 1/4-inch felt for relief of plantar fasciitis. B, Two-inch adhesive tape covering over pad.

drugs (NSAIDs). Relief from a combination treatment lasts for 6–8 weeks. Padding alone offers relief for only 3–5 days.

Toenail Debridement

Indications

Toenail debridement can relieve pain and pressure caused by toenail growth and hypertrophy, especially in patients with diabetes, sight impairment, severe arthritis, and peripheral vascular disease.

Contraindications: severe diabetes or severe peripheral vascular disease.

Procedure

Proper treatment of the toenails involves cutting the nail straight across (Fig. 9) and maintaining a clean nail groove. The nail grooves are on the medial and lateral borders of the nail and extend from the base of the nail to the distal end of the toe. Cutting the nail too short or angling the distal end of the nail causes the distal nail groove to close or narrow. Excessively tight socks or stockings may compress the distal tuft of the toe, pushing the skin proximally and flattening it up against the nail. When the nail grows out, it is forced to grow into the skin, causing ingrown toenails and possibly infection. In proper debridement technique, the nail splitter is held parallel to the distal edge of the nail and perpendicular to the toe (Fig. 10). Once debridement is completed, the nail grooves must be cleaned with a nail curette. The curette has a cutting edge, so care must be taken not to cut the skin (Fig. 11).

Outcome/Prognosis

Proper nail care insures against ingrown or infected ingrown toenails. Treatment should be repeated every 6–8 weeks.

Electric Burring/Grinding

Indications

Burring and grinding smooth the rough edges of debrided nails and reduce thick nails caused by trauma or fungus. **Contraindications:** hypersensitivity and infected toenails.

Procedure

After much of the toenail is debrided with a clipper, the remaining debridement is accomplished with an electric burr (Fig. 12). The dominant hand firmly holds the drill, bracing against the foot with the fourth of fifth finger. The other hand holds the digit from the plan-

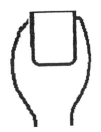 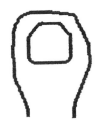

Figure 9. The proper way to cut toenails is straight across (*left*), not short and angled (*right*).

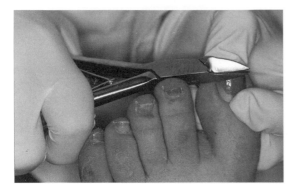

Figure 10. Proper technique for toenail debridement.

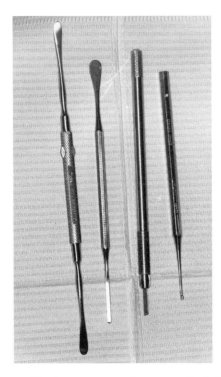

Figure 11. Instruments for toenail debridement (*left to right*): nail curette, Beaver No. 61 blade and handle, spatula packer, elevator.

tar aspect. The burr is moved from medial to lateral or vice versa, repeatedly, until the desired amount of nail is removed. Note that burring generates heat; therefore, the burr must not be held in one area for long periods.

Outcome/Prognosis

This technique affords 6–8 weeks of relief and should be repeated after that time.

Laser Waffling

Indications

Laser waffling is a conservative method of curing fungal toenails. **Contraindications:** diabetes or peripheral vascular disease.

Procedure

A CO_2 laser burns numerous small holes in the affected nail. The laser beam is set so that it will not completely penetrate the toenail and cause damage or burns to the underlying soft tissue. Topical antifungal medications are then applied daily by the patient (see Chapter 4, Table 1). Topical medications alone do not work well on fungal nails because they are unable to penetrate the thick nail. Laser waffling allows better penetration of the medications.

Outcome/Prognosis

The waffling technique is repeated every 2 weeks. With patient compliance, the fungal toenail is cured in 4–6 months.

Nail Surgery

Indications

Nail surgery is undertaken for temporary or permanent removal of the entire nail or part of the nail. **Contraindications:** diabetes, peripheral vascular disease, bleeding disorders.

Procedure

After local anesthesia has been administered and the foot and lesion have been scrubbed carefully with povidone-iodine (Betadine) or hexylresorcinol (PHisoHex) solution, the necessary amount of nail is removed. In **total nail removal,** an elevator is used to free the proximal nail fold (Fig. 13). Once it is completely free the elevator is reversed and slipped under the proximal edge of the nail. The nail is then lifted up and off, using the elevator as a lever. The exposed nail matrix can be cauterized or destroyed with phenol or laser, or surgically excised for permanent removal.

In **partial nail removal,** after local anesthesia has been administered and a rubber tourniquet has been applied, a spatula packer is used to free the proximal nail fold on the affected side (Fig. 14). (Note that the tourniquet also can be used in the total nail procedure. A tourniquet should not be applied in the elderly or in patients with diabetes or poor circulation.) A

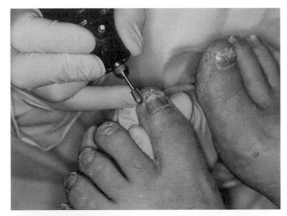

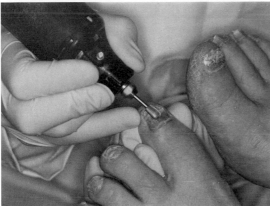

Figure 12. Technique for burring toenails.

nail splitter or an English Anvil splitter then is inserted and positioned to remove the desired amount of nail (Fig. 15). Once this is complete, a hemostat is employed to grab the freed nail and remove it. Excessive granulation tissue can be further removed by trimming with scissors or cauterizing with a silver nitrate stick. As in total nail removal, the exposed nail matrix can be destroyed or cauterized with phenol or laser, or surgically excised for permanent removal. For both removal procedures, 88% phenol is administered with sterile applicator sticks to the exposed nail matrix for 1–2 minutes (Fig. 16). Care must be taken not to get any phenol on surrounding skin. After the applicator is removed, the area is flushed with alcohol to neutralize any remaining phenol. The phenolized area should turn a greyish white; if this color is not observed, the procedure should be repeated. Range of total application varies from 90 seconds to 5 minutes.

The latest technique, an alternative to phenol application, is laser cautery of the exposed nail matrix (Fig. 17). The procedure is techni-

cally more difficult than the phenol procedure; it requires a steady hand. Once completely cauterized with laser, the exposed tissue turns a brownish-white color. The procedure should be repeated until this point is reached.

Surgical matricectomy often is preferred for young, healthy patients. It is accomplished by subcutaneous dissection of the nail bed underlying the excised portion of nail, from proximal to distal, using a No. 15 blade. Remove matrix fragments with a rongeur and soft tissue remnants with a Buck bone curette. Excessive tissue voids should be closed with sutures.

Outcome/Prognosis

For partial and total nail removal without destruction of the nail matrix, the recovery period is 2 or 3 weeks. An aseptic dressing should be worn until the wound is dry. It is important that the toe box of the shoe is adequately sized. It may be necessary to prohibit both weight bearing and the wearing of a shoe for several days. Modification of the current shoe often is required. The nail grows back in 3–6 months.

The phenol technique for matrix destruction works well but has some drawbacks. The wounds drain for weeks, and there is associated pain. Also, phenol accidentally applied to surrounding skin causes painful burns and skin slough. The laser technique, if not done properly, has a higher incidence of recurrence, although there is minimal drainage and little pain. The postoperative course is much better for the patient with laser. Surgical matricectomies are generally painful. Suture removal is in 10–14 days, depending on wound condition.

The recovery period for nail surgery is 4–6 weeks, with evaluation in 4–6 months for nail regrowth. There is a 3–5% incidence of regrowth of nail spicules and/or portions of ingrown nail with chemocautery; surgical matricectomy has a 1% recurrence or regrowth rate. Postoperative analgesics may be necessary.

Strapping

Indications

Strapping is beneficial for mild sprains, tendonitis, and fasciitis. It can improve foot function and serve in a prophylactic capacity prior to athletic activities. **Contraindications:** allergy to tape or adhesives, severe sprains, fractures, dislocations.

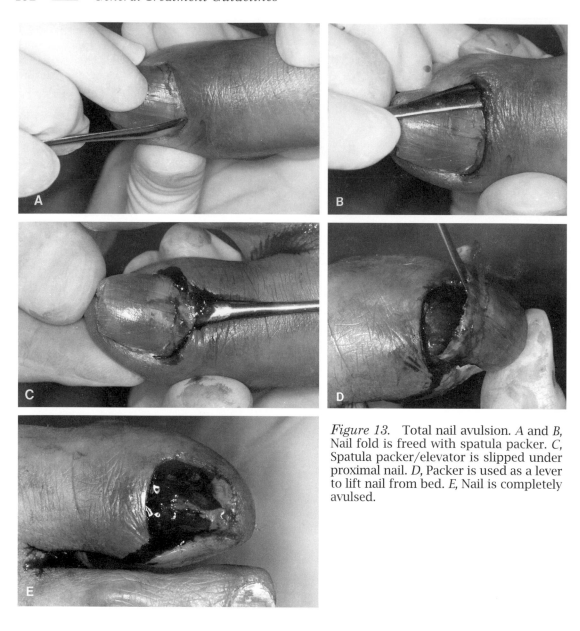

Figure 13. Total nail avulsion. *A* and *B,* Nail fold is freed with spatula packer. *C,* Spatula packer/elevator is slipped under proximal nail. *D,* Packer is used as a lever to lift nail from bed. *E,* Nail is completely avulsed.

Procedures

Plantar rest strap. This technique is used to relieve the symptoms of fasciitis (Fig. 18). It is applied as follows: first measure the amount of tape needed. Using a roll of one-inch tape, apply the end of the *nonadherent* side against the skin overlying the head of the first metatarsal. Extend the tape proximally around the heel along the lateral aspect of the foot to the head of the fifth metatarsal. Tear the tape at this point and stick it to the examination table so that it can hang freely. Measure two more pieces the exact same length. Now using two-inch tape and the same method of mea-

suring, measure four pieces of tape from the medial aspect of the metatarsal plantarly to the lateral. Place this tape nearby. Using the one-inch strips, begin medially at the first metatarsal head and apply the tape all the way around the foot to the head of the fifth metatarsal. Apply a second one-inch strip on top of the first, overlapping 1/4 inch plantarly. The tape should be bowstrung in the arch area. The two-inch tape is now applied from medial to lateral, starting just proximal to the metatarsal heads. The two-inch tape should be based on both sides of the one-inch tape from medial to lateral, and overlapping by 1/2 inch from distal to proximal. Once all the two-inch

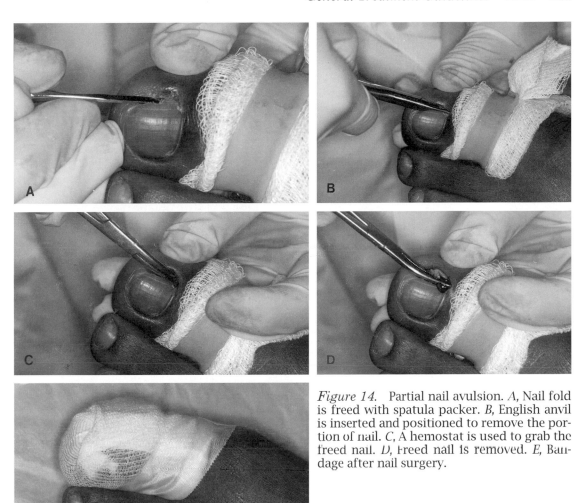

Figure 14. Partial nail avulsion. *A*, Nail fold is freed with spatula packer. *B*, English anvil is inserted and positioned to remove the portion of nail. *C*, A hemostat is used to grab the freed nail. *D*, Freed nail is removed. *E*, Bandage after nail surgery.

tape is in place, the final piece of one-inch tape is applied, as a binder, exactly over the first two pieces of one-inch tape. This strapping will last 3–5 days if it doesn't get wet.

J strap. This is a common strapping employed by practitioners and athletic trainers (Fig. 19). It is used to stabilize the subtalar joint and limit either inversion or eversion. It is applied as follows: after applying prewrap to the foot and leg, measure out two-inch tape from the inferior aspect of the medial malleolus to the middle of the lateral aspect of the leg. Three pieces of tape this length are necessary. Have the patient sit on the examining table with his/her foot hanging off the side. To prevent subtalar inversion, with the foot perpendicular to the leg, have the patient evert the foot and hold it in this position. (If the patient is unable to do this, you may need an assistant to hold the foot in position.) Apply the tape

just inferior to the medial malleolus around the plantar aspect of the heel and up the lateral side of the leg. Repeat this with the second and third strips of two-inch tape. Binders are placed across the anterior aspect of the leg where the tape is bow strung, using one-inch tape. (The binders should not circumscribe the leg.) This strapping is reversed to prevent subtalar eversion. It also can be done on both sides, termed the double J, to limit subtalar motion completely.

Louisiana heel lock. This technique prevents the symptoms of excessive pronation, ankle sprains and strains, and shin splints (Fig. 20). Protect the anterior of the ankle and both malleoli using Webril or gauze. Start the wrap with one-inch tape on the dorsal lateral surface of the ankle. Roll the tape around the foot under the arch toward the lateral and proximal aspect on the plantar heel. The tape then

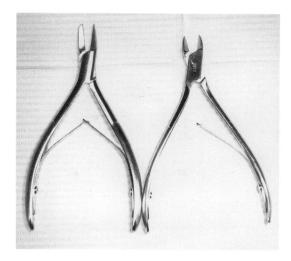

Figure 15. English anvil (*left*) and nail splitter (*right*).

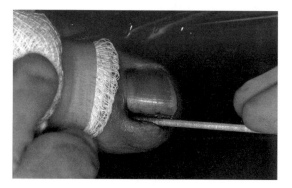

Figure 16. Application of 88% phenol to cauterized nail matrix.

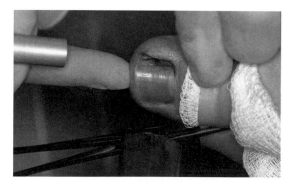

Figure 17. Positioning of laser beam for laser cautery of nail matrix.

comes up hooking the lateral side of the heel and is directed superiorly, posterior to the ankle. The tape runs on the posterior aspect of the calcaneus or over the Achilles insertion

headed medially. The tape then crosses over the medial malleolus and ends as it crosses over the starting point. With a second piece of tape, perform the procedure in the opposite direction for the medial heel lock. Use one-inch tape as anchors over any free edges.

Gibney ankle strap/basketweave. The Gibney procedure allows dorsiflexion and plantarflexion of the ankle and limits inversion and eversion of the subtalar joint (Fig. 21). Place the calcaneus parallel to the ground and the foot perpendicular to the leg. Using one-inch tape, start the first strip of tape on the medial aspect of the leg close to the Achilles tendon, about five inches above the medial malleolus. Carry the tape down the leg, under the heel, up the lateral border of the leg to the same height as the medial side. The second strip is started just proximal to the first metatarsal head, follows the medial border of the foot around the heel, and is ended proximal to the head of the fifth metatarsal. The third and subsequent perpendicular strips are placed parallel to and overlapping the previous strips by about 1/4 inch. The fourth and subsequent horizontal strips are placed parallel to and overlapping the previous strips by 1/4 inch. The size of the ankle determines the number of strips used.

Injection Therapy

Indications

Injection therapy is employed in any area where pain and inflammation are localized and are not relieved by NSAIDs and conservative physical therapy. Conditions that typically benefit include capsulitis, arthritis, bursitis, sesamoiditis, and, most commonly, heel spur syndrome. **Contraindications:** diabetes, pe-

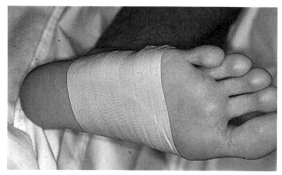

Figure 18. Plantar rest strap to relieve symptoms of fasciitis.

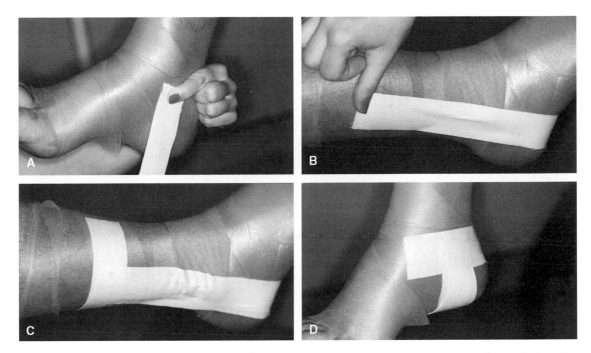

Figure 19. J strap. *A*, Tape extends from the medial side of the foot just interior to the medial malleolus. *B*, Boundaries extend to the lateral aspect of the leg. *C* and *D*, Medial and lateral binders.

ripheral vascular disease, overlying infections, fractures, and known allergies to injectable solutions.

Procedure

Using an 18-gauge drawing needle on a 3-ml syringe, 2 ml of a 50/50 mixture of 1% lidocaine hydrochloride plain and .5% bupivacaine hydrochloride plain is drawn. A small amount of a long-acting steroid is then added (e.g., dexamethasone 0.8–1 mg). Surgically prepare the area to be injected with povidone-iodine and numb with ethyl chloride spray. Now switch to a 25-gauge 1 1/4-inch needle, and thoroughly mix the syringe. Determine the area of tenderness by palpation prior to injecting (e.g., medial tubercle of calcaneus for heel spur). The injection should be directed at the area of most tenderness. With a dart-like motion, advance the needle, aspirate, and infiltrate the area with the mixture. Never inject tendons. To assure that the sheath or peritendinous tissue is being infiltrated, ask the patient to move the muscle tendon unit. Movement of the syringe indicates that the needle is in the tendon. After withdrawal of the needle, massage the area slightly to insure dispersion of the agents.

Outcome/Prognosis

The relief should last from 1–7 days, at which time a subsequent injection may be necessary. If the pain is not relieved by four injections, surgery should be considered.

Methods For Diagnosing Infection

Probe

Using a probe such as found in routine surgical debridement kits (MedCare Custom Packing, West Swanzey, New Hampshire), probe into the ulcer. Grayson, et al. note that a rock-hard, often gritty structure at the ulcer base without the apparent presence of any intervening soft tissue is a positive test for osteomyelitis.

Fungal Tissue Cultures

Using a sterile scalpel, scrape the superficial tissue into a sterile, sealable transport container, such as a urine or culture and sensitivity cup. Add a small quantity of sterile nonbacteriostatic normal saline. Send the sealed container to the microbiology lab.

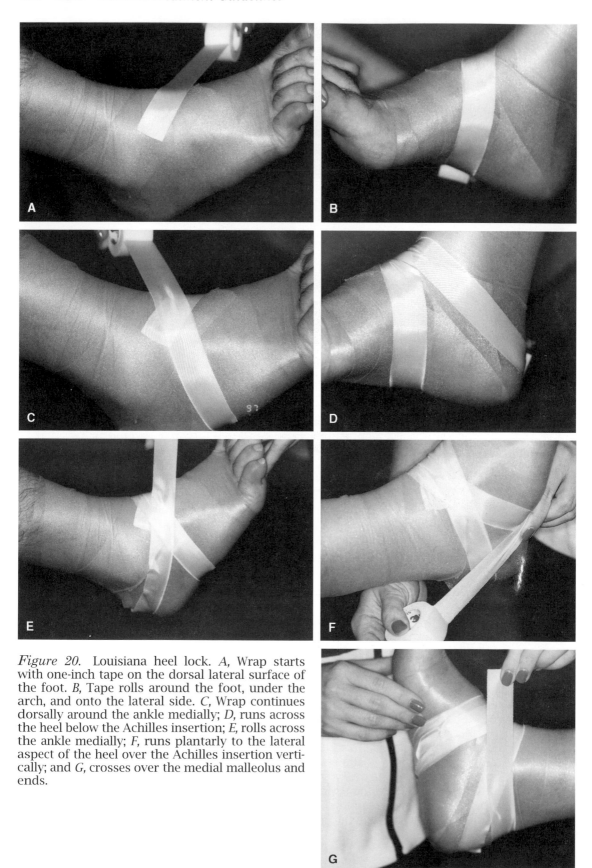

Figure 20. Louisiana heel lock. *A*, Wrap starts with one-inch tape on the dorsal lateral surface of the foot. *B*, Tape rolls around the foot, under the arch, and onto the lateral side. *C*, Wrap continues dorsally around the ankle medially; *D*, runs across the heel below the Achilles insertion; *E*, rolls across the ankle medially; *F*, runs plantarly to the lateral aspect of the heel over the Achilles insertion vertically; and *G*, crosses over the medial malleolus and ends.

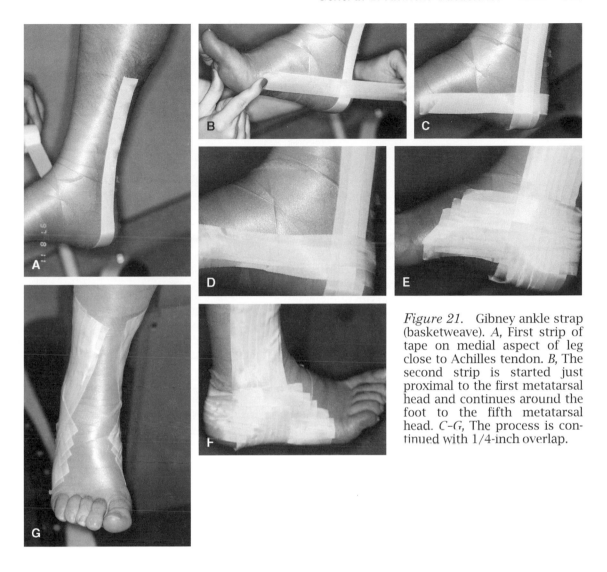

Figure 21. Gibney ankle strap (basketweave). *A,* First strip of tape on medial aspect of leg close to Achilles tendon. *B,* The second strip is started just proximal to the first metatarsal head and continues around the foot to the fifth metatarsal head. *C–G,* The process is continued with 1/4-inch overlap.

Culture

Cultures can be obtained either as aspirates, swab cultures of the wound, or debrided tissue after superficial tissue debridement.

Aspirate

Clean the intact superficial skin near the leading edge of the cellulitis with Betadine. Using a tuberculin syringe and 25-gauge needle, inject 0.1–0.2 ml sterile nonbacteriostatic saline into the tissue, then aspirate; wet a rayon-tipped swab with the aspirate and break the swab-tip end into a transport medium (e.g., BBL Port-A-Cul, which provides aerobic and anaerobic medium), and send the sealed tube to the microbiology lab.

Tissue

Using a sterile scalpel, debride the superficial tissue away from the wound/ulcer. Obtain a small quantity of exposed tissue (either by punch biopsy or additional debridement) and place it into a sterile, sealable container with a small amount of sterile nonbacteriostatic saline. Send the sealed container to the microbiology lab.

Swab Culture

Using a rayon-tipped swab, contact the deep or purulent tissue (with some vigor), then break the swab tip end into transport medium, e.g., BBL Port-A-Cul. Send the sealed tube to the microbiology lab.

Orthotics

Indications

Orthotics reduce impact, cushion the foot, relieve pressure and pain, and correct biomechanic abnormalities. **Contraindications:** No significant contraindications. Rigid materials should be avoided in patients with diabetes or peripheral vascular disease.

Procedure

An extensive biomechanic evaluation must be completed prior to casting for these devices (see Chapter 2). **Functional orthotics** are rigid or semirigid and generally only extend to the metatarsal heads. They are used to correct biomechanic abnormalities. **Accommodative orthotics** are made to disperse pressure or accommodate bony prominences on the plantar aspect of the foot (e.g., plantar corns, heel spurs). They are made of softer materials like leather or plastazote and can extend to the sulcus or to the tip of the toes. Although accommodative orthotics wear out relatively quickly, they afford the patient months of relief (Table 1).

The casting technique described here appears simple, but unless the foot is positioned exactly right, the results will be unacceptable. Any hyperkeratotic lesions are marked prior to the application of plaster; povodine-iodine solution works well as a marker. The casting takes 30–45 minutes.

The patient lies prone on the examining table with both feet hanging over the edge. Determine the neutral position of the subtalar joint by repeatedly supinating and pronating the joint while holding the fourth and fifth metatarsal heads. The other hand feels for the talar head and positions the foot exactly in neutral. Once a neutral position is found, ask the patient to hold that position. A five-inch-wide plaster splint, pre-cut to the length of the patient's foot, is dipped in cool water, wrung out, and applied to the medial side of the foot from distal to proximal. The plaster splint should not extend to the dorsum of the foot. Rub the plaster in thoroughly so it conforms well to the foot. A second splint is then applied to the lateral side in the same manner, again working the plaster in well. Once the plaster has dried, the slipper cast is removed. (Shaking the foot or having the patient wiggle the toes makes removal easier. Application of petroleum jelly to the foot prior to casting also can aid removal.) This procedure is then repeated for the other foot.

These cast impressions of the feet are called the negative casts. Positive casts made from these negatives serve as templates for the fabrication of the orthotics. The casts are sent to an orthotics laboratory for fabrication of the specified orthotic (Fig. 22 and Table 2).

Outcome/Prognosis

The treatment of pathomechanics is a difficult and challenging endeavor. Functional devices limit pathologic pronation at the subtalar joint, realigning the foot in relation to the supporting surface and re-establishing a normal propulsive sequence. Accommodative devices increase the weight-bearing surface of the foot by bringing the supportive surface up to the foot. This improves weight distribution and symptomatology without necessarily establishing a propulsive gait. In general, accommodative devices are indicated for the more subluxed and deformed foot.

Efficiency of foot orthoses depends on their shape, fabrication, and composition, which should be devised and prescribed with specific goals for total body mechanics. When the body compensates for the new position induced by the orthotics, problems such as iliotibial band syndrome, hip rotator strain, greater trochanteric bursitis, exacerbated low back pain, and plantar fasciitis may arise. Solutions include decreasing the control and prescribing exercises to increase the range of motion of all lower extremity joints.

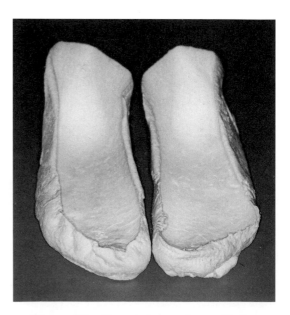

Figure 22. Negative casts for orthotics.

Table 1. Orthoses

General Type/Examples	Indications
Soft	Elderly patients with metatarsalgia beyond the age of
Spenco	surgical correction
Steinmold	To determine whether permanent orthoses are needed
Professional Protective	Pain from overuse injuries
Technology	
Sorbothane (no cast needed)	
Semiflexible	Athletes
(neutral cast needed)	Unidirectional sports
	Multidirectional sports
	Skiing
	Control of abnormal pronation and supination
	Decrease overuse and/or acute injuries associated with
	abnormal foot positioning
Rigid*	Everyday activity (i.e., walking)
Rohadur	Edge-control sports
	Use of high heeled shoes (can decrease shock of contact at
	heel strike)

*Avoid in patients with diabetes or peripheral vascular disease.

Upon dispensing the orthotic, the patient should be instructed about the break-in period. The orthotics should be worn 1–2 hours for the first day, 2–3 hours the second day, and so on, until they can be worn all day. The break-in period is generally 2 weeks. The orthotics may need adjustments by the lab if casting techniques were improper.

Total-Contact Plaster Cast

Patients with diabetes and peripheral sensory neuropathy are at great risk of plantar ulcer development. These ulcers are difficult to treat and cure. Gravity-dependent edema and pressure from a weight-bearing surface increase both the duration of a chronic condition and likelihood of a poor prognosis and eventual lower extremity amputation.

Bed rest and daily dressing changes achieve healing of plantar ulcers. However, patients usually abandon this modality before healing is complete. Moreover, compliancy of *complete* bed rest is poor; patients tend to rise for short periods to accomplish daily activities such as bathing and eating. A total-contact plaster cast eliminates the problems of bed rest and allows the patient to be mobile.

Total-contact casting alleviates the pressure and edema around plantar ulcers. However, secondary ulcers and problems can occur in these plaster casts due to friction and shear forces rather than from direct pressure. Proper casting technique prevents the foot from moving within the cast; there should be no padding between the sole of the foot and the molded plaster. The cast is applied in the following manner:

1. Position the patient in the prone position with the knee flexed, the leg below the knee vertical, and the sole of the foot horizontal. Steady the foot in this position—avoid changing the angle of the foot while the plaster is still wet and moldable.

2. Apply a simple gauze dressing over the ulcer and secure it with paper adhesive tape.

3. Apply stockinette up the leg.

4. Apply one broad area of padding (four-inch-wide pieces of orthopaedic felt or multiple layers of webril) extending from the lateral malleolus to the medial malleolus, then across the dorsum of the foot. This padding softens the contours of any prominences and guards against the possibility of pressure sores on the dorsum of the foot at the angle between the foot and the leg.

5. Apply a strip of felt down the front of the tibia to the toes to simplify cast removal.

6. Apply a single roll of fast-setting plaster bandages (i.e., Gypsona) around the foot, ankle, and lower leg. Do not add any plaster until the first layer has been molded and set. Rub a thin, egg-shell layer to every contour and hollow and around every prominence of the foot and ankle. Meticulous molding assures

Table 2. General Prescription Guidelines For Foot Orthotics

Width	Length	Flanges	Posting*

Normal
Wide
Slim/thin
	Metatarsal head:
	    Device ends just proximal
	    to metatarsal heads
	Sulcus: Device ends at
	    level of plantar sulcus,
	    just distal to metatarsal
	    heads
	Full foot: Covering over
	    orthotic shell extends to
	    full foot as captured
	    by cast
	Extra long: Covering
	    over orthotic shell
	    extends beyond cast
		Medial: Orthotic shell
		    continues up longitudinal
		    arch superiorly (for an
		    overly pronated foot)
		Lateral: Orthotic shell
		    continues superiorly up
		    lateral border of foot (for
		    global rigid cavus foot
		    type)
			Extrinsic: Additions of
			    different materials to
			    bottom of orthotic shell
			    to balance/control foot
			    function
			Intrinsic: Bending/
			    twisting of orthotic
			    shell to balance
			    cast to control foot
			    function
			Neutral: No
			        extrinsic/intrinsic
			        posting
			    Post-to-cast: Extrinsic
			    posting placed upon
			    exterior of cast as it is
			    placed in its neutral
			    position
			Negative heel: A
			    hollowed-out heel cup

* The balancing of a cast to the best functioning position of the foot.

smooth plaster in total contact with the skin. Wrap plaster well around the heel and into the hollows of the sole.

7. Apply the remainder of the cast in the conventional way, working fast and applying a posterior slab, and finish with a circumferential bandage.

8. Apply a strip of plywood to the underside of the sole, and fill gaps between it and the plaster with a rumpled plaster bandage.

9. Walk with a rubber walking heel on this plywood at or just behind the center of the foot. *Note:* to insure cast setting, the patient should rest for 24 hours before weight bearing.

The cast is changed at intervals of 24 hours, 3 days, 5 days and then once a week until the ulcer has resolved. It is recommended that casting be continued for 2 weeks because newly formed granulation tissue on a weight-bearing surface is extremely vulnerable. Walkers or other devices also are advisable during the transition period from total-contact casting to return to shoe gear.

Total-contact casting greatly reduces the healing time in the sensory-deprived diabetic patient. The average time to heal a plantar ulcer with this technique is 8 weeks. Careful monitoring, shoe modifications, and even con-

tinued use of ankle-foot orthotic devices may be required to prevent recurrence of plantar ulcers.

Shoe Modification/Molded Shoes

Indications

Modification of existing shoes and construction of molded shoes are conservative treatments for foot ailments, particularly those due to diabetes, arthritis, vascular disease, or chronic ulceration. **Contraindications:** fractures, dislocations, or other traumatic injuries.

Procedures

Modification. Athletic running shoes (i.e., sneakers) prevent pronation and are a socially acceptable solution for painful, dysfunctional feet. They have wide soles, medial-lateral stability, good arch support, and heel support. Velcro closures improve the ease of opening and closing. Other helpful features include cushioning of the sole, soft tops, and a lower heel. Athletic shoes should be part of a comprehensive treatment program that features muscle-strengthening exercises, biomechanical support, pain relief, weight loss in the obese, and physical therapy.

Modifications can be added inside or outside the shoe. Custom-molded orthotic devices can be inserted into the shoe. Plastazote inserts are used in diabetics and ulcer patients to relieve pressure. The depth-inlay shoe or extra-depth shoe allows easy insertion of orthotic devices. For adult shoes, most external modifications come in the form of accommodations. Bunion-last shoes have a modification in the last providing more space for the dorsomedial eminence of the bunion and a higher toe box for hammer toes. For regular last shoes, shoemakers have a device called a swan that stretches the shoe leather overlying the painful bunion. Submetatarsal pain can be relieved with a metatarsal bar placed proximal to the metatarsals on the sole of the shoe. Limb length deformities also can be accommodated with additions to the sole and the heel.

Casting. Custom-molded shoes can be used to accommodate painful foot conditions (Fig. 23). Prosthetics and braces also can be incorporated when necessary. The technique for casting is as follows: The patient is seated, and a foam pad covered with plastic is placed under the foot. Petroleum jelly is applied to the foot. Five-inch-wide plaster splints are applied to the plantar aspect of the foot, extending medially and laterally but not dorsally, one inch above the posterior aspect of the ankle. The foot is placed in a neutral subtalar position and then positioned semi-weight bearing on the foam pad. The plaster is allowed to dry. Petroleum jelly is applied to the edge of the plaster. The dorsal plaster then is applied, covering the remaining area of the foot completely. Once the plaster is dry, pencil marks are made from the plantar to the dorsal plaster splints for reference points for realignment later. The cast then is removed and sent to a lab for fabrication.

Outcome/Prognosis

The practitioner should keep in mind that once the shoe is modified, the patient is limited to that shoe for relief. Also, when the condition has resolved, the modified shoe may have to be discarded. Shoe modification and molded shoes offer an alternate method of relief for the nonsurgical candidate. The average shoe lasts from 8 months to 2 years.

Surgery: General Guidelines

Indications

Elective foot surgery is indicated for painful conditions not relieved by conservative ther-

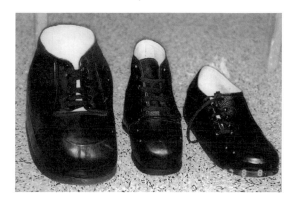

Figure 23. Custom molded shoes.

apy. **Contraindications:** severe diabetes and peripheral vascular disease.

Procedures

Foot surgery has become very popular over the past few decades. Two options exist: closed surgery (minimal incision) and open surgery. Both require extensive knowledge of foot pathology and anatomy, and both can be done on an ambulatory basis either in a hospital or in an office setting.

Prior to any surgical procedure, the patient should be informed of the risks and benefits. See Appendix V for an example of a standard surgical consent form. This form should be read and discussed in detail with the patient and his or her family. The surgery along with the postoperative course should be discussed because the medicolegal ramifications of operating without informed consent can be very costly.

Sterile technique is paramount in any surgical procedure. All articles used in the operation must be sterile, including gloves, gowns, instruments, sponges, and drapes.

Minimal incision involves small stab incisions, rotary burrs, and drills to grind and cut bone. The bony structures are never directly visualized in this type of surgery. The practitioner must rely on knowledge of surface and structural anatomy and an extensive examination of the joint, including x-rays. X-rays or fluoroscopy often are used intraoperatively to insure proper positions of instruments. Osteotomies can be made with specialized burrs. Fixation of osteotomies is seldom done; bandages hold them in place. The skin incisions require only one or two sutures for closure and afford minimal scar formation. Tourniquets are not used in this type of surgery.

In open foot surgery, 3–12 cm incisions are made overlying the deformities. Tissues are dissected in layers down to bone. Knowledge of deep anatomic tissues and vessels is mandatory. The bones and joints are directly visualized, and osteotomies are fixated using screws, wires, and pins according to A.O.* methods. Closure of wounds requires deep-tissue closure in layers and skin closure with numerous sutures. Tourniquets often are used in this type of surgery to afford the surgeon a bloodless field.

Local anesthesia. Once the patient is on the operating table, local anesthesia must be administered. Lidocaine hydrochloride 1% with bupivacaine hydrochloride .5% in a 50/50 mix gives long-lasting anesthesia. Mixing lidocaine with warmed sterile bicarbonate in a 9:1 ratio makes the injection almost painless. (The surgeon should be aware of the toxic dose of each anesthetic and not exceed this limit. 175 mg of bupivacaine is toxic; each cc of .5% solution contains 5 mg. For lidocaine the toxic dose is 350 mg; each cc of 1% solution contains 10 mg).

In a hallux digital block, 3 cc of anesthetic solution are injected with a 25-gauge, 1 1/4-inch needle (Figure 24). The initial puncture is at the base of the proximal phalanx laterally. After aspiration a wheal is raised at this site. The needle is advanced plantarly, again aspirating and raising a wheal. As the needle is slowly withdrawn, anesthesia is injected. The needle is not removed completely from the first injection site. After aspiration it is advanced to the medial aspect of the digit where, after aspiration again, another wheal is raised. (Avoid injecting into the extensor tendons. Dorsiflexion of the toe allows the needle to pass underneath them.) Remove the needle completely, injecting anesthesia slowly. The second puncture is at the site of the medial wheal (wait until the skin is numb). Advance plantarly and repeat the procedure, aspirate, raise a wheal, inject slowly while withdrawing. The third puncture is at the plantar medial wheal. The needle is advanced laterally, and the procedure is repeated for the last time. For the lesser digits, the third puncture is not used. A similar technique can be used proximally at the metatarsal level to block for bunion surgery.

Preparation and draping. Once the surgical site is numb, it is "prepped" and draped for surgery. Prepping consists of a 10-minute antiseptic scrub with povidone-iodine. The entire foot should be scrubbed, not just the operative site. The foot is dried with a sterile towel and draped. The patient is asked to raise the operative foot, leaving the other foot on the table. The bottom drape is then placed over the nonoperative foot and the operating table. The operative foot is lowered to the table. A top drape is applied over the patient, exposing only the operative foot. The drape at the patient's head should be raised, screening the operation. After the drapes are in place, the foot is painted with Betadine solution, and the patient is ready for surgery.

Tourniquet. Tourniquets expedite the surgical procedure by providing a bloodless field. For nail surgery, a Penrose drain or heavy elastic band can be used as a tourniquet. It is applied to the proximal aspect of the toe, pulled tight, and clamped with a hemostat. A pneumatic tourniquet is used for more proximal surgery and bone surgery. Applied to the ankle, over some cast padding, the tourniquet generally is inflated to 250 mmHg. This pressure is tolerable for about 90 minutes. Caution should be taken when procedures last longer.

Suturing. Sutures are used to approximate and hold skin or subcutaneous tissues together until the tissue has enough strength to withstand stress. The technique for simple skin closure requires 4-0 nylon on a half-circle cutting needle. A sterile needle holder, pickup, and scissors also are necessary. For simple sutures, grasp with a pickup (forceps with teeth) the skin to be sutured, everting it. While holding the skin with the pickup, insert the needle. To insert the curved needle, exert a turning force on the needle holder. This pressure in the line of the needle allows it to slip through the skin more easily. Tie a square knot, and cut the end of the suture material approximately 1/4 inch. The technique is continued, spacing the sutures approximately 1/4 inch apart, until the wound is closed. The sutures should remain clean, dry, and intact for 10–14 days.

For suture removal, cleanse the area with Betadine. Grasp one of the sutures with a pickup or hemostat, and cut the suture where it dips beneath the skin with scissors or a No. 15 scalpel blade. After it is cut, gently pull it out. Repeat the process until all sutures are removed. Apply a sterile dressing to the site for 2–3 days until the suture holes close over.

Outcome/Prognosis

The postoperative course is similar for both closed and open surgery, and recovery takes 8–12 weeks.

*Arbeitgemeinschaft fur Osteosynthesisfragen

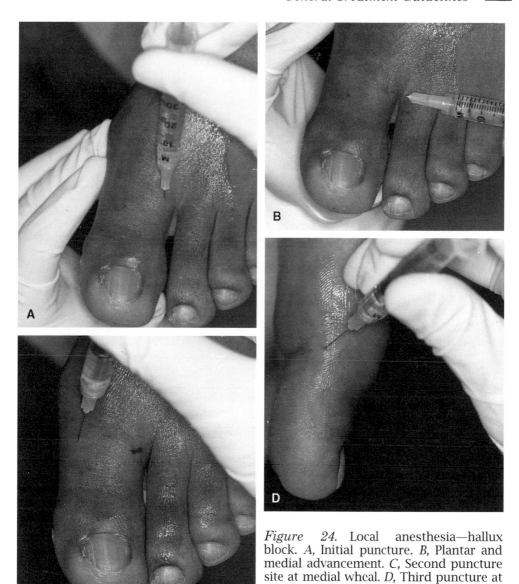

Figure 24. Local anesthesia—hallux block. *A,* Initial puncture. *B,* Plantar and medial advancement. *C,* Second puncture site at medial wheal. *D,* Third puncture at plantar medial wheal.

Surgery: Specific Procedures

The procedures described below are intended to increase the reader's understanding of advanced surgical management of common foot problems. Such techniques are not normally part of the primary care physician's armamentarium. Additional procedural training is required.

Hammer Toe Procedure/Arthroplasty

As stated in the section on corns and calluses, surgery is indicated for permanent correction of painful corns. A standard, open-technique arthroplasty is described here. After satisfactory anesthesia, the patient is prepped and draped in the usual manner, and a tourniquet is applied. Two converging, semielliptical incisions are centered over the proximal interphalangeal joint (PIP) (Fig. 25A). The incision is deepened, and the skin wedge is removed. Dissection is continued down through the subcutaneous tissue until the tendon overlying the PIP joint is identified. A transverse incision is made in the tendon and capsule at this level. Then all capsular and ligamentous structures are dissected free from the head of the proximal phalanx, and the head is delivered dorsally.

A double-action bone cutter is used to resect the head of the proximal phalanx (Fig. 25B). This is excised in toto. The wound is flushed, the tendon is reapproximated using 3-0 Dexon, and the skin is closed with 4-0 nylon (Fig. 25C). The toe is then bandaged with gauze and roll bandages (e.g., Kling). Next, the tourniquet is released, and capillary return is evaluated to assure that the bandage is not on too tightly. Postoperative x-rays are taken. The patient is given a postsurgical shoe and allowed to ambulate. The first redressing is 3-4 days after surgery. Sutures are removed in 10-14 days, and the patient should be completely out of compression bandages in 3 weeks.

Metatarsal Osteotomy

The indications for a metatarsal osteotomy include submetatarsal bursitis, anterior metatarsal head bursitis, and tailor's bunions. After the osteotomy is made, it generally is fixated with either a screw, pin, or wire.

Second, third, and fourth metatarsals. The procedure for a metatarsal osteotomy for submetatarsal bursitis to the second, third, and fourth metatarsals is as follows: after satisfactory anesthesia, the patient is prepped and draped in the usual sterile manner; a tourniquet is applied to the ankle and inflated to 250 mmHg. A dorsal skin incision overlying the metatarsophalangeal (MTP) joint, extending from the base of the proximal phalanx proximally to the distal third of the metatarsal shaft, is made. The physician makes the incision deep, down through the subcutaneous tissue, taking note of all vital structures. All bleeders are clamped and ligated in the usual manner.

Dissection is continued until the extensor tendons are identified and isolated. Retracting these tendons laterally exposes the joint capsule to the MTP joint. A dorsal incision is made in the capsule, and then all remaining capsule and ligamentous structures are dissected free, exposing the surgical neck of the metatarsal. A through-and-through osteotomy from dorsal to plantar is made at this level. The displaced capital fragment is then positioned 1-2 mm dorsal and is fixated in place. A .045 Kirschner wire is inserted from dorsal proximal to distal plantar. (The wire enters the metatarsal shaft at a 45° angle and is advanced into the capital fragment to the level of subchondral bone.) The wire is left protruding through the skin dorsally for easy removal in 3-4 weeks.

Deep closure is with 3-0 Dexon, skin clo-

sure is with 4-0 nylon simple sutures. Dry, sterile dressings of 4 × 4 gauze and Kling are applied. The tourniquet is released, and capillary return is evaluated. The postoperative course allows the patient to ambulate in a postoperative shoe. The first redressing is 3-4 days after surgery. The sutures are removed in 10-14 days. The pin is removed in 3-4 weeks, depending on the x-ray findings.

This procedure can be done by minimal incision as follows: a stab incision is made at the

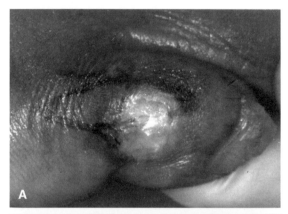

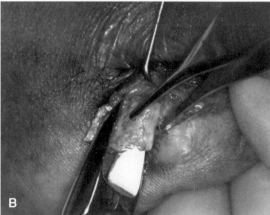

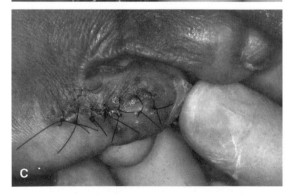

Figure 25. Arthroplasty of the fifth toe. *A,* Skin incision outline. *B,* Bone cutter resects the head of the proximal phalanx. *C,* Skin closure.

surgical neck of the metatarsal. The incision is deepened down to bone. A periosteal elevator is inserted in the incision to free soft tissue from bone. Once this is completed, a side-cutting burr is inserted, and a through-and-through osteotomy is made at the surgical neck. The skin is then closed with 4-0 nylon. Dry, sterile dressings of 4×4 and Kling are applied. The postoperative course allows the patient to ambulate in a postoperative shoe. The first redressing is 3-4 days after surgery, and the sutures are removed in 10-14 days. The patient is followed with x-ray evaluations until bone healing is noted.

Fifth metatarsal. The initial part of the procedure for an open osteotomy is the same as above. Once down to bone, a dorsolateral exostosis is noted; this must be resected to conform to the normal contours of the shaft. After resection, a through-and-through osteotomy is made at the surgical neck. The osteotomy is angled from dorsal distal to proximal plantar, and distal lateral to proximal medial. The capital fragment is shifted medially 3-4 mm and dorsally 1-2 mm and fixated in place with a Kirschner or monofilament wire (Fig. 26). For monofilament wire, drill holes are made through the dorsal aspect of the metatarsal to the plantar aspect through the osteotomy. A 2-0 wire is then passed through this hole and tightened onto itself. The wire is cut short and covered over with joint capsule.

Deep closure is with 3-0 Dexon; skin closure with 4-0 nylon. Dry, sterile dressing is with 4×4 and Kling. The tourniquet is released, and capillary return is evaluated. The postoperative course is the same as for lesser metatarsal osteotomy. There is no pin removal if monofilament wire is used.

Bunion Surgery

Bunion surgery is a complex procedure requiring extensive knowledge of anatomy, biomechanics, and surgical principles. Four of the more common procedures are described.

Head osteotomy. After satisfactory anesthesia, the patient is prepped and draped in the usual manner. A tourniquet is applied to the ankle and inflated to 250 mmHg. A skin incision is then made, extending from the base of the proximal phalanx proximally to the distal third of the metatarsal shaft. There are four landmark points: distal is the base of the proximal phalanx, proximal is the distal third of the metatarsal shaft, medial is the dorsomedial eminence, and lateral is the extensor tendon

(Fig. 27A). The skin incision is from the distal to proximal points, in between the medial and lateral points. The incision is deepened through the skin and into the subcutaneous tissue, taking note of all vital structures. All bleeders are cut and ligated in the usual manner.

Dissection is continued down until the capsule of the first MTP joint is identified. A dorsomedial linear capsular is then made. All capsular and ligamentous structures are dissected free from the dorsomedial aspect of the metatarsal head. The dorsomedial bump is resected with an osteotome and mallet to conform to the normal contours of the shaft (Fig. 27B and C).

Attention is directed into the first interspace where, by means of sharp and blunt dissection, the conjoint tendon is identified, isolated, and tenotomized. Returning medially, an L-shaped, through-and-through osteotomy is made at the head. The apex of the osteotomy is midway between the proximal ends of the articular cartilage. The plantar cut is made first and then the dorsal wing. The capital fragment is then moved laterally and fixated in place (Fig. 27D). A Kirschner wire can be used, as described in the lesser metatarsal osteotomy (a .062-inch wire is used instead of a .045).

After the osteotomy is fixated, the remaining prominent medial shaft is burred smooth, and the area is flushed and closed in layers. Capsule and deep structures are closed with 2-0 and 3-0 Dexon (Fig. 27E); skin closure is with 4-0 nylon (Fig. 27F). The postoperative course is the same as for the lesser metatarsal osteotomy.

Base osteotomy. Base osteotomy is used when head osteotomy will not lower the intermetatarsal angle enough. The skin incision is extended proximally to the base of the metatarsal. The procedures done at the metatarsal head are exactly the same as previously described without the osteotomy.

Once attention is directed to the base of the metatarsal, dissection is down through the subcutaneous tissue until the extensor tendons are identified. After retracting them laterally, the underlying capsule of the metatarsal cuneiform joint is exposed. A dorsal linear incision is made at the base of the metatarsal. The periosteum and capsule in this area are reflected with a periosteal elevator. A wedge osteotomy is then made 1.5 cm distal to the metatarsal base. The apex of the wedge is medial and the base is lateral (Fig. 28A).

This is *not* a through-and-through os-

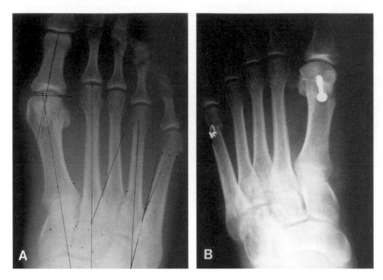

Figure 26. Metatarsal osteotomy. *A,* Preoperative x-ray of bunion and tailor's bunion. *B,* Postoperative. Note correction of fifth metatarsal with monofilament wire fixation.

teotomy; only the lateral cortex is cut completely. The medial cortex must be left intact. A wedge of bone is removed from this site, without breaking through the medial cortex. (The amount of bone to be removed is determined preoperatively on weight-bearing radiographs.) The osteotomy is then closed down and fixated either with a screw or Kirschner wire (Fig. 28B and C). Deep closure and skin closure are the same as for head osteotomy. The postoperative course has the patient off weight bearing in a below-knee cast for 4-6 weeks. A longer course of postoperative physical therapy also may be necessary.

Keller procedure. The Keller procedure is a joint destructive procedure wherein the distal part of the first MTP joint is removed (Fig. 29). Therefore, it is reserved for severely arthritic joints with no possibility of normal function. The procedure starts off the same as the head osteotomy. Once down to capsule, the capsular incision is extended distally onto the base of the proximal phalanx. All capsule and ligamentous structures are dissected free from the base of the proximal phalanx and the dorsomedial aspect of the metatarsal shaft. The dorsomedial bump is removed with an osteotome and mallet.

Attention is then directed to the base of the proximal phalanx where the proximal one-third of the phalanx is resected and excised in toto. The area is flushed and closed as above. The postoperative course allows the patient to ambulate in a postoperative shoe. The first re-

dressing is in 3-4 days, and sutures are removed in 10-14 days. Generally, the patient is completely recovered in 4-6 weeks.

Keller with implant. Total joint implants are used to restore joint motion and decrease shortening of the hallux caused by the Keller procedure (Fig. 30). The procedure is the same as the Keller, with the following additions: the articular cartilage of the head of the metatarsal is resected, perpendicular to the shaft; the medullary canal of the metatarsal and the remaining proximal phalanx are reamed to accommodate the implant; and the implant is inserted. Special reamers are available for this procedure. The postoperative course is the same as for the Keller. Implants can be used in any of the distal joints of the foot (Fig. 31).

Rehabilitation and Physical Therapy

The "golden period" consists of the first 30-60 minutes following trauma. During this period there is much pathologic and histochemical activity (biochemical mediators of processes such as inflammation, chemotaxis, vascular permeability) but relatively no or minimal clinical findings. The treatment for all stabilized trauma is RICE. The R represents rest, which is a relative term (i.e., the injured component is rested whereas the noninjured areas can still be trained). I stands for ice and immobilization. C is for compression, and E represents elevation. This time-honored formula is a sim-

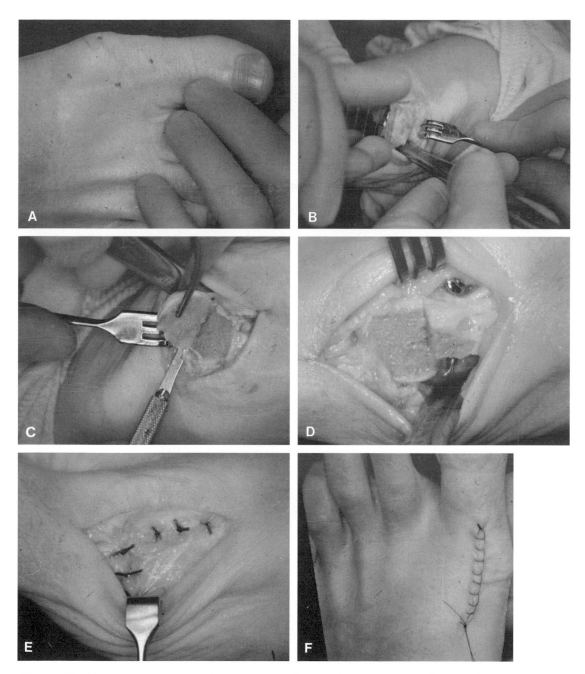

Figure 27. Bunion surgery—head osteotomy with screw fixation. *A,* Four landmark points for skin incision. *B* and *C,* Removal of dorsomedial exostosis. *D,* Screw fixation. *E,* Deep capsule closure. *F,* Skin closure.

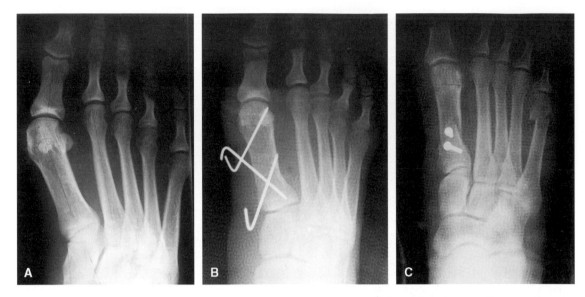

Figure 28. Base osteotomy. *A,* Preoperative x-ray of bunion deformity requiring base wedge osteotomy. *B,* Fixation with cross Kirschner wire. Note head osteotomy of metatarsal, also fixated with Kirschner wire. *C,* Fixation with screws.

ple, cost-effective technique for minimizing inflammatory response and maximizing functional return.

In treating pain, swelling, and muscle spasm of the lower extremity, long-term use of NSAIDs or oral narcotics is contraindicated. Physical therapy modalities, alone or as an adjunct to oral or injected medications, are an excellent method of treating chronic and acute foot pain with few negative effects.

The advantages of using physical therapy are:

1. Local treatment to the affected area
2. Noninvasive and nonsystemic approach; therefore, not causing stomach upset or allergic reaction
3. Immediate response in acute conditions (e.g., ice for an ankle sprain)
4. Nonhabit-forming treatment that can be used as often and as long as necessary.

Figure 29. Keller procedure with head osteotomy. *A,* Preoperative and *B,* postoperative radiographs.

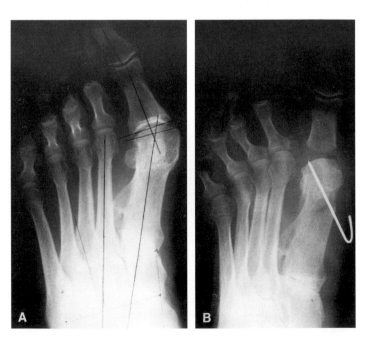

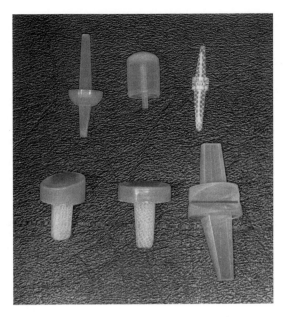

Figure 30. Various implants used in foot surgery.

The object of physical therapy is to increase or decrease blood flow to an area. Heat modalities cause the physiologic response to vasodilation. Vasodilation increases blood flow, which increases inflammation and pain. Cold modalities do the exact opposite: they vasoconstrict. Vasoconstriction decreases blood flow, which in turn decreases the inflammatory response and edema.

Heat Modalities

Heat modalities work well on subacute and chronic conditions. They should not be used in the acute condition because they increase inflammatory response and pain. The general rule for acute conditions is cold for the first 24–48 hours and then heat. Heat therapy is indicated for pain and swelling due to rheumatoid arthritis, osteoarthritis/traumatic arthritis, myositis, surgery/trauma, and muscle spasm.

Heat modalities are contraindicated for patients with circulatory impairments, malignancies, ulcerations or any open wounds, pregnancy, sensory-impairment (e.g., diabetes, alcoholism), acute conditions, fractures, apophyseal centers, postsurgical areas with metal screws, plates, and wires, and infections.

Conductive heat is a superficial heat modality that penetrates to a depth of 1–2 mm after direct application to the skin. Hot packs, paraffin, and hydrotherapy (whirlpool) are some examples of conductive heat. The temperature must be monitored and should never exceed 106–108° F. Most professional whirlpool and paraffin baths have thermometers or thermostats for easy monitoring.

Whirlpool baths allow the patient to receive therapy and perform active range-of-motion exercises at the same time (Fig. 32). The ankle, subtalar joints, MTP joints, and digits can be rehabilitated using hydrotherapy. Treatments are generally 10–15 minutes, two to three times weekly until symptoms resolve.

Paraffin is another excellent superficial heat modality. It relieves symptoms of all the joints in the foot. The foot is dipped quickly in the paraffin bath five to ten times. A plastic bag is then applied over the foot, and the patient elevates the foot until the wax cools. This procedure can be repeated once or twice per treatment, occurring twice weekly.

Radiant heat, a type of convection, is another form of superficial heating. There is no contact with the skin; a heat lamp or infrared lamp is used from a distance. Again, careful monitoring of the skin temperature is important. Skin thermometers may be used for this purpose. This modality works well on all inflammatory conditions of the feet. The patient should be lying supine with the feet elevated. Treatment should be given twice weekly.

Conversion heating is a deep heat modality in which electric energy is converted to heat in the deeper tissues. The penetration is much greater than conductive or radiant heat and can exceed 5 cm. Ultrasound is the most common form of conversion heat that is applied directly to the skin (Fig. 33). There are two basic settings: continuous and pulse. The continuous mode is used over soft tissue areas, and the ultrasound transducer must be moved constantly. Conduction jelly must be applied to the skin prior to therapy. There is a large buildup of heat with ultrasound, and burns are a complication. The pulse mode allows the ultrasound head to be left in one position, making it useful over bone prominences. The pulse mode does not heat the skin; it only affects deep tissue.

Contraindications for ultrasound include any metal on the skin or in the deep tissues or bone (i.e., screws, wires, and pins). Metal absorbs heat faster than body tissues and may cause unnecessary burns. Ultrasound is excellent for rehabilitation of all parts of the foot. Treatments are generally 8–10 minutes, two to three times weekly.

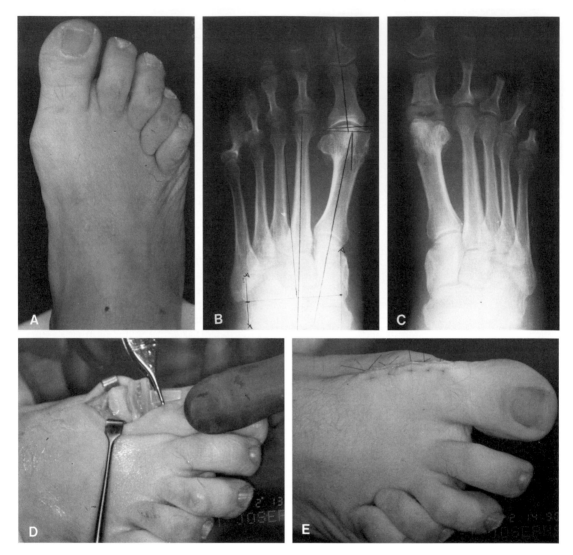

Figure 31. Implant surgery. *A,* Clinical appearance of foot. *B,* Preoperative x-ray (note the arthritic first metatarsophalangeal joint and osteophytes). *C,* Postoperative x-ray. *D,* Insertion of the total implant into the first metatarsophalangeal joint. *E,* Skin closure after total joint implant.

Cold Modalities (Cryotherapy)

Cold modalities work well in acute conditions. They are indicated for acute trauma, pain (topical anesthetic), pruritus, the immediate postoperative period, acute spasm, and shin splints.

They are contraindicated for circulatory disorders, especially vasospastic; sensory-impaired patients (e.g., diabetes, alcoholism); ulcerations; infections; and stiff joint conditions (e.g., arthritis).

Cold modalities are administered solely by conduction. Either the affected foot is placed in a cool tank of water or an ice pack is applied. The therapy is given for 10–20 minutes con-tinuously, at a temperature less than 15° C, alternating with 20–30 minutes off until acute inflammation has subsided. Cryotherapy is best combined with RICE for an acute injury. Cool whirlpools used postsurgically rehabilitate the joint without increasing edema. Treatment is for 10–15 minutes, three times weekly for 2 weeks. Cold therapy is generally a short-term treatment for acute inflammation but may be used in conjunction with heat for a longer term (e.g., contrast bath therapy).

Exercise

After the acute inflammatory reaction has subsided, range-of-motion (ROM) exercises

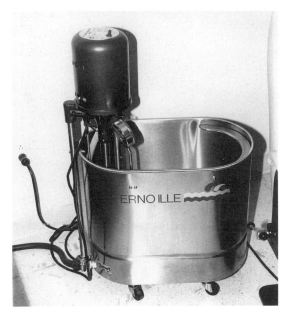

Figure 32. Whirlpool bath.

With the affected foot alongside the door, the patient is instructed to close and open the door with just the foot. Increased resistance can be placed on the foot by holding the door manually. This exercise is excellent for strengthening chronic ankle instability. To strengthen the ankle joint, the patient should be seated on a high table or chair with the foot dangling. A pocketbook is hung over the forefoot area. The ankle is dorsiflexed as much as possible and held for a count of 10 seconds; this is repeated 10-15 times. The exercise strengthens the anterior ankle muscles. To strengthen the posterior muscles of the ankle, heel raises are recommended. Have the patient stand flatfooted on the floor and raise the heels as far off the ground as possible. The patient may need to hold onto a chair or wall for balance. These exercises should be repeated 10-15 times.

More complex rehabilitative protocols are available and should be handled in conjunction with a physical therapist and physiatrist.

within the limits of pain are begun. Once painless ROM is achieved, progressive resistance exercises, consisting of gradual load increases to a 80-repetition maximum load, are started. These isotonic exercises can be supplemented with isometric (fixed-length) and isokinetic (fixed-speed) exercises.

To rehabilitate the MTP joints and digits, have patients try to pick up marbles or a pencil with their toes. Extension and flexion of the digits repeatedly 10-15 times also is effective. To rehabilitate the subtalar joints, inversion and eversion exercises are useful. Have the patient sit in a chair in front of an open door.

====

References

1. Albom MJ: Avulsion of a nail plate. J Dermatol Surg Oncol 3:1,34–35, 1977.
2. Albom MJ: Digital block anesthesia. J Dermatol Surg 2:366–367, 1976.
3. Bordelon RL: Orthotics, shoes, and braces. Orthop Clin North Am 20(4):751–757, 1989.
4. Bunch WH (ed): Atlas of Orthotics, 2nd ed. St. Louis, C.V. Mosby Co., 1985.
5. Grayson ML, et al: Probing to the bone in infected pedal ulcers. JAMA 273(9):721–723, 1995.
6. Marshall P: The rehabilitation of overuse foot injuries in athlete and dancers. Clin Sports Med 7(1):175–192, 1988.
7. Molnar ME: Rehabilitation of the injured ankle. Clin Sports Med 7(1):193–205, 1988.
8. Subotnick SI: Foot orthoses: An update. Phys Sports Med 11(8):103–109, 1983.
9. Yale I (ed): Podiatric Medicine, 2nd ed. Baltimore, Williams & Wilkins, 1980.

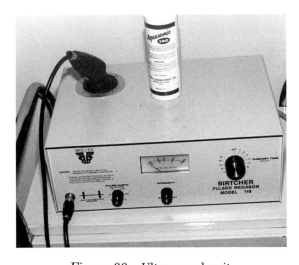

Figure 33. Ultrasound unit.

■
■

The Podiatry Cabinet and Supplies

The three critical elements for the successful management of office podiatric patients are: an adjustable examination table, a bright operating light, and an adjustable stool. Though an electrically maneuverable podiatry chair provides the greatest flexibility, the standard office examination table is satisfactory.

The majority of podiatric pathologies can be treated and managed with the physician sitting or standing. The examiner's stool should be mobile, on sturdy rollers, flexible to allow for leg length adjustments, and sufficiently comfortable to provide for prolonged sitting.

Office Supplies Useful in the Management of Common Podiatric Problems

Item	Quantity	Item	Quantity
Cold sterilization tray and solution	1	Nail clippers, small and large	1 each
Electric burr	1	1% and 2% lidocaine (Xylocaine)	1 each
Scalpel blades Nos. 10, 11, 15, and 20	Several	0.5% bupivacaine (Marcaine)	1
No. 3 or No. 4 Bard-Parker scalpel handle	1	Dressing materials: Adhesive surgical tape ½, 1, and 2-inch	Several each
Flat-jawed tissue forceps*	1	Paper tape (hypo-allergenic) ½, 1, and 2-inch	
Curette excavator with 1.5-and 2.5-mm holes*	1 each	Cotton balls	
		Gauze 2×2, 4×4	
Medium-size chisel ¼-inch and ⅜-inch	1 each	Roll bandages (Kling)	
Straight nail splitter (thin)*	1	Felt adhesive and nonadhesive ⅛ and ¼-inch	
Suture material: 000 Dexon/Vicril 2-0 Monofilament 4-0 Monofilament	Several each	Moleskin Cotton/wool ⅛ and ¼-inch Rubber, polyurethane foam	
Straight surgical scissors	1	Plaster of Paris (fast dry) 2, 3, and 4-inch	Several rolls each
Splinter forceps*	1	Plaster splints 5-inch	
		Solutions: Povidone-iodine Benzoin tincture Ethyl chloride Phenol	One bottle each

* These surgical instruments can be sterilized in a glass bead apparatus in 5 seconds at 232 ° C or 450° F.

▬
▬

Guidelines for the Patient With Diabetes or Peripheral Vascular Disease

DO

1. Inspect feet daily. Contact your physician at the first sign of redness, swelling, inflammation, infection, prolonged pain, numbness, tingling, or inability to move a foot or a leg.
2. Wash feet daily in lukewarm water (check temperature with hand or elbows) and mild soap; use soft brush.
3. Dry feet with a soft towel by blotting gently, not rubbing, especially between the toes.
4. Keep feet moist by applying an emollient or lanolin, particularly at the heel margins after a bath or shower. Use lamb's wool between overriding toes.
5. Use nonmedicated talc powder or corn starch if your feet sweat easily.
6. Use socks or stockings made from unmercerized cotton or wool that are not wrinkled and are half an inch longer than the longest toe; avoid stretch (nylon) socks, those with an elastic band/garter at the top, or socks with internal seams.
7. Beware of new shoes. Choose a shoe according to the following guidelines: soft leather, Blucher type, and a rigid shank or wedge. Or be fitted for a custom-molded shoe—round with a high toe box.
8. Break in new shoes slowly and only after they have been approved by your doctor.
9. Inspect shoes daily for foreign bodies such as gravel, protruding nails, and torn linings.
10. Loosen bedclothes to ensure reduced pressure on toes, heels, and bony prominences.
11. Keep feet warm and avoid extreme temperatures.
12. If feet hurt at night, raise head of bed six to ten inches (15 to 25 cm) on blocks.

DON'T

1. Use any instruments on the feet.
2. Cut your calluses or corns or use chemicals/medications to remove them.
3. Soak your feet.
4. Use hot water, a heating pad, massage, or an electrical or mechanical device.
5. Contact hot surfaces.
6. Go barefoot.
7. Use adhesive tape or other chemicals on skin.
8. Use inserts or pads without medical advice.
9. Tear or rub nails or skin.
10. Walk when your shoes are wet.
11. Expose your feet to cold weather.
12. Wear sandals or cutout shoes.
13. Wear shoes that are uncomfortable or that rub, blister, or cut your foot.
14. Cross your legs when sitting.
15. Put cream or lotion between toes.
16. Wear shoes without socks.
17. Use tobacco.

Common Podiatric Terminology

Athlete's foot—tinea pedis, Hong Kong foot.

Ball—area of the foot defined by the widest part of the sole and anatomically consisting of the metatarsal heads and overlying tissue.

Bar (e.g., metatarsal)—a transverse bar consisting of synthetic material (e.g., rubber) across the bottom of the shoe sole with the apex proximal to the metatarsal heads.

Black toe—a black or purple toenail due to subungual hematoma, partial nail avulsion, or both. Caused by increased pressure or friction to the toe.

Blucher oxford—a front-laced shoe pattern with the posterior part of the upper extending just below the malleoli and consisting of a tongue extending from the shoe forepart and tie laces along the sides of the shoe.

Bunion—inflammation of the bursa overlying the metatarsophalangeal joint of the first toe.

Callus—see *Tyloma.*

Corn—see *Heloma.*

Clubfoot—talipes equinovarus. Adducted forefoot, inverted rearfoot, equinus, and subluxation of the talocalcaneal navicular joints.

Counter-reinforcement—a variety of synthetic or natural materials used to preserve the shape of a particular portion of the shoe (e.g., heel counter, lateral or medial counter).

Dancer's foot—inflammatory swelling of the bursa of the first metatarsus associated with high-heeled dancers.

Flare—modification of a last to accommodate a natural foot shape or provide correction for an underlying pathology (e.g., in-flares, out-flares).

Golfer's foot—weakness of the anterior arch in association with plantar fasciitis occurring in golfers and other sports enthusiasts.

Hallux valgus—deviation of the first toe curved toward the outer or lateral portion of the foot.

Hammered hallux—dorsal contraction of the hallux at the interphalangeal joint.

Hammer toe—dorsal contraction of the lesser toe at the proximal interphalangeal joint.

Heel—solid, supporting portion of the posterior shoe that projects downward (e.g., Cuban, military, flat, spring heels).

Heloma—a localized, inflammatory focus consisting of a core of hyperkeratotic cells composed of impacted, desquamated, dead cells at the site of focal pressure and friction. Helomata may be soft (molle) or hard (durum). Synonym—corn.

Inlay—any type of device that can be inserted into a shoe (e.g., mold, arch support).

Instep—the dorsal, arched, middle portion of the human foot; that portion of the foot covering the anatomic instep.

Jogger's foot—see *Runner's foot.*

Last—a synthetic or natural model of the weight-bearing aspect of the foot from which a shoe is formed (e.g., straight, combination, bunion lasts).

March foot—fracture of the shaft of the second metatarsal in association with a tender, rounded, dorsal swelling which may be diffusely cyanotic. The condition originally was described in soldiers, though it is now more commonly seen as stress fractures in runners and joggers.

Orthoposer—a stand to hold an x-ray cassette.

Pes planus—flat foot or splay foot.

Runner's foot—medial calcaneal nerve entrapment.

Runner's toe—see *Black toe.*

Shank—the area of the last extending from the ball of the foot to the anterior portion of the heel.

Splay foot—a type of flat foot.

Toe box—that area of the shoe forepart that contains the toes.

Toe off—to use the toes to push off during ambulation.

Trench foot—the chronic sympathetic neurovascular changes associated with frostbite affecting the feet of soldiers required to stand for prolonged periods in cold water. Synonym—immersion foot.

Turf toe—toe sprain caused by the toe, usually the hallux, jamming in a shoe and hyperextending.

Tyloma—a generalized area of hyperkeratotic skin due to diffuse irritation, friction, or pressure typically at the ball of the foot. Synonym—callus.

Supplier and Resource Organizations

AliMed
68 Harrison Avenue
Boston, MA 02111
Telephone: (617) 350-6783, 1-800-225-2610

American Podiatric Medical Association
9312 Old Georgetown Road
Bethesda, MD 20814
Telephone: (301) 571-9200

Apex Foot Health Industries
170 Wesley Street
South Hackensack, NJ 07606
Telephone: (201) 487-2739

Doctor's Choice
671 Third Place South
Garden City, NY 11530
Telephone: 1-800-556-5011

Fillauer Orthopaedic
1480 East Third Street
Chattanooga, TN 37401
Telephone: (423) 698-8971

Gill Podiatry Supply
7803 Freeway Circle
Middleburg Heights, OH 44130
Telephone: 1-800-321-1348

Knit-Rite
2020 Grand Avenue
Kansas City, MO 64141
Telephone: (816) 221-5200

Medasonics, Inc.
47233 Fremont Blvd.
Fremont, CA 94538
Telephone: 1-800-227-8076

Moore Medical
389 John Downey Drive
New Britain, CT 06050
Telephone: 1-800-234-1464

M-PACT (previously Summit Medical)
1040 OCL Parkway Drive
Eudora, KS 66025
Telephone: 1-800-821-2527

Pedifix
4 Columbus Avenue
Mt. Kisco, NY 10549
Telephone: 1-800-424-5561

Rubatex Corporation
906 Adams Street
Bedford, VA 24523
Telephone: (540) 586-2611

Silipos
2150 Liberty Drive
Niagra Falls, NY 14304
Telephone: 1-800-229-4404

Spenco Medical Corporation
P.O. Box 2501
Waco, TX 76710
Telephone: 1-800-877-3626

Universal Foot Care Products
300 Wainwright Drive
North Brook, IL 60062
Telephone: 1-800-323-5110

U.S. Public Health Services
Gillis W. Long
Hansen's Disease Center
Carville, LA 70721
Telephone: (504) 642-4722

Consent for Medical or Surgical Procedure

Patient's Name: _____ Date of Surgery: _____

Time of Surgery _____A.M. _____P.M.

1. I, (or _____ for _____) hereby authorize Dr._____, and/or such assistants as may be selected to treat the following condition: _____

_____

(Explain the nature of the condition and the need to treat such.)

2. The procedure(s) necessary to treat my condition has (have) been explained to me by Dr._____, and I understand the nature of the procedure to be: _____

_____

(A description of the procedures in layman's language.)

3. I have been made aware of certain risks and consequences that are associated with the procedure(s) described in Paragraph 2 such as, but not limited to, **postoperative infections, delayed healing, numbness around the operative site(s), postoperative swelling, excessive and/or painful scar formation, recurrence of the problem.** Dr. _____has also explained possible alternative methods of treatment. I hereby acknowledge that I understand the information given me.

4. I understand that the explanation of the risks and consequences that I have received is not exhaustive and that other, more remote risks and consequences may arise. I have been advised that these more remote risks and consequences will be explained to me upon request. I acknowledge that I have been given the opportunity to ask questions concerning this procedure and its risks and consequences, and my questions, if any, have been answered to my satisfaction.

5. It has been explained to me that during the course of the procedure, unforeseen conditions may be involved that necessitate an extension of the original procedure(s) or different procedures and that Dr. _____, the assistants, or the designees may perform such surgical or medical procedures as are necessary and desirable in the exercise of their professional judgment. The authority granted under this paragraph (5) shall extend to treating all conditions that require treatment and are not known to Dr. _____at the time that the operation or procedure is commenced.

☐ 6. I consent both to the administration of anesthesia to be applied by or under the direction of the surgeon, Dr. _____or the designees and to the use of such anesthesia as they may deem advisable.

☐ 7. I acknowledge that I have received no guarantee concerning the medical or surgical procedure to which I am consenting.

☐ 8. I hereby authorize Dr. _____ either to dispose of any tissues or organs removed as a result of the procedure authorized above or to preserve such tissues or organs, at discretion, for scientific or teaching purposes.

☐ 9. I acknowledge that I have read this document in its entirety, that I fully understand it, and that all blank spaces have been either completed or crossed off prior to my signing.

_____ _____ _____

Witness   Signature of Patient   Date

(If patient is unable to sign or is a minor, complete the following.)

Patient is a minor _____ years of age or is unable to sign because: _____

_____

_____ _____ _____

Witness   Relative or Legal Guardian   Date

Index

Page numbers in **boldface** indicate complete chapters.

3